Companion Animal End-of-Life and Loss

Veterinary, Caregiver, and Organizational Perspectives

Companion Animal End-of-Life and Loss

Veterinary, Caregiver, and Organizational Perspectives

Edited by:

Lori R. Kogan

CABI

CABI is a trading name of CAB International

CABI
Nosworthy Way
Wallingford
Oxfordshire OX10 8DE
UK

Tel: +44 (0)1491 832111
E-mail: info@cabi.org
Website: www.cabi.org

CABI
200 Portland Street
Boston
MA 02114
USA

T: +1 (617)682-9015
E-mail: cabi-nao@cabi.org

A catalogue record for this book is available from the British Library, London, UK.

ISBN-13: 9781836994022 (hardback)
9781836994039 (ePDF)
9781836994046 (ePub)

DOI: 10.1079/9781836994046.0000

Commissioning Editor: Victoria Taylor
Editorial Assistant: Theresa Regueira
Production Editor: Rosie Hayden

Typeset by Exeter Premedia Services Pvt Ltd, Chennai, India
Printed and bound in the UK by CPI Group (UK) Ltd, Croydon, CR0 4YY

Contents

Supplementary Content

https://www.cabidigitallibrary.org/doi/book/10.1079/9781836994046.0000

Chapter 4 includes supplementary material:

- Appendix 1. Course Evaluation Survey Questions 2019–2021
- Appendix 2. Student Perceptions of Teaching (SPOT) Survey Questions (2022–2024) Questions asked in SPOT surveys

Chapter 6 includes supplementary material:

- Demographics of EOL Mobile Veterinarians
- Survey of EOL Mobile Veterinarians

Original Publication Details

1 **The Evolution, Challenges, and Future of Veterinary Hospice and Palliative Care**
Coleen Ellis, Kellie Littrell, Tyler Carmack and Karin Christopher
https://doi.org/10.1079/hai.2024.0033

2 **Veterinary Professionals' Experiences with Human Caregivers when Providing Animal Hospice and Palliative Care**
Heath C. Hoffmann and George E. Dickinson
https://doi.org/10.1079/hai.2021.0019

3 **One Owner's Perspective After a Pet Hospice Journey**
Allison C. Hudock
https://doi.org/10.1079/hai.2025.0027

4 **Compassionate End-Of-Life Care: Development, Implementation, and Evaluation of a Comprehensive Euthanasia Course in Veterinary Education From 2019–2024**
Virginia K. Corrigan, Kathleen Cooney and Raeann Foster
https://doi.org/10.1079/hai.2025.0025

5 **The Untapped Potential of Registered Veterinary Technicians in Hospice Care**
Emily Piche
http://dx.doi.org/10.1079/hai.2025.0034

6 **Veterinary End-Of-Life Mobile Practitioners: Motivators, Challenges, Job Fulfillment, and Burnout**
Lori R. Kogan, Jennifer Currin-McCulloch, Kellie Littrell and Emma Brown
https://doi.org/10.1079/hai.2025.0018

7 **A Time to Say Goodbye: Empathy and Emotion Regulation Predict Timing of End-of-Life Decisions by Pet Owners**
Jennifer Vonk, Esther Maria Corina Bouma and Arie Dijkstra
https://doi.org/10.1079/hai.2022.0013

8 Predictors of Opting for Advanced Medical Care versus Euthanasia for Companion Animals with Severe Cardiac Disease
Samantha Siess, George A. Kramer, Dar Ozer, Nikki Gaudette, Brienne Williams, Brittany Antal and Anne Moyer
https://doi.org/10.1079/hai.2021.0013

9 Overcoming the Social Stigma of Losing a Pet: Considerations for Counseling Professionals
Michelle Kay Crossley and Colleen Rolland
https://doi.org/10.1079/hai.2022.0022

10 Older Adults and Companion Animal Death: A Survey of Bereavement and Disenfranchised Grief
Cary A. Brown, Donna M. Wilson, Eloise Carr, Douglas P. Gross, Maxi Miciak and Jean E. Wallace
https://doi.org/10.1079/hai.2023.0017

11 When Support is "Pawsed": Increased Attachment Mediates the Association Between Loss of Support and Pet Bereavement During the Pandemic
Victoria L. O'Connor, Jennifer Vonk and Katherine Compitus
https://doi.org/10.1079/hai.2022.0020

12 "We Lost a Member of the Family": Predictors of the Grief Experience Surrounding the Loss of a Pet
Anna Maria C. Behler, Jeffrey D. Green and Jennifer Joy-Gaba
https://doi.org/10.1079/hai.2020.0017

13 Dealing with Death: The Role of Animal-Themed Literature in Supporting Children with Grief and Loss
Elaine Smit and Bradley P. Smith
https://doi.org/10.1079/hai.2023.0002

14 How to Care for the Caregiver: The Power of Ritual
Loretta Truman
https://doi.org/10.1079/hai.2025.0022

15 Supporting Clients Through Loss: A Qualitative Review of Current Practices of Accredited Assistance Dog Organizations
Dena DeSantis and Janet Hoy Gerlach
https://doi.org/10.1079/hai.2025.0009

16 The Loss of a Service Dog Through Retirement: Experiences and Impact on Human Partners
Jennifer Currin-McCulloch, Cori Bussolari, Wendy Packman, Lori R. Kogan and Phyllis Erdman
https://doi.org/10.1079/hai.2022.0017

17 "My Lifeline is Gone": An Exploration of the Experiences of Veterans Following the Loss of their Psychiatric Service Dog(s)
Maryellen Gibson, Darlene Chalmers and Siyu Ru
https://doi.org/10.1079/hai.2022.0009

18 Animal Loss and Grief in Zoos: Qualitative Insights to Inform Organizational Support for Zoo Professionals and Volunteers
Nichole Louise Nageotte, Jennifer Currin-McCulloch, Shelby McDonald, Abigail Walker and Lori R. Kogan
https://doi.org/10.1079/hai.2025.0004

Contributors

Brittany Antal: Department of Cardiology, Atlantic Coast New York Veterinary Specialists, Bohemia, NY, USA

Anna Maria C. Behler, PhD: North Carolina State University, NC, USA

Esther Maria Corina Bouma: Department of Social Psychology, Faculty of Behavioral and Social Sciences, University of Groningen, Netherlands

Cary A. Brown: Department of Occupational Therapy, Faculty of Rehabilitation Medicine, University of Alberta, Edmonton, Alberta, Canada

Emma Brown: Department of Sociomedical Sciences, Columbia University, New York, NY, 10027, USA

Cori Bussolari: University of San Francisco, Department of Clinical Psychology, San Francisco, CA, USA

Tyler Carmack: Caring Pathways, Denver, CO, USA

Eloise Carr: Faculty of Nursing, University of Calgary, Calgary, Alberta, Canada

Darlene Chalmers: Faculty of Social Work, University of Regina, Saskatchewan, Canada

Karin Christopher: Pet Quietus, Corpus Christi, TX, USA

Katherine Compitus: Silver School of Social Work, New York University, New York, NY, USA

Kathleen Cooney: Companion Animal Euthanasia Training Academy (CAETA), Lutz, FL, USA

Virginia K. Corrigan: University of Tennessee College of Veterinary Medicine, Departments of Academic Affairs and Small Animal Clinical Sciences, University of Tennessee Institute of Agriculture, Knoxville TN, USA

Michelle Kay Crossley: Counseling, Educational Leadership, and School Psychology, Rhode Island College, RI, USA

Jennifer Currin-McCulloch: School of Social Work, Colorado State University, Fort Collins, CO, USA

Dena DeSantis: The University of Alabama, Tuscaloosa, AL, USA

George E. Dickinson: College of Charleston, Charleston, SC, USA

Arie Dijkstra: Department of Social Psychology, Faculty of Behavioral and Social Sciences, University of Groningen, Netherlands

Coleen Ellis: Two Hearts Pet Loss Center, Indianapolis, IN, USA

Phyllis Erdman: Washington State University, College of Education, Pullman, WA, USA

Raeann Foster: Virginia Maryland College of Veterinary Medicine, Department of Small Animal Clinical Sciences, Virginia Tech, Blacksburg, VA, USA

Nikki Gaudette: Department of Cardiology, Atlantic Coast New York Veterinary Specialists, Bohemia, NY, USA

Janet Hoy Gerlach: Director of Veterinary Social Work, Open Door Veterinary Collective, Grand Rapids, OH, USA

Maryellen Gibson: Department of Sociology, University of Saskatchewan, Canada

Jeffrey D. Green, PhD: Virginia Commonwealth University, VA, USA

Douglas P. Gross: Department of Physical Therapy, Faculty of Rehabilitation Medicine, University of Alberta, Edmonton, Alberta, Canada

Heath C. Hoffmann: College of Charleston, Charleston, SC, USA

Allison C. Hudock: Independent Researcher, 189 N. Marengo Ave., Apt 210 Pasadena, CA 91101, USA

Jennifer Joy-Gaba, PhD: Virginia Commonwealth University, VA, USA

Lori R. Kogan: Colorado State University, College of Veterinary Medicine and Biomedical Sciences, Department of Clinical Sciences, Fort Collins, CO, USA

George A. Kramer: Department of Cardiology, Atlantic Coast New York Veterinary Specialists, Bohemia, NY, USA

Kellie Littrell: Caring Pathways, Denver, CO, USA; Texas Tech University School of Veterinary Medicine, Lubbock, TX, 79409, USA

Shelby McDonald: School of Social Work, Colorado State University, Fort Collins, CO, USA

Maxi Miciak: Faculty of Rehabilitation Medicine, University of Alberta, Edmonton, Alberta, Canada

Anne Moyer: Department of Psychology, Stony Brook University, NY, USA

Nichole Louise Nageotte: Department of Community Research and Evaluation, Denver Zoo Conservation Alliance, Denver, CO, USA

Victoria L. O'Connor: Department of Psychology, Oakland University, Rochester Hills, MI, USA

Dar Ozer: Department of Cardiology, Atlantic Coast New York Veterinary Specialists, Bohemia, NY, USA

Wendy Packman: Professor Emerita, Palo Alto University, Department of Psychology, Palo Alto, CA, USA

Emily Piche: The Art of Goodbye – Hospice and Euthanasia Training Institute, 40 Concession Road 8, East, Tiny Township, Ontario, L0L-2J0, Canada

Colleen Rolland: Association for Pet Loss and Bereavement Albany, NY, USA

Siyu Ru: Department of Sociology, University of Saskatchewan, Canada

Samantha Siess: Department of Psychology, Stony Brook University, NY, USA

Elaine Smit: College of Psychology, School of Health, Medical and Applied Sciences, Central Queensland University, Adelaide, Australia

Bradley P. Smith: College of Psychology, School of Health, Medical and Applied Sciences, Central Queensland University, Adelaide, Australia

Loretta Truman: Argus Institute, Colorado State University, Veterinary Teaching Hospital, 300 West Drake Road, Fort Collins, CO, 80523, USA

Jennifer Vonk: Department of Psychology, Oakland University, Rochester Hills, MI, USA

Abigail Walker: School of Social Work, Colorado State University, Fort Collins, CO, USA

Jean E. Wallace: Faculty of Arts, University of Calgary, Calgary, Alberta, Canada

Brienne Williams: Department of Cardiology, Atlantic Coast New York Veterinary Specialists, Bohemia, NY, USA

Donna M. Wilson: Faculty of Nursing, University of Alberta, Edmonton, Alberta, Canada

Introduction

Lori R. Kogan
Colorado State University, USA

The field of animal assisted services (AAS), and equine-assisted services (EAS) specifically, has grown exponentially over the last couple of decades, emerging as a popular intervention to help support human health and well-being (Fine and Andersen, 2021). Multitudes of studies have validated what we have intuitively known for years: interactions with animals can have a profound positive impact on human health and functioning. In recent years, the breadth of animal-involved interventions has expanded in numerous areas, offering a wide array of options for human–animal teams. Although most of the AAS studies have focused on dog-assisted interventions (Bert *et al.*, 2016), EAS represent an emerging field within AAS. As the field of EAS has grown, it has become apparent that standardized terminology is needed to have a common language for horse-related services to facilitate collaboration across professional disciplines, reduce terminological confusion, and create the framework needed to implement and study EAS (Wood *et al.*, 2021). To this end, a consensus document was published in 2020 that provides guidance regarding optimal terminology for the diverse services that incorporate horses to benefit people (Wood *et al.*, 2021). This optimal terminology began with suggesting the use of the term Equine-assisted services (EAS) to reference the multiple services in which professionals incorporate equines to benefit people. Twelve types of EAS were subsequently categorized under three large umbrellas: therapy, learning and horsemanship. Under the umbrella of therapy, five types were identified including counseling, occupational therapy, physical therapy, psychotherapy, and speech-language pathology. Counseling is performed by licensed therapy professionals and refers to the incorporation of horses into mental health counseling to address psychological and emotional challenges. Occupational therapy refers to the inclusion of horses to support functional skill development and improving daily living and work-related capabilities. Physical therapy uses equine movement to support rehabilitation, physical functioning, and overall health and wellness. Psychotherapy refers to the integration of horses into psychological treatment. Speech-language pathology utilizes horse-related activities to support the development of communication skills by providing sensory and interactive experiences that target speech and language development (Wood *et al.*, 2021). Regardless of the type of therapy, each one involves licensed professionals who work within the scope of practice of their particular discipline. In addition, it is strongly recommended that these professionals obtain specialized training focused on incorporating horses into their treatments (Wood *et al.*, 2021). The umbrella of learning includes three types of services including equine-assisted learning in education, organizations, and personal development.

Over the past several decades, research related to companion animal end-of-life (EOL), loss, and bereavement has grown exponentially. This expanding body of work reflects the fact that companion animals are increasingly recognized as valuable family members (Carmack, 1985; Archer, 1997; Walsh, 2009; Hudock, 2025; Li and Wong, 2025; Northrope *et al.*, 2025). In parallel, companion animal EOL care within veterinary medicine has evolved substantially (Ellis *et al.*, 2024). Historically framed as a technical or procedural task centered on euthanasia, EOL care is now often conceptualized as an ethically complex process involving animals, caregivers, and veterinary teams (Rollin, 2011; Villalobos and Kaplan, 2017; Kogan and Cooney, 2023; Corrigan *et al.*, 2025; Northrope *et al.*, 2025).

The growth of veterinary hospice and palliative care reflects this broader conceptual shift, emphasizing comfort, quality of life, and support for the entire family. Organizations such as the International Association for Animal Hospice and Palliative Care (IAAHPC) have played a pivotal role in professionalizing the field through education and credentialing, including the Certified Hospice and Palliative Care Veterinarian (CHPV®) program and related credentials for veterinary technicians and advocates. The organization has also demonstrated a sustained commitment to advancing research in the field through initiatives such as its sponsorship of the *Human–Animal Interactions* special issue, "Veterinary Hospice, Palliative Care, and the Human–Animal Bond", and the IAAHPC Research Grant Program.

As the field has developed, research examining EOL care and its impact on veterinary professionals' well-being has emerged as an increasingly important area of inquiry. This work highlights the emotional labor inherent in EOL practice, as well as risks for moral distress and compassion fatigue (Moses *et al.*, 2018; Fournier and Mustful, 2019; Hoffmann and Dickinson, 2021; Kogan and Cooney, 2023; Piche, 2025). Compassion fatigue is defined and described as it may affect animal welfare agents (AWAs) who advocate in animal-welfare work, and who engage in animal activism. The demographics of this group are described, as well as the nature of the work and its challenges. At the same time, some studies challenge simplistic narratives that equate repeated exposure to euthanasia with inevitable burnout. Emerging evidence suggests that meaning-centered, relationship-focused EOL work may instead enhance professional fulfillment (Kogan and Rishniw, 2024).

EOL care research has also increasingly focused on the emotional impact of animal caregiving and loss for pet owners and other animal caretakers (Vonk *et al.*, 2022; McDonald *et al.*, 2024; Hudock, 2025; Truman, 2025; Hyland, 2026). Companion animal death is now widely understood as a significant life event with implications for individual mental health and family functioning (Packman *et al.*, 2011; Behler *et al.*, 2020; Crossley and Rolland, 2022; Brown *et al.*, 2023; Smit and Smith, 2023). Their loss frequently elicits grief responses comparable to human bereavement (Field *et al.*, 2009; Packman *et al.*, 2011; Behler *et al.*, 2020; Kogan *et al.*, 2022; O'Connor *et al.*, 2022). Yet, unlike human death, animal loss is often minimized, resulting in disenfranchised grief - grief that is not socially recognized, validated, or supported (Doka, 1989). This lack of recognition can intensify distress and limit access to both formal and informal support (Bussolari *et al.*, 2021; Park *et al.*, 2021; Kogan *et al.*, 2023).

Recent studies demonstrate that multiple factors shape pet owners' grief, including attachment strength, anthropomorphism, guilt, and shame (Packman *et al.*, 2014; Testoni *et al.*, 2019; Behler *et al.*, 2020; Siess *et al.*, 2021; Wu and Song, 2025). This body of work challenges assumptions that pet grief is less serious or shorter-lived than grief related to human loss, while highlighting the centrality of meaning-making and continuing bonds (Klass *et al.*, 1996; Field *et al.*, 2009; Packman *et al.*, 2011; Kogan *et al.*, 2022).

More recently, scholarship has extended into professional, service, and organizational contexts. Service and assistance dogs, therapy and emotional support animals, and animals in captive care (e.g., zoos) often occupy dual roles as emotionally significant partners and working colleagues, making their loss both personal and functional (Brooks *et al.*, 2018; Currin-McCulloch *et al.*, 2022; Gibson *et al.*, 2022; Kogan *et al.*, 2023; DeSantis and Gerlach, 2025). In these settings, grief is frequently compounded by ambiguous loss, role strain, and institutional pressures, particularly within organizational cultures that discourage emotional expression or recovery time (Leonhardt-Parr and Rumble, 2024; McDonald *et al.*, 2024).

Although these contexts vary widely, they converge around several shared themes: companion animal EOL and loss are best understood as ongoing processes rather than discrete events; grief is relational and shaped by social context; and uneven access to recognition, education, and institutional support continues to leave some caregivers well supported while others grieve alone.

However, these shared insights have developed largely in parallel, leaving the field fragmented across disciplinary and professional silos. This volume responds to that gap by bringing together veterinary medicine, mental health, human–animal interaction, and organizational scholarship.

The first section, "Veterinary Hospice, Palliative, and EOL Care", centers on the clinical, educational, and professional contexts in which companion animal EOL decisions occur. These chapters, many of which come from the special HAI issue sponsored by the International Association for Animal Hospice and Palliative Care (IAAHPC) explore the historical evolution and contemporary practice of veterinary hospice and palliative care, the emotional, ethical, and relational demands placed on veterinarians and veterinary teams, and the training structures that shape preparedness for this work. Collectively, the section positions EOL care as a core veterinary competency with far-reaching implications for animal welfare, caregiver experience, and clinician well-being.

The second section, "Pet Loss, Grief, and Bereavement (Individuals and Families)", shifts attention to the lived experience of loss across the lifespan. These chapters examine disenfranchised grief following companion animal death, the vulnerabilities of older adults and children, and the psychological processes that shape grief intensity, guilt, and meaning-making. The contributions underscore the need for validation, ritual, and developmentally and contextually responsive support for individuals and families navigating animal loss.

The final section, "Service, Professional, and Organizational Grief", broadens the lens to examine loss within working partnerships and institutional settings. Chapters in this section explore grief following the retirement or death of service and psychiatric service dogs, the compounded losses experienced by veterans and disabled partners, and organizational responses to animal death in assistance dog programs and zoos.

Taken together, this volume advances a comprehensive, biopsychosocial understanding of companion animal EOL and loss. By integrating clinical practice, empirical research, lived experience, and organizational analysis, the book offers both conceptual frameworks and practical guidance for supporting animals, caregivers, and professionals through one of the most profound aspects of the human–animal bond.

Part 1: Veterinary Hospice, Palliative, and EOL Care

The first chapter, "The Evolution, Challenges, and Future of Veterinary Hospice and Palliative Care" provides a comprehensive overview of the historical development, current landscape, and ongoing barriers shaping hospice and palliative care within veterinary medicine. The chapter traces the origins of veterinary hospice and palliative care to early advocates in the late 1980s and early 2000s, highlighting key conceptual milestones such as the introduction of "pawspice" care and the founding of the International Association for Animal Hospice and Palliative Care (IAAHPC). The authors describe how these developments catalyzed a philosophical shift from a cure-focused model toward one that prioritizes comfort, quality of life, and support for the entire family.

The chapter also reviews major professional advancements, including the development of EOL care guidelines, accreditation programs, and species-specific hospice recommendations, all of which have contributed to increased professional legitimacy and visibility for hospice care.

Despite these advances, the authors identify persistent challenges limiting broader adoption. These include resistance among some veterinarians to hospice philosophy, limited integration of hospice training within veterinary and veterinary technician curricula, and ongoing misconceptions among pet caregivers regarding hospice care and euthanasia. The authors also highlight structural barriers, such as gaps between research and clinical implementation and limited funding for veterinary palliative care research.

Looking forward, the chapter emphasizes the need for enhanced interdisciplinary collaboration, expanded education and training, and proactive public communication to normalize EOL discussions and improve access to hospice services. The authors also underscore the potential benefits of hospice care for veterinarian well-being, suggesting that hospice models may reduce emotional burden and compassion fatigue by fostering continuity of care and deeper client relationships. In summary, the chapter positions veterinary hospice and palliative care as an evolving, bond-centered approach with significant implications for animal welfare, caregiver support, and professional sustainability.

The second chapter in this section, "Veterinary Professionals' Experiences with Human Caregivers when Providing Animal Hospice and Palliative Care" examines veterinarians' perspectives on providing hospice, palliative, and end-of-life (EOL) care for companion animals. Drawing on veterinarians' responses to open-ended questions, the study explores what veterinarians wish clients understood prior to seeking EOL services, as well as the most challenging and most rewarding aspects of this work.

A central theme involved the ongoing need to educate clients about the goals, scope, and value of hospice and palliative services. Closely related challenges included being contacted too late to meaningfully alleviate animal suffering, limited time available per client, and the demands of operating a financially sustainable practice. Participants described the emotional complexity of entering clients' homes during highly charged moments, navigating expectations shaped by prior veterinary advice, and balancing clinical realities with clients' readiness for decision-making.

Burnout and self-care emerged as another prominent theme. Veterinarians described compassion fatigue, emotional exhaustion, and the cumulative strain of supporting grieving families while managing their own sorrow. Financial pressures further compounded these challenges, particularly given the labor-intensive nature of hospice care.

Despite these challenges, veterinarians overwhelmingly described EOL care as deeply meaningful and professionally rewarding. Relieving animal suffering, facilitating a peaceful death, and witnessing gratitude and relief from families were frequently mentioned. For some, hospice work restored professional fulfillment and reaffirmed their commitment to veterinary medicine.

The next chapter in this section, "One Owner's Perspective After a Pet Hospice Journey" presents a first-person narrative describing a caregiver's experience navigating hospice and EOL care for her cat diagnosed with advanced gastrointestinal lymphoma. Through the story of Peaches, the author offers a detailed and emotionally grounded account of receiving a life-limiting diagnosis, making treatment and hospice decisions, and managing the realities of caregiving during the final months of her companion animal's life.

The chapter begins with the shock of diagnosis following emergency surgery and the author's sudden immersion into unfamiliar oncology terminology, prognostic information, and EOL options. After weighing treatment options, the author chose hospice care, prioritizing quality of life over aggressive intervention. Although the decision was made without regret, it carried significant emotional weight and responsibility.

As Peaches' condition declined, the author relied on quality-of-life tracking tools, online research, and peer support communities to regain a sense of control. The sudden onset of new symptoms ultimately led to a rapid euthanasia decision, described as both necessary and profoundly disorienting. In reflection, the author identifies unmet needs that could have improved the hospice experience, including earlier hospice referrals, clearer care planning, education on pain and quality-of-life assessment, and accessible tele-hospice support. The chapter powerfully illustrates the depth of caregiver burden in animal hospice and underscores the need for veterinary professionals to recognize, validate, and support the emotional labor inherent in EOL caregiving.

The following chapter, "Compassionate EOL Care: Development, Implementation, and Evaluation of a Comprehensive Euthanasia Course in Veterinary Education from 2019–2024" examines the creation and assessment of a specialized veterinary elective designed to address longstanding gaps in EOL education. The chapter focuses on a third-year veterinary course developed at the Virginia–Maryland College of Veterinary Medicine (VMCVM) in collaboration with the Companion Animal Euthanasia Training Academy (CAETA), integrating technical euthanasia skills with communication, ethics, and emotional competencies.

The authors discuss the course within broader concerns about inadequate EOL preparation in veterinary curricula, noting that euthanasia, despite being one of the most common procedures in veterinary practice, remains underrepresented in formal training. A distinctive feature of the course is embedded micro-credentialing, allowing students to earn certification as a Certified Peaceful Euthanasia Veterinarian (CPEV).

Course evaluation data were drawn from multiple sources, including structured surveys completed by students enrolled between 2019 and 2021 and longitudinal Student Perceptions of Teaching (SPOT) evaluations collected from 2022 through 2024. Quantitative and qualitative findings consistently indicated improved student confidence in euthanasia techniques, enhanced communication skills, and increased preparedness for managing emotionally complex EOL situations. Hands-on cadaver laboratories were identified as particularly valuable, while the hybrid format was praised for balancing flexibility with experiential learning. The authors conclude that the course offers a replicable model for integrating comprehensive EOL education into veterinary curricula.

The next chapter, "The Untapped Potential of Registered Veterinary Technicians in Hospice Care" presents a systematic review examining the roles, barriers, and opportunities for Registered Veterinary Technicians (RVTs) within veterinary hospice and palliative care. As demand for EOL services continues to increase, the chapter argues that RVTs represent an underutilized yet well-positioned workforce capable of expanding access to compassionate hospice care.

The author reviewed veterinary literature published between 2000 and 2024. Searches across PubMed, CAB Abstracts, and Google Scholar yielded 86 articles, of which 21 met inclusion criteria focused on RVT roles, training, scope of practice, clinic economics, and access to care. Thematic analysis identified six recurring themes shaping RVT involvement in hospice care.

Across the literature, RVTs were consistently described as underutilized, with misunderstandings about their training and scope of practice limiting their integration into hospice services. Several studies highlighted the promise of technician-led hospice models, noting improved continuity of care, enhanced client communication, and increased patient comfort. However, a lack of formal dedicated hospice and palliative care training for RVTs emerged as a persistent barrier, alongside regulatory ambiguity and cultural resistance within veterinary teams.

The review also emphasized the role RVTs could play in addressing access-to-care challenges. By assuming leadership in hospice coordination, client education, symptom monitoring, and follow-up care, RVTs could help alleviate veterinarian workload, reduce burnout, and allow practices to offer more timely and sustained EOL support.

Drawing parallels to expanded nursing roles in human healthcare, the authors conclude that clarifying scope of practice, closing training gaps, and supporting technician-led models are critical steps toward strengthening veterinary hospice delivery.

The next chapter, "Veterinary EOL Mobile Practitioners: Motivators, Challenges, Job Fulfillment, and Burnout" examines the professional experiences of veterinarians who specialize in mobile EOL care. As EOL services have grown as a distinct area of veterinary practice, this study addresses a notable gap in the literature by exploring why veterinarians choose mobile EOL work and how this specialization relates to professional fulfillment and burnout.

Using an anonymous, cross-sectional online survey, the authors collected data from 162 mobile EOL veterinarians across the United States. Results indicated that veterinarians are primarily drawn to mobile EOL practice by the opportunity to make a meaningful difference for pets and families, provide individualized care in familiar home environments, and gain greater control over scheduling and workload. Although participants identified logistical and business-related challenges—such as lack of health benefits, administrative burden, unpredictable income, and travel demands—few reported these factors as highly challenging. Importantly, emotional strain related to euthanasia itself was not identified as a primary source of distress.

Measures of professional well-being revealed relatively high levels of fulfillment and comparatively low burnout. Nearly 70% of participants met criteria for professional fulfillment, while approximately 15% met criteria for burnout—rates notably lower than those reported in studies of veterinarians in traditional clinical settings.

The authors conclude that engagement in euthanasia, when conducted within a supportive, client-centered, and self-directed practice model, does not inherently compromise veterinarians' mental health. Instead, mobile EOL practice appears to offer a viable and fulfilling alternative career pathway for some veterinarians, with important implications for workforce sustainability and EOL care delivery.

The chapter "A Time to Say Goodbye: Empathy and Emotion Regulation Predict Timing of EOL Decisions by Pet Owners" addresses a critical but understudied aspect of veterinary EOL care: how pet owners decide *when* to euthanize a companion animal. Drawing on survey data from 1,542 dog and cat owners in North America and Europe who had previously made euthanasia decisions, this study examines whether individual differences in empathy for animals, emotion regulation, and attitudes toward pets predict the timing of EOL decisions and associated feelings of guilt.

Contrary to the authors' original hypotheses, higher empathy was associated with *later* euthanasia decisions rather than earlier ones. Emotion regulation did not interact with empathy to predict decision timing; however, both higher empathy and greater emotion dysregulation independently predicted increased guilt for *both* early and late decisions. These findings suggest that highly empathetic owners may experience heightened moral and emotional burden regardless of when the decision is made, complicating assumptions about "optimal" decision-making.

The authors highlight the complexity of EOL decision-making and note that individual psychological traits explain only a small portion of variability in timing. They emphasize the importance of veterinarians recognizing how empathy, guilt, and emotional coping shape owner experiences.

This section ends with the chapter "Predictors of Opting for Advanced Medical Care versus Euthanasia for Companion Animals with Severe Cardiac Disease". This chapter examines how psychological factors and client–veterinarian communication influence treatment decisions for critically ill companion animals. Focusing on owners of dogs and cats diagnosed with severe cardiac disease, this study explores why some owners pursue intensive hospitalization while others decline treatment or elect euthanasia.

Eighty pet owners were recruited from a specialty referral hospital. Owners and veterinarians independently estimated the animal's chance of two-year survival and anticipated quality of life with intensive treatment. Consistent with prior research, owners demonstrated a significant optimistic bias when interpreting *poor* prognoses—overestimating survival when the veterinarian estimated less than a 50% chance—while no such bias emerged for quality-of-life assessments. This suggests that optimistic bias may function as a self-protective response to the threat of imminent loss rather than a misunderstanding of welfare.

Contrary to expectations, neither optimistic bias nor attachment to the companion animal predicted whether owners approved intensive treatment. Instead, client satisfaction with veterinarian communication and financial transparency emerged as the strongest predictors of decision-making. These findings underscore the ethical and emotional consequences of communication failures, highlighting the important role that effective communication plays in improving patient outcomes.

Part 2: Pet Loss, Grief, and Bereavement (Individuals and Families)

The first chapter in this section, "Overcoming the Social Stigma of Losing a Pet: Considerations for Counseling Professionals"explores the social, relational, and psychological consequences of losing a companion animal.

Drawing on attachment theory, grief and bereavement literature, and human–animal bond research, the chapter highlights how the strength and role of the pet–owner relationship shape the intensity and trajectory of grief. The chapter also addresses non-death losses including relinquishment, divorce-related separation, disaster-related abandonment, and lifestyle transitions as legitimate sources of grief and distress.

A central focus of the chapter is the role of counseling professionals in supporting clients experiencing pet loss. Counselors are encouraged to critically examine their own assumptions, assess human–animal attachments during intake, and validate pet loss as a significant emotional event. The chapter reviews grief models relevant to pet loss, emphasizing adaptation, meaning-making, and continuing bonds, and outlines counseling interventions including group support, narrative and expressive therapies, bibliotherapy, and online grief communities.

The next chapter, "Older Adults and Companion Animal Death: A Survey of Bereavement and Disenfranchised Grief" presents an empirical examination of bereavement experiences and disenfranchised grief among community-dwelling older adults following the death of a companion animal. Drawing on survey data from 98 adults aged 60 years and older, the study findings indicate high levels of attachment to companion animals and moderate levels of bereavement distress, with approximately one-third of participants reporting reluctance to disclose their grief due to anticipated lack of social support. Participants who perceived their grief as unsupported exhibited significantly higher bereavement distress and were more likely to report declines in physical health following the death.

Qualitative findings further illustrate the ways in which companion animal loss affects older adults' emotional health, daily routines, social engagement, and sense of identity. Invalidating responses such as minimizing the loss, encouraging replacement of the animal, or discouraging expressions of grief were seen as contributing factors for social withdrawal and private grieving. In contrast, being listened to, having the loss acknowledged as meaningful, and engaging in memorialization practices were identified as supportive and healing.

Overall, this chapter posits grief following companion animal death as a consequential yet under-recognized public health and aging issue. The findings highlight critical gaps in social recognition, clinical assessment, and bereavement support for older adults, highlighting the need for improved screening tools, professional training, and tailored interventions to support grief resolution and well-being following companion animal loss.

The next chapter, "When Support Is 'Pawsed': Increased Attachment Mediates the Association Between Loss of Support and Pet Bereavement During the Pandemic", examines how pandemic-related stressors shaped pet attachment and grief following companion animal loss during COVID-19. Situated within the broader context of widespread social disruption, isolation, and cumulative loss, this chapter explores whether reduced social support and increased isolation intensified attachment to pets, thereby exacerbating grief.

Drawing on survey data from 244 community and college participants who experienced pet loss during the height of the pandemic, the study found increased isolation and cumulative loss did not significantly predict stronger attachment to pets. However, cumulative loss was directly associated with greater grief following pet loss, even though it did not significantly predict stronger attachment to pets. This pattern suggests that grief intensity may be shaped by broader emotional burden during the pandemic, rather than by increased compensatory reliance on pets.

Unexpectedly, perceived social support was positively associated with pet attachment, which in turn mediated the relationship between support and grief. Individuals who perceived greater social support also reported stronger attachment to their pets, and this heightened attachment was linked to more intense grief following loss. These findings complicate common assumptions that reduced social support drives increased pet attachment during crises, instead highlighting the intertwined nature of human and animal social bonds.

Overall, this chapter underscores the complexity of grief experiences during collective crises. It reinforces prior evidence that stronger attachment predicts more intense pet bereavement, while demonstrating that social support may simultaneously buffer distress and deepen bonds with companion animals. The findings call for more nuanced, pet-specific approaches to understanding grief and the need for tailored bereavement support.

The next chapter, "'We Lost a Member of the Family': Predictors of the Grief Experience Surrounding the Loss of a Pet", examines the psychological mechanisms that shape the intensity, duration, and character of grief following companion animal loss. Drawing on an internet-based survey of 328 dog and cat owners, this chapter investigates how anthropomorphism, attachment, social support, guilt, and shame interact to produce grief experiences that closely mirror bereavement following human loss.

The findings demonstrate that grief over the loss of a pet is profound and multifaceted, with many participants reporting emotional closeness to their pets comparable to that felt toward human loved ones. Central to this process is anthropomorphism which not only predicted greater grief but significantly mediated the relationship between attachment and bereavement, clarifying why stronger bonds translate into more intense loss reactions.

The chapter also provides further evidence of disenfranchised grief, with participants reporting significantly lower perceived social support following pet loss than after human loss, despite similar levels of emotional closeness. Social support, when present, however, played a protective role. In contrast, guilt and shame, particularly surrounding euthanasia or unexpected death, were associated with heightened grief.

Together, these findings reinforce the need to recognize pet loss as a significant psychosocial event and to develop grief supports that reflect the depth and complexity of human–animal bonds.

The next chapter, "Dealing with Death: The Role of Animal-Themed Literature in Supporting Children with Grief and Loss", explores how mental health practitioners use animal-themed bibliotherapy to help children understand death and process grief. Drawing on a mixed-methods online survey of Australian psychologists, counselors, and psychotherapists who specialize in childhood grief, the chapter examines when, how, and why animal characters are incorporated into therapeutic work.

Findings show that animal-themed death literature is a commonly used tool, preferred by just over half of practitioners and most often employed with younger children (ages 2–7). Its perceived usefulness declines with age, with practitioners viewing it as least effective for adolescents. Importantly, animal-themed bibliotherapy was rarely considered a standalone intervention: instead, it was most often used as an adjunct to other modalities, such as play therapy, drawing, storytelling, and family-based work.

Thematic analysis revealed three central functions of animal-themed literature. First, practitioners described animal characters as creating a safe emotional bridge, allowing children to explore grief indirectly. Second, animals were seen as familiar figures that help children conceptualize death as permanent and universal, drawing on their observations of animal life cycles. Third, the use of animal-themed books was described as highly individualized, shaped by children's age, interests, neurodevelopmental profiles, the therapist's preferences, and available resources.

Overall, this chapter positions animal-themed bibliotherapy as a tool that can facilitate emotional expression, normalize grief, and support early death understanding, particularly in younger children.

The last chapter in this section, "How to Care for the Caregiver: The Power of Ritual", centers on the emotional labor of caring for a terminally ill companion animal and the critical need to support human caregivers through both anticipatory grief and bereavement. Written from the perspective of a licensed clinical social worker embedded within a veterinary teaching hospital, the chapter offers a clinically grounded, practice-oriented exploration of how intentional rituals can help families navigate EOL decision-making, minimize regret, and move through grief with greater self-compassion and meaning.

Drawing on grief theory and clinical experience, the chapter distinguishes between grief as an internal emotional experience and mourning as its outward expression, positioning ritual as a bridge between emotion and meaning-making. Rituals are described as structured, meaningful actions that provide containment for overwhelming emotions, foster mindfulness, and restore a sense of agency during periods of uncertainty and loss. The chapter highlights the particular relevance of ritual in companion animal loss, where formalized mourning practices are often absent.

Through case examples, the author illustrates how rituals can be integrated before loss to ground caregivers in the present moment and create meaningful shared experiences, as well as after loss to sustain continuing bonds, honor the animal's life, and facilitate healing. These rituals range from daily mindful walks and shared "bucket list" experiences to journaling, memorial practices, letter writing, and culturally or spiritually rooted ceremonies.

Collectively, the chapter underscores ritual as a deeply personal, powerful clinical tool that supports both caregiving and grief processing. It calls on veterinary teams and allied professionals to actively encourage and normalize ritualized practices as part of holistic, family-centered EOL care.

Part 3: Service, Professional and Organizational Grief

The first chapter in this section, "Supporting Clients Through Loss: A Qualitative Review of Current Practices of Accredited Assistance Dog Organizations", is a qualitative investigation of how assistance dog organizations support clients through the death or retirement of an assistance dog. Drawing on semi-structured interviews with representatives from 21 Assistance Dogs International–accredited organizations in the United States, the chapter documents the grief-support services offered to their clients. Participants described a continuum of services ranging from personal outreach, psychoeducation, peer support, acknowledgment rituals, counseling services, and memorialization initiatives. At the same time, the chapter reveals substantial variability in how grief support is offered across organizations, influenced by organizational size, resources, and staffing. Despite accreditation standards emphasizing "lifetime support," the absence of explicit guidance regarding grief and bereavement contributes to inconsistent practices and gaps in care.

Building on this variability, the study's findings suggest that the quality of the ongoing relationship between the organization and the client functions as a key protective factor during periods of loss and transition. In addition, it stresses the importance of proactive preparation through psychoeducation, retirement planning, and anticipatory guidance in reducing distress and supporting clients through the grief process. When grief support is integrated across the lifespan of the partnership—rather than introduced only at its end—clients appear better equipped to navigate both the emotional and functional disruptions associated with loss. The chapter concludes by identifying assistance dog organizations as critical in supporting clients through the profound personal, functional, and identity-related losses associated with the end of an assistance dog partnership.

The next chapter, "The Loss of a Service Dog Through Retirement: Experiences and Impact on Human Partners", presents a qualitative exploration of the often-overlooked experience of service dog retirement and its emotional, functional, and identity-related consequences for human partners. Drawing on interviews with 22 service dog partners whose dogs had retired within the previous five years, the chapter examines how retirement constitutes a distinctly unique and frequently misunderstood form of loss, often generating profound, disenfranchised grief.

Findings highlight that partners experience retirement as the loss of an interdependent working relationship. Participants described intense distress surrounding decision-making about timing, rehoming, caregiving capacity, and the integration of successor dogs, many times while their retired dog remained physically present but no longer able to fulfill its former role. The pressure to quickly acquire a successor dog, combined with concerns about bonding and diminished independence further complicated the grieving process.

The chapter also underscores the social invisibility of retirement-related grief. Participants frequently reported feeling misunderstood or silenced by family, colleagues, and broader society, exacerbating feelings of isolation and limiting opportunities for mourning. At the same time, some partners found meaning and comfort through continuing bonds and reciprocal acts of care for their retired dogs. Drawing on these findings, the chapter emphasizes the need for greater awareness among service dog organizations, veterinarians, and mental health professionals regarding the unique challenges of retirement-related loss. By recognizing retirement as a significant event rather than merely a transition, the chapter calls for proactive psychoeducation, systemized support, and interdisciplinary care to better support service dog partners navigating this complex and often invisible grief.

The next chapter, "'My Lifeline Is Gone': An Exploration of the Experiences of Veterans Following the Loss of Their Psychiatric Service Dog(s)", presents an exploratory qualitative examination of grief among Canadian military veterans who experienced the loss of a psychiatric service dog (PSD) through death, retirement, or relinquishment. Drawing on in-depth interviews with four veterans living with posttraumatic stress disorder (PTSD), the chapter centers the lived experience of losing a dog that functioned not only as a companion, but as a critical source of emotional regulation, safety, and daily functioning. The findings reveal that the loss of a PSD represents a relational, functional, and identity-based loss.

Analysis identified a recurring grief cycle consisting of four interrelated stages: the development of a profound bond with the PSD, an intense grief response following loss, a period of coping and healing, and a transitional stage involving the introduction of a new PSD. Participants described their dogs as "lifelines," and their loss as comparable to losing a close family member or combat companion. Grief was frequently compounded by disenfranchisement, with participants reporting limited societal understanding, minimal formal support from service providers, and a lack of socially sanctioned rituals to acknowledge their loss.

Despite these challenges, veterans identified meaning-making strategies that supported healing, including reminiscence, continuing bonds through objects and memories, and peer connection with others who had experienced similar losses. The introduction of a new PSD was described as emotionally complex, requiring readiness, time, and space to grieve before forming a new bond.

The chapter underscores the need for mental health professionals, veterinarians, and service dog organizations to better recognize and respond to the unique grief experiences of veterans with PSD. By legitimizing this loss, providing anticipatory guidance, and integrating grief-informed practices, providers can play a critical role in supporting veterans through the transition of a service dog partnership.

The chapter "Animal Loss and Grief in Zoos: Qualitative Insights to Inform Organizational Support for Zoo Professionals and Volunteers" examines how zoo professionals and volunteers experience animal-related grief and how organizational cultures and policies shape their ability to cope with these losses. Drawing on qualitative responses from 182 U.S.-based zoo professionals and volunteers, this study highlights grief as a pervasive yet often unsupported occupational stressor within zoo settings.

Thematic analysis identified three central areas for organizational improvement. First, participants emphasized the need for a grief-affirming organizational culture that legitimizes emotional expression. Many described cultures of silence and shame that discourage mourning, contributing to feelings of isolation, guilt, and burnout. Second, participants called for stronger organizational responses and resources, including clear communication protocols following animal deaths or transfers, opportunities for memorialization and ritual, and equitable acknowledgment of loss across all species and roles. Third, respondents highlighted the importance of enhanced human resource policies, such as flexible scheduling, task redistribution, paid time off to grieve, and access to mental health supports tailored to zoo-specific losses.

Across roles, participants stressed that meaningful bonds with animals are central to both animal welfare and professional fulfillment, yet these bonds can intensify grief when losses occur. The absence of formal support systems often forced individuals to suppress grief while continuing high-risk, emotionally demanding work. Conversely, examples of supportive leadership, peer solidarity, and ritualized acknowledgment of loss were associated with greater well-being and organizational commitment.

The chapter concludes with actionable recommendations for zoo leaders and institutions, emphasizing low- to moderate-cost interventions that can foster compassionate, trauma-informed workplaces. By normalizing grief, training leaders in empathic responses, and integrating structured support practices, zoos can better protect staff and volunteer well-being while sustaining ethical, effective animal care.

References

Archer, J. (1997). Why do people love their pets? *Evolution and Human Behavior*, 18(4), 237–259. DOI: 10.1016/S0162-3095(99)80001-4.

Behler, A.M.C., Green, J.D. and Joy-Gaba, J. (2020). "We lost a member of the family": Predictors of the grief experience surrounding the loss of a pet. *Human-Animal Interaction Bulletin*, 8(3), 54–70.

Bert, F., Gualano, M.R., Camussi, E., Pieve, G., Voglino, G, and Siliquini, R. (2016). Animal assisted intervention: A systematic review of benefits and risks. *European Journal of Integrative Medicine*, 8(5), 695–706.

Brooks, H.L., Rushton, K., Lovell, K., Bee, P., Walker, L. *et al*. (2018). The power of support from companion animals for people living with mental health problems: A systematic review and narrative synthesis of the evidence. *BMC Psychiatry*, 18(1), 31. DOI: 10.1186/s12888-018-1613-2.

Brown, C.A., Wilson, D.M., Carr, E., Gross, D.P., Miciak, M. *et al*. (2023). Older adults and companion animal death: A survey of bereavement and disenfranchised grief. *Human-Animal Interactions*, 2023.

Bussolari, C., Habarth, J.M., Phillips, S., Katz, R. and Packman, W. (2021). Self-compassion, social constraints, and psychosocial outcomes in a pet bereavement sample. *OMEGA - Journal of Death and Dying*, 82(3), 389–408. DOI: 10.1177/0030222818814050.

Carmack, B.J. (1985). The effects on family members and functioning after the death of a pet. *Marriage & Family Review*, 8(3–4), 149–161. DOI: 10.1300/J002v08n03_11.

Corrigan, V., Cooney, K. and Foster, R. (2025). Compassionate end-of-life care: Development, implementation, and evaluation of a comprehensive euthanasia course in veterinary education from 2019–2024. *Human-Animal Interactions*. DOI: 10.1079/hai.2025.0025.

Crossley, M.K. and Rolland, C. (2022). Overcoming the social stigma of losing a pet: Considerations for counseling professionals. *Human-Animal Interactions*, 2022. DOI: 10.1079/hai.2022.0022.

Currin-McCulloch, J., Bussolari, C., Packman, W., Kogan, L. and Erdman, P. (2022). The loss of a service dog through retirement: Experiences and impact on human partners. *Human-Animal Interaction Bulletin*, 2022. DOI: 10.1079/hai.2022.0017.

DeSantis, D. and Gerlach, J.H. (2025). Supporting clients through loss: A qualitative review of current practices of accredited assistance dog organizations. *Human-Animal Interactions*, 13(1), 0009. DOI: 10.1079/hai.2025.0009.

Doka, K. (1989). *Disenfranchised Grief: Recognizing Hidden Sorrow*. Lexington Books, Maryland.

Ellis, C., Littrell, K., Carmack, T. and Christopher, K. (2024). The evolution, challenges and future of veterinary hospice and palliative care. *Human-Animal Interactions*, 12(1). DOI: 10.1079/hai.2024.0033.

Field, N.P., Orsini, L., Gavish, R. and Packman, W. (2009). Role of attachment in response to pet loss. *Death Studies*, 33(4), 334–355. DOI: 10.1080/07481180802705783.

Fine, A.H. and Andersen, S.J. (2021). A commentary on the contemporary issues confronting animal assisted and equine assisted interactions. *Journal of Equine Veterinary Science*, 100, 103436.

Fournier, A.K. and Mustful, B. (2019). Chapter 27 - Compassion Fatigue: Presenting Issues and Practical Applications for Animal-Caring Professionals. In L. Kogan and C. Blazina (eds.), *Clinician's Guide to Treating Companion Animal Issues* (pp. 511–534). Academic Press. DOI: 10.1016/B978-0-12-812962-3.00027-7.

Gibson, M., Chalmers, D. and Ru, S. (2022). "My Lifeline is Gone": An exploration of the experiences of veterans following the loss of their psychiatric service dog(s). *Human-Animal Interaction Bulletin*, 2022. DOI: 10.1079/hai.2022.0009.

Hoffmann, H. and Dickinson, G. (2021). Veterinary professionals' experiences with human caregivers when providing animal hospice and palliative care. *Human-Animal Interaction Bulletin*. DOI: 10.1079/hai.2021.0019.

Hudock, A. (2025). One owner's perspective after a pet hospice journey. *Human-Animal Interactions*. DOI: 10.1079/hai.2025.0027.

Hyland, P. (2026). No pets allowed: Evidence that prolonged grief disorder can occur following the death of a pet. *PloS One*, 21(1), e0339213. DOI: 10.1371/journal.pone.0339213.

Klass, D., Silverman, P. and Nickman, S. (1996). *Continuing Bonds | New Understandings of Grief | Dennis Klass, Phyllis*. Taylor & Francis. https://www.taylorfrancis.com/books/edit/10.4324/9781315800790/continuing-bonds-dennis-klass-steven-nickman-phyllis-silverman

Kogan, L.R. and Cooney, K.A. (2023). Defining a "Good Death": Exploring veterinarians' perceptions of companion animal euthanasia. *Animals : An Open Access Journal from MDPI*, 13(13), 2117. DOI: 10.3390/ani13132117.

Kogan, L.R., Packman, W., Bussolari, C., Currin-McCulloch, J. and Erdman, P. (2022). Pet death and owners' memorialization choices. *Illness, Crisis & Loss*, 10541373221143046. DOI: 10.1177/10541373221143046.

Kogan, L.R., Packman, W., Currin-McCulloch, J., Bussolari, C. and Erdman, P. (2023). The loss of a service dog through death or retirement: Experiences and impact on partners. *Illness, Crisis & Loss*, 31(2), 244–270. DOI: 10.1177/10541373211054168.

Kogan, L.R. and Rishniw, M. (2024). Relief and mobile veterinary careers may offer a path towards improved quality of life. *Journal of the American Veterinary Medical Association*, 262(2), 209–215. DOI: 10.2460/javma.23.07.0422.

Leonhardt-Parr, E. and Rumble, B. (2024). Coping with animal companion loss: A thematic analysis of pet bereavement counselling. *Omega*, 89(1), 362–378. DOI: 10.1177/00302228211073217.

Li, J. and Wong, N.M.L. (2025). The mediating role of loneliness in the relationship between pet ownership and human well-being. *Scientific Reports*, 15, 35899. DOI: 10.1038/s41598-025-19692-2.

McDonald, S.E., Kogan, L.R., Nageotte, N.L., Currin-McCulloch, J. and Dickler-Mann, R. (2024). Zoo professionals and volunteers in the U.S: Experiences and prevalence of burnout, mental health, and animal loss. *Frontiers in Psychiatry*, 15. DOI: 10.3389/fpsyt.2024.1373525.

Moses, L., Malowney, M.J. and Boyd, J.W. (2018). Ethical conflict and moral distress in veterinary practice: A survey of North American veterinarians. *Journal of Veterinary Internal Medicine*, 32(6), 2115–2122. DOI: 10.1111/jvim.15315.

Northrope, K., Shnookal, J., Ruby, M.B. and Howell, T.J. (2025). The relationship between attachment to pets and mental health and wellbeing: A systematic review. *Animals*, 15(8), 1143. DOI: 10.3390/ani15081143.

O'Connor, V.L., Vonk, J. and Compitus, K. (2022). When support is "pawsed": Increased attachment mediates the association between loss of support and pet bereavement during the pandemic. *Human-Animal Interactions*, 2022.

Packman, W., Carmack, B.J., Katz, R., Carlos, F., Field, N.P. and Landers, C. (2014). Online survey as empathic bridging for the disenfranchised grief of pet loss. *OMEGA - Journal of Death and Dying*, 69(4), 333–356. DOI: 10.2190/OM.69.4.a.

Packman, W., Field, N.P., Carmack, B.J. and Ronen, R. (2011). Continuing bonds and psychosocial adjustment in pet loss. *Journal of Loss and Trauma*, 16(4), 341–357. DOI: 10.1080/15325024.2011.572046.

Park, R.M., Royal, K.D. and Gruen, M.E. (2021). A Literature Review: Pet bereavement and coping mechanisms. *Journal of Applied Animal Welfare Science*. DOI: 10.1080/10888705.2021.1934839.

Piche, E. (2025). The untapped potential of Registered Veterinary Technicians in hospice care. *Human-Animal Interactions*. DOI: 10.1079/hai.2025.0034.

Rollin, B.E. (2011). Euthanasia, moral stress, and chronic illness in veterinary medicine. *Veterinary Clinics of North America: Small Animal Practice, Palliative Medicine and Hospice Care*, 41(3), 651–659. DOI: 10.1016/j.cvsm.2011.03.005.

Scotney, R.L., McLaughlin, D. and Keates, H.L. (2019). An investigation of the prevalence of compassion fatigue, compassion satisfaction and burnout in those working in animal-related occupations using the Professional Quality of Life (ProQoL) Scale. *The Veterinary Nurse*, 10(5). DOI: 10.12968/vetn.2019.10.5.276.

Siess, S., Kramer, G.A., Ozer, D., Gaudette, N., Williams, B. *et al*. (2021). Predictors of opting for advanced medical care versus euthanasia for companion animals with severe cardiac disease. *Human-Animal Interaction Bulletin*, 11(3), 1–22.

Smit, E. and Smith, B.P. (2023). Dealing with death: The role of animal-themed literature in supporting children with grief and loss. *Human-Animal Interactions*, 2023. DOI: 10.1079/hai.2023.0002.

Testoni, I., De Cataldo, L., Ronconi, L., Colombo, E.S., Stefanini, C. *et al*. (2019). Pet grief: Tools to assess owners' bereavement and veterinary communication skills. *Animals : An Open Access Journal from MDPI*, 9(2), 67. DOI: 10.3390/ani9020067.

Truman, L. (2025). How to care for the caregiver: The power of ritual. *Human-Animal Interactions*, 13(1), 0022. DOI: 10.1079/hai.2025.0022.

Villalobos, A. and Kaplan, L. (2017). *Canine and Feline Geriatric Oncology: Honoring the Human-Animal Bond*. Wiley-Blackwell. https://www.wiley.com/en-us/Canine+and+Feline+Geriatric+Oncology%3A+Honoring+the+Human-Animal+Bond%2C+2nd+Edition-p-9781119290469

Vonk, J., Bouma, E. and Dijkstra, A. (2022). A time to say goodbye: Empathy and emotion regulation predict timing of end-of-life decisions by pet owners. *Human-Animal Interaction Bulletin*. DOI: 10.1079/hai.2022.0013.

Walsh, F. (2009). Human-Animal Bonds II: The role of pets in family systems and family therapy. *Family Process*, 48(4), 481–499. DOI: 10.1111/j.1545-5300.2009.01297.x

Wood, W., Alm, K., Benjamin, J., Thomas, L., Anderson, D. *et al*. (2021). Optimal terminology for services in the United States that incorporate horses to benefit people: A consensus document. *The Journal of Alternative and Complementary Medicine: Paradigm, Practice, and Policy Advancing Integrative Health*, 27(1), 88–95.

Wu, Y. and Song, J. (2025). The relationship between pet attachment and pet loss grief in Chinese undergraduates: A conditional process model. *Behavioral Sciences*, 15(4), 431. DOI: 10.3390/bs15040431.

1 The Evolution, Challenges, and Future of Veterinary Hospice and Palliative Care

Coleen Ellis[1], Kellie Littrell[2], Tyler Carmack[2] and Karin Christopher[3]*
[1]Two Hearts Pet Loss Center, Indianapolis, IN, USA; [2]Caring Pathways, Denver, CO, USA; [3]Pet Quietus, Corpus Christi, TX, USA

Keywords: hospice, palliative care, end-of-life, euthanasia, veterinary

Veterinary hospice and palliative care have undergone significant evolution, responding to increased life spans in companion animals (Montoya *et al.*, 2023) and the growing recognition of pets as beloved family members (McConnell *et al.*, 2011). This increase in pet life expectancy, combined with the strengthening of the human–animal bond, necessitates the need to provide end-of-life comfort, dignity, and support for critically ill or aging animals, principles that parallel human hospice care. The animal hospice mentality revolves around a holistic, compassionate approach to end-of-life care. It prioritizes the pet's comfort, pain management and emotional well-being, while also supporting the grieving family. Although considerable advancements have been made, gaps in knowledge among veterinary professionals, researchers and pet caregivers, coupled with persistent misconceptions, hinder the broader adoption and implementation of veterinary hospice strategies imperative to an animal's quality of life.

The roots of veterinary hospice and palliative care trace back to the late 1980s when veterinary pioneers Dr. Eric Clough and his wife, Jane, Dr. Guy Hancock, Dr. James Harris and Dr. Bonnie Mader began advocating for compassionate end-of-life care (Marocchino, 2011). Prior to this shift, euthanasia was often the primary option for terminally ill animals. Dr. Alice Villalobos introduced the concept of "pawspice" care in 2000, emphasizing comfort and quality-of-life above extending the lifespan at all costs (Villalobos, 2011). In 2009, the International Association for Animal Hospice and Palliative Care (IAAHPC) was founded to provide needed high-quality end-of-life education, research, and increase professional and public discourse (Shanan and Shearer, 2023). This movement has since gained momentum, integrating the principles of pain management, emotional support, and a dignified farewell. The philosophies of treating the entire family unit, rather than just the animal patient, and shifting from a "cure" to a "care" mentality are fundamental principles of veterinary hospice and palliative care.

Today, veterinary hospice and palliative care are widely recognized within the veterinary profession, largely due to the efforts of the IAAHPC. In 2013, the IAAHPC developed the

*Corresponding author: karin@petquietus.com

first End-of-Life Care Guidelines, and in 2016, in collaboration with the American Animal Hospital Association (AAHA), it created the updated AAHA/ IAAHPC End-of-Care Guidelines (Bishop *et al.*, 2016). These guidelines have been endorsed by the American Veterinary Medical Association (n.d). In 2020, AAHA announced its End-of-life Care accreditation program to recognize veterinary practices that provide compassionate, respectful, and efficient end-of-life care for pets and their human companions (End-of-Life Care Accreditation, n.d). In 2023, the American Association of Feline Practitioners (AAFP), in collaboration with the IAAHPC, released hospice care guidelines specific to felines (Eigner *et al.*, 2023). In addition, veterinary hospice and palliative care books and peer-reviewed articles and reviews have added to the growing body of literature for both professionals and pet caregivers.

Despite these advances, wider recognition, acceptance, and implementation of animal hospice philosophy and care among veterinarians and pet caregivers remain limited. Some veterinarians resist the hospice philosophy, preferring curative treatments even when palliative care would better serve the animal's quality of life (Downing, 2011). A recent paper noted some of the common challenges to palliative care in both veterinary and human medicine, which include, but are not limited to; dealing with chronic illness, unresolved grief, lack of support and absence of specialized care providers (de Costa *et al.*, 2024). While instruction and continuing education in animal hospice and palliative care via conferences, certification programs and other virtual and in-person learning modalities are offered to veterinarians, technicians and paraprofessionals, integrating this content into veterinary and veterinary technician curricula has proven more difficult. Two veterinary schools, Colorado State University and Michigan State University, launched hospice programs in 2019 (Gore *et al.*, 2019; Yaxley, 2019), yet at the time of this writing, neither appear as stand-alone services on their respective websites.

The lack of knowledge and comfort level among veterinary professionals regarding animal hospice and palliative care means many pet caregivers are unaware of these options, often discovering them only when confronted with a dire prognosis, rather than early in the course of the disease (Paz *et al.*, 2024). Although awareness and demand are increasing, it is still unclear what caregivers know about end-of-life care for their pets (Heuberger and Pierce, 2017). Even when informed, resistance and misconceptions persist. Some people may perceive hospice care as merely prolonging suffering, unclear that it focuses on alleviating pain and stress. Other owners fear being judged for choosing hospice over immediate euthanasia, reflecting a societal discomfort with death and dying. Still, others may decline veterinary hospice due to finances, unaware that as less money is spent on diagnostics and cure, more can be applied to managing and treating symptoms to provide comfort. It is imperative for the veterinary community to address this knowledge gap through public education and proactive communication (Shaw and Lagoni, 2007). In alignment with the spectrum-of-care approach, pet owners should be compassionately educated about the benefits and availability of veterinary hospice and palliative care early in their pets' healthcare journey. This can be accomplished through informational brochures, social media campaigns, and discussions during routine veterinary visits.

In addition to the gaps in hospice knowledge among veterinary professionals and pet caregivers, a noticeable disconnect between veterinary practitioners and researchers exists. Veterinarians in clinical practice may lack exposure to the latest research and methodologies, while researchers might not fully comprehend the practical challenges faced in veterinary clinics. Available evidence-based literature on veterinary palliative care is also lacking, contributing to this gap (de Costa *et al.*, 2024). In addition, funding may not be adequate to stimulate the kind of studies needed to provide evidence-based research to sufficiently explore and validate the concepts of veterinary hospice and palliative care. Enhanced collaboration and communication between researchers and veterinarians in clinical practice, more high-quality evidence-based studies, along with grants and other funding focused on the hospice and palliative care model, could lead to a more cohesive approach and improved care standards.

Addressing misconceptions and resistance to veterinary hospice and palliative care will require a shift in the broader veterinary culture.

Potential strategies to reduce misunderstanding and promote end-of-life animal welfare include normalizing conversations about death, training veterinarians to discuss hospice care sensitively, and emphasizing the core goal of enhancing the quality of life rather than simply extending it. Through continued education and evidence-based research, veterinary hospice models within veterinary clinics, mobile veterinary practices or those guided by case managers, will be best served by collaborating through an interdisciplinary team (IDT) and maintaining a bond-centered approach focus (Shanan and Shearer, 2023).

One of the most profound benefits of integrating hospice and palliative care into veterinary practice, besides improving the quality of life of animals, is the positive impact on mental health for both veterinarians and their clients. The emotional toll of euthanasia on veterinary personnel is significant, contributing to high stress, compassion fatigue, and burnout (Scotney *et al.*, 2015). Offering veterinary hospice and palliative care could help to minimize this burden, allowing veterinarians to provide ongoing care and support while fostering deeper relationships with clients. For pet guardians, the availability of animal hospice care can provide peace of mind and reassurance that their beloved companions can experience a dignified and comfortable end-of-life journey. This emotionally supportive environment nurtures healthier outcomes to cope with grief.

Veterinary hospice and palliative care represent the continual evolution of the deep bonds we share with our animal companions. By addressing gaps in knowledge, misconceptions, and fostering a culture of compassionate care, we can enhance the well-being of pet caregivers and veterinarians alike and advance veterinary hospice and palliative care through evidence-based research and broader communication. Embracing this holistic approach promises a future where end-of-life care is as dignified as the life that precedes it. Through continued education, collaboration, and cultural shifts, the veterinary profession can fully realize the profound potential of hospice and palliative care, ensuring that every pet's final chapter is written with love and tenderness.

Conflict of Interest

The authors have no conflicts of interest to declare.

Funding

This research received no external funding.

Ethics Statement

The authors confirm that the research meets any required ethical guidelines, including adherence to the legal requirements of the study country.

Author Contributions

All authors contributed equally to the development of this article.

References

American Veterinary Medical Association (n.d) Veterinary End-of-Life Care. Available at: https://www.avma.org/resources-tools/avma-policies/veterinary-end-life-care (accessed 4 August 2024).

Bishop, G., Cooney, K., Cox, S., Downing, R., Mitchener, K. *et al.* (2016) 2016 AAHA/IAAHPC end-of-life care guidelines. *Journal of the American Animal Hospital Association* 52(6), 341–356. DOI: 10.5326/JAAHA-MS-6637.

de Costa, J.M., Barroso, T.G. and Prata, J.C. (2024) Research priorities in veterinary palliative care. *Veterinary Journal (London, England: 1997)* 306, 106184. DOI: 10.1016/j.tvjl.2024.106184.

Downing, R. (2011) Pain management for veterinary palliative care and hospice patients. *The Veterinary Clinics of North America. Small Animal Practice* 41(3), 531–550. DOI: 10.1016/j.cvsm.2011.03.010.

Eigner, D.R., Breitreiter, K., Carmack, T., Cox, S., Downing, R. *et al.* (2023) 2023 AAFP/IAAHPC feline hospice and palliative care guidelines. *Journal of Feline Medicine and Surgery* 25(9), 1098612X231201683. DOI: 10.1177/1098612X231201683.

End-of-Life Care Accreditation (n.d) AAHA. Available at: https://www.aaha.org/about-accreditation/earn-aaha-accreditation/end-of-life-care-accreditation/ (accessed 5 August 2024).

Gore, M., Lana, S.E. and Bishop, G.A. (2019) Colorado state university, pet hospice program. *The Veterinary Clinics of North America. Small Animal Practice* 49(3), 339–349. DOI: 10.1016/j.cvsm.2019.01.002.

Heuberger, R.A. and Pierce, J. (2017) Companion-animal caregiver knowledge, attitudes, and beliefs regarding end-of-life care. *Journal of Applied Animal Welfare Science* 20(4), 313–323. DOI: 10.1080/10888705.2017.1321483.

Marocchino, K.D. (2011) In the shadow of a rainbow: The history of animal hospice. *The Veterinary Clinics of North America. Small Animal Practice* 41(3), 477–498. DOI: 10.1016/j.cvsm.2011.03.008.

McConnell, A.R., Brown, C., Shoda, T., Stayton, L. and Martin, C. (2011) Friends with benefits: On the positive consequences of pet ownership. *Journal of Personality and Social Psychology* 101(6), 1239–1252.

Montoya, M., Morrison, J.A., Arrignon, F., Spofford, N., Charles, H. *et al.* (2023) Life expectancy tables for dogs and cats derived from clinical data. *Frontiers in Veterinary Science* 10, 1082102. DOI: 10.3389/fvets.2023.1082102.

Paz, B.F., Ferreira, M.G.P.A., Martins, K.R., Uccella, L. and Barboza de Nardi, A. (2024) Practical principles of palliative care in veterinary oncology: Alleviating the suffering of the animal, owner, and veterinarian. *Veterinary Medicine International* 2024, 5565837. DOI: 10.1155/2024/5565837.

Scotney, R.L., McLaughlin, D. and Keates, H.L. (2015) A systematic review of the effects of euthanasia and occupational stress in personnel working with animals in animal shelters, veterinary clinics, and biomedical research facilities. *Journal of the American Veterinary Medical Association* 247(10), 1121–1130. DOI: 10.2460/javma.247.10.1121.

Shanan, A. and Shearer, T. (2023) What is animal hospice and palliative care? In: Shanan, A., Pierce, J. and Shearer, T. (eds) *Hospice and Palliative Care for Companion Animals*, 1st edn. Wiley, Hoboken, NJ, pp. 6–15. DOI: 10.1002/9781119808817.ch2.

Shaw, J.R. and Lagoni, L. (2007) End-of-life communication in veterinary medicine: Delivering bad news and euthanasia decision making. *The Veterinary Clinics of North America. Small Animal Practice* 37(1), 95–108; abstract viii–ix. DOI: 10.1016/j.cvsm.2006.09.010.

Villalobos, A.E. (2011) Assessment and treatment of nonpain conditions in life-limiting disease. *The Veterinary Clinics of North America. Small Animal Practice* 41(3), 551–563. DOI: 10.1016/j.cvsm.2011.03.003.

Yaxley, P.E. (2019) Michigan state university veterinary hospice care: An academic hospice practice 2011 to 2014. *The Veterinary Clinics of North America. Small Animal Practice* 49(3), 351–362. DOI: 10.1016/j.cvsm.2019.01.003.

2 Veterinary Professionals' Experiences with Human Caregivers When Providing Animal Hospice and Palliative Care

Heath C. Hoffmann* **and George E. Dickinson**
College of Charleston, Charleston, SC, USA

Abstract
A significant role in veterinary medical practices is the provision of end-of-life (EOL) care to pets and their clients. Yet, U.S. veterinarians report being dissatisfied with the level of training they receive on EOL issues in their veterinary medical programs (Dickinson *et al.*, 2011). At the same time, the ubiquity of veterinary information on the Internet (e.g., "Dr. Google") has the potential for instilling pet owners with a false sense of expertise that veterinarians must then negotiate when providing EOL care. In this context, we surveyed 86 veterinary members of the International Association for Animal Hospice and Palliative Care (IAAHPC) to explore whether and/or how veterinary medical information clients obtain from the Internet impacts the veterinarians' delivery of EOL care to those clients' pets; we similarly investigate the information that veterinarians prefer their clients knew before meeting with them to provide EOL care. In light of the inherent challenges of EOL veterinary care outlined above, we learn from veterinarians what they feel are the most challenging and rewarding aspects of providing palliative and hospice care. Using qualitative thematic coding, our results show, in sum, that veterinary information from the Internet is both helpful and harmful to veterinarian interactions with clients; veterinarians wished clients understood the value of hospice and palliative care as an EOL care option and that grief is normal; and veterinarians report a most positive aspect of dealing with these issues is the gratitude clients show for helping their pets die peacefully.

Keywords: veterinarians, end-of-life knowledge of clients, rewards of animal hospice and palliative care

"Euthanasia is sometimes the last arrow in our quiver, the last act of love we can give."
Dr. Mike Paul, DVM (Paul, 2019)

As Dr. Paul suggests above, euthanasia is a normative part of the end-of-life (EOL) care veterinarians provide. However, advances in hospice and palliative care provide additional arrows to the veterinarians' quiver in caring for pets at the end of their lives. Hospice is the philosophy of care that regards death as a natural process and prioritizes comfort and quality of life over quantity of life as death draws near and supports the cultural and spiritual aspects of dying (Goldberg, 2016). Animal hospice involves advanced pet comfort care, client expectation

*Corresponding author: hoffmannh@cofc.edu

management and education (Gregersen, 2016). The establishment of hospice and palliative care as distinct areas of veterinary practice is a relatively recent phenomenon (Goldberg, 2016).

Animal hospice care began in the 1980s, following the hospice model for humans which started in the United Kingdom in the late 1960s, before moving to the US in the early 1970s (Dickinson and Hoffmann, 2019). Palliative care also came into existence in the 1970s and is designed to give the patient as pain-free an experience as possible. Hospice is basically palliative care at the EOL (Goldberg, 2016). The prominence of EOL in the work of veterinarians is problematic. A minority (33%) of U.S. veterinarians, for example, report being well-prepared by their veterinary medical school training to deal with EOL issues (Dickinson *et al.*, 2011). As a result, veterinarians and staff have developed competence on EOL issues from on-the-job training (Gregersen, 2016). The dearth of formal training in veterinary EOL is troubling. Veterinary burnout and compassion fatigue are at least partially linked to the frequent exposure to trauma or "critical incidents" (see Mitchener and Ogilvie, 2002) and the difficult emotional work associated with administering euthanasia and other EOL care (Gardner and Hini, 2006; Huggard and Huggard, 2008; Bartram *et al.*, 2009; Platt *et al.*, 2012; Tran *et al.*, 2014; Hart and Yamamoto, 2017). In fact, the increased frequency of practicing euthanasia is associated with an increased likelihood of depression and an increased suicide risk (Tran *et al.*, 2014). A growing body of research shows that suicide rates among veterinarians are 2–4 times higher than among the general population across different countries and continents (Mellanby, 2005; Bartram and Baldwin, 2008; Jones-Fairnie *et al.*, 2008; Bartram and Baldwin, 2010; Milner *et al.*, 2015; Tomasi *et al.*, 2019).

The grief and stress experienced by the owners of dying pets may itself impact veterinarians' well-being (Spitznagel *et al.*, 2017). Thus, providing EOL care is challenging for veterinarians and their staff. This is particularly concerning given that 75% of American veterinarians agree that veterinary medical schools should place more emphasis on communication skills with owners of terminally ill animals (Dickinson *et al.*, 2011). The client-veterinarian interaction is the domain in which clients' knowledge and expectations about EOL veterinary care complements or collides with what veterinarians can realistically do for the clients' pets. As such, this research draws from the experiences of veterinarian members of the International Association of Animal Hospice and Palliative Care (IAAHPC) to examine the issues veterinarians specializing in EOL care encounter with their clients. Specifically, we explore whether and/or how veterinary medical information clients obtain from the Internet impacts the veterinarians' delivery of EOL care to those clients' pets. We similarly investigate the information that veterinarians prefer their clients knew before meeting with them to provide EOL care to their companion animal. In light of the inherent challenges of EOL veterinary care outlined above, we learn from veterinarians what they feel are the most challenging and rewarding aspects of providing palliative and hospice care. This study will attempt to address these queries in the hopes of helping to make the entire EOL experience with the client and the pet more tolerable and satisfying for all concerned—the veterinarian, the client, and the pet.

Method

Survey solicitation was distributed via email list-serve on February 6, 2017, to approximately 400 members of the International Association of Animal Hospice and Palliative Care (IAAHPC) regarding their experiences and preferences in providing EOL care to companion animals. Approximately 95% of those members are practicing veterinarians or veterinary technicians, and thus, 380 of the IAAHPC members were eligible to participate in this study. A follow-up email solicitation was distributed via email on March 2, 2017. A solicitation to this survey was also posted on the IAAHPC's Facebook page on February 2, 2017 as well as the Facebook page for VetTechLife.com.

Survey solicitations included a hyperlink to an electronic survey in Qualtrics. While the survey contains approximately 30 questions, this paper examines respondents' answers to the following four open-ended questions: (1) How interaction with clients is enhanced or complicated by the proliferation of veterinary medical information on the Internet; (2) what the veterinarian wishes all pet owners knew before calling on the veterinarian to provide EOL care to their pet; (3) what the most challenging aspect is of providing palliative and hospice care; and (4) what the most rewarding part is of providing palliative and hospice care.

Qualitative thematic coding procedures were used to analyze participants' answers to the above questions and is a standard analytical process employed in the social, behavioral and health sciences (see Nowell *et al.*, 2017). The analytical process involved the following stages:

1. The data were organized vertically in a column of an Excel sheet—one Excel sheet for each of the four questions. Columns to the right of the data column are used for successive rounds of coding and a "Notes" column serves as a repository for observations, thoughts, analytical questions and to highlight quotable material that can be integrated into the manuscript.
2. The analytical process began by becoming familiar with the data, reading through all responses to all four questions, noting preliminary themes and observations by reading through all responses to all four questions.
3. The data were read again to generate initial codes and to develop preliminary labels for the themes appearing in each response. At this stage, each response will likely contain several initial codes (e.g. a single response to a question might reference "Dr. Google," "frustrated with client," "grief management"). In this stage, the data and initial codes were read through a second time to double-check consistency across initial codes.
4. The initial codes were reviewed to identify, inductively, larger themes that reflect commonalities in these initial codes. At the same time, the published literature and our previous conversations with, and surveys of veterinarians, pointed to themes into which these initial codes might coalesce. For example, our interest in the rewarding aspects of providing veterinary EOL care was based in part on conversations with veterinarians indicating that compassionate EOL care helps to relieve human's suffering as well as the pet's—thus that was a deductive theme into which initial codes can begin to be grouped.

After engaging in the above process through successive iterations, we reached a point of saturation where continued reading and analysis of the data and scrutinization of the codes and emerging themes yielded no new insights. The product of this process is the themes appearing below as subheadings in each of the major sections.

This research study was reviewed and approved (IRB-2015-4-28-114909) by the College of Charleston's Institutional Review Board (FWA 00000772).

Results

The survey was accessed electronically by 214 individuals, 137 of whom submitted a partially or fully completed survey. Of those, 86 respondents answered one or more of the four questions that are the subject of the analysis below. That only 86 veterinarians completed the open-ended questions is not atypical in survey research given that the open-ended questions appeared at the end of the survey and, in general, survey respondents are least likely to complete open-ended questions due to time constraints and the survey fatigue that is plaguing the social science research world today. Because the survey solicitation was posted and shared via the IAAHPC's Facebook page, it is not possible to calculate a response rate as the population size cannot be finitely measured. The demographic profile of those responding to the survey is summarized in Table 2.1.

Respondents completed their veterinary medical or veterinary technician training at 36 different institutions in seven countries (U.S., Canada, Italy, England, Australia, Scotland and St. Kitts and Nevis). Most respondents were trained at U.S. universities and those mentioned most often are the University of California, Davis (n=8), Colorado State University (n=7), Ontario Veterinary College (n=6) and Texas A&M (n=6). The veterinary programs at the University of Georgia and the University of Minnesota were

Table 2.1. Demographic profile of survey respondents.

Female	92%
Age[a]	73%
25–34 years old	1%
35–44 years old	26%
45–54 years old	37%
55–64 years old	21%
65 and older	6%
Year Veterinary Training Completed[a]	
1970–1979	2%
1980–1989	18%
1990–1999	34%
2000–2009	33%
2010–2017	13%
Professional Status	
Full-time veterinarian	74%
Part-time veterinarian	14%
Veterinary technician	8%
Other	4%
Veterinary Practice Type	
Mobile veterinary practice	53%
Clinic-based practice	25%
Mobile veterinary and clinical practice	13%
Other	9%
Regional Location	
West	36%
South	28%
Midwest	13%
Northeast	13%
Outside U.S.	10%

[a]Percentages might not add up to 100% due to rounding

each mentioned by four respondents. Cornell, Iowa State University, Kansas State University, The Ohio State University, Ross University and the University of Florida were each mentioned by three respondents.

The participants in this study have extensive experience providing EOL care. The average number of animals euthanized by respondents in a typical year was 239 (with a range between 4 and 1000), with dogs (62%) and cats (36%) constituting the majority of animals euthanized. Thirty percent of respondents felt that they knew the animal and its family well. Sixty-two percent of those responding report that euthanasia was typically performed in the client's home, 21% in the veterinary clinic, and 6% in the emergency veterinary clinic. That clinic-based euthanasia procedures are performed relatively infrequently by our respondents reflects the fact that a majority of them (53%) work in a mobile-veterinary practice or a mobile and clinical practice (13%). Below we summarize these veterinarians' views on the impact the Internet has on their practice of veterinary medicine, what they wish their clients knew or understood when providing EOL care to their clients' pets and the most challenging and rewarding aspects of providing EOL veterinary care.

"Dr. Google"

We asked veterinary professionals how their interactions with clients have been complicated and/or enhanced by pet owners consulting Internet information sources before bringing their pet to the clinic. For some there is a love-hate relationship with the Internet as noted by one veterinarian who wrote, "Oh, Dr. Google, how I despise and appreciate you... this is a mixed bag. Of course, it is wonderful for clients to be well informed; however, the down sides to misinformation are numerous." The nuance around this issue is likely why only 13 of the 81 veterinary professionals who answered this question focus entirely on the negative consequences of clients consulting the Internet before soliciting their services. For example, one veterinarian succinctly expressed a view with, "Hate Dr. Google!!!" Another wrote, "...after the client has first consulted 'Dr Google', I wind up having to work even harder than usual to gain my client's trust, undo the Internet damage and educate the client correctly." Still another veterinarian wrote, "Owners go on the Internet prior to a consultation and become very stressed about 'worst case' scenarios by the time they come to the veterinarian. I don't find anyone is better equipped by googling [sic] their animal's symptoms." Another veterinarian outlined the myriad problems with information clients obtain online but concludes with a statement of support for the "education" their clients generally receive from the Internet:

> Probably the biggest complication is in compliance with medications. I have some clients that research drugs and side effects to the nth degree and ALWAYS see those side effects in their pets. Forums can also complicate, as my clients read about other peoples [sic] experiences with the same disease. Many of these discussions are quick to blame or give credit where it is not due (Miracle supplements, etc.). There are also companies/veterinarians promising miracles with their products. In general, I love the education that the internet can provide for my clients.

In spite of the difficulty of ensuring that clients are accessing accurate and valid veterinary information online, negative evaluations of "Dr. Google" is a minority view among those we surveyed. In fact, one veterinarian reframed the "Dr. Google" dilemma around the attitude of the clinician, writing, "The complication or enhancement of such consultations depends entirely on the attitude of the clinician. Only the most judgmental, arrogant DVMs bemoan 'Dr. Google.'" The overwhelming consensus among those in our study is that veterinary information obtained by clients presents both positive and negative challenges to them professionally (approximately 13% said the Internet is not problematic at all). Having to correct misinformation clients have obtained from the Internet was mentioned most often by respondents as a challenge (approximately 20%), including clients who had developed inaccurate expectations of what euthanasia would be like for their pet, medication compliance (because clients had read about side effects that were exceedingly rare or not clinically accurate) and having to tactfully contradict and correct their clients' misdiagnosis of their pet's condition that was obtained from "Dr. Google."

The dominant theme that emerges among veterinary professionals is that the wealth of veterinary information available online better prepares clients for the provision of EOL care to their pets, the dying process and how to recognize changes in their pets' well-being. For example, one veterinarian wrote:

> They generally are more informed or misinformed. Those who research ahead of time want more detailed explanations of what is going on with their pet and what we are doing. Some need detailed explanations of why what they found online isn't accurate. It feels like a detriment at times, but if I don't fight it and use it as a teaching experience instead of getting offended that they consulted Dr. Google; it can enhance the trust and relationship.

A second veterinarian made a similar point in the following statement:

> I think the internet has given clients (guardians) a wealth of information and they are more invested in doing what is right for themselves and the pet than they were in the past. They don't leave it up to the doctor to decide (which I think is right)—sometimes they need more guidance than the internet can give them which is where I come in.

The latter veterinarian's view was echoed by several respondents, including veterinarians who explicitly noted that clients regularly consulted with them for clarification of veterinary information they had obtained from an Internet source. In fact, respondents regularly mentioned directing their clients to "approved" veterinary websites (e.g. veterinarypartner.com) or to websites and blogs that they themselves had created to help clients better care for their pets, illustrating the powerful role of Internet veterinary information to reinforce veterinary medical practice. Further, that the Internet can be harnessed to support veterinary practitioners is evidenced by the fact that approximately 16% of respondents indicated in our survey that their clients had found their practice online (especially among respondents whose practices consist entirely of providing at-home euthanasia services). As a result, veterinarians regularly indicated in this study that they purposely invested significant resources to developing their clinic's websites in order to attract clients as well as offer a platform for educating their clients.

What veterinarians wish their clients knew

We asked veterinary professionals what they wished all pet owners knew and/or understood before they were called upon to provide EOL care to their pets. Seventy-two respondents answered this question. Four issues emerged as the most common and concerning to these veterinarians: 1) pet owners' understanding of the euthanasia process and how animals experience death; 2) that grief is a normal experience for pet owners who should not feel guilty for making the decision to euthanize a family pet; 3) pet owners' understanding of how to gauge a pet's quality of life and how animals display pain; and 4) that pet owners seek help sooner rather than later and, in doing so, be aware of and fully understand the role veterinary hospice and palliative care can play in facilitating a "good death" for pets; We discuss each of these below alongside less often mentioned themes that did not fit into these general categories.

The euthanasia process

Approximately 23 of our respondents expressed a desire for their clients to understand the euthanasia process (e.g. how clients' experience at the clinic will be organized), what death looks like for the pet (e.g. the pet's eyes will not close and the animal's bowels and bladder will release), that "death can be peaceful and painless" and occurs quickly but euthanasia also does not always go as planned (e.g. "veins don't always cooperate"). The following quote is illustrative of this category, encapsulating each of these themes while emphasizing the more mechanical steps of the euthanasia procedure:

> In my initial consult I describe potentially unsettling things that can occur during the process. I stress these are individual differences and do not mean anything is going wrong: react to the first sedation injection, any potential drug reactions, necessity of trying more than once to get venipuncture and place butterfly IV catheter, agonal breathing, muscular twitching, eyes open, urination/defecation.

A second veterinarian's response offers a less mechanical view of the euthanasia process that might help clients prepare for the end of their pet's life, writing,

> The experience is intended to be peaceful, intimate, respectful and unrushed. It allows the pet to be surrounded by those that love him/her and not be scared or panicked being in a noisy, rushed clinic. It is a time to honor the pet's life.

Grief

Over 20 respondents highlighted the importance of clients' awareness of the grief they will experience after their pet's death, that they should not feel guilty about deciding to euthanize their pets and that the decision to do so is actually a gift to a pet suffering and in pain. In speaking of an at-home euthanasia, one veterinarian writes about both the euthanasia process and how it can ameliorate feelings of guilt:

> I wish they knew how beautiful the experience could be with music and storytelling and crying together and respect of the pet's body afterward and the relief they will feel that they provided their pet with the best possible 'good' death that is available. That we talk about possible triggers of guilt that may come upon them afterwards and dispelling the reasons for guilt and how we talk about what is normal to feel and that they are not alone in these feelings. How we discuss losing a pet can be harder emotionally than losing a person.

That clients are making a really difficult decision that is in their pet's best interest is, according to several respondents, critical for clients to acknowledge to help ameliorate the guilt and grief they experience. Clients may perceive euthanasia as the "final gift they can give their pet" or, as a decision their pets would be "okay with." The latter is evidenced by one veterinarian who wrote,

> There is no objective right or wrong time to do this. Each time we make this decision it must be made in the moment (surely informed by past experiences and others' insights). Yet one can never know exactly what the decision is until we make it. AND Whatever the decision is our nonhuman companion will BE OK with it.

Finally, grief is clearly not reserved for the clients but a central part of the veterinarian's professional life, as illustrated by one veterinarian who wrote, "I wish they know that sometimes it is very difficult for me, especially if I have known the pet for a long time and/or have tried to 'heal or cure' them and have been unsuccessful."

Quality of life and pain displays

Another prominent theme among veterinarians is the desire for clients to know how to gauge their pets' quality of life and how animals display pain to aid in the EOL decision-making for their pets. Approximately 16 veterinarians referenced some version of this concern. For example, one respondent wrote,

> Age does not determine quality of life. Death comes slowly if they elect to just 'wait it out' and often the pet is suffering silently. Something as simple as pain management can greatly improve a pet's quality of life. Just because they are not crying in distress, does not mean they are pain free.

Similarly, another veterinarian wrote,

> I wish more family's [sic] sought help for their painful pets before calling us to schedule euthanasia. I wish family's [sic] had a better idea of how to know if their pet is in pain (we provide an article on this to hospice patients & on our website).

Early help-seeking and the role of hospice and palliative care

The quotes in the preceding section illustrate how clients' awareness of their pets' quality of life is directly connected to veterinarians' wish that clients call them sooner rather than later to ensure pets have access to appropriate care throughout the dying process and not just the euthanasia experience. By seeking help sooner, veterinarians can better help control their non-human clients' pain but only if their clients were aware of hospice and palliative care services. These are themes mentioned by 28 veterinarians. One veterinarian exemplifies this point writing:

> I really wish clients were aware of and used palliative care/hospice services. I also wish clients were better educated about how animals display pain and what constitutes good quality of life. I see so many patients who have suffered greatly before finally becoming so bad the owners realized they needed to be euthanized. It's a serious welfare issue that I think we as a profession have an obligation to address.

The consequence of delayed care for a pet is not just the potential for the pet's unnecessary suffering but the veterinarian is placed in a precarious position weighing the needs of the pet versus those of the pet owner:

> I wish that owners were aware that I provide in-home hospice/palliative care. Many of my patients could have had a significantly better quality of life prior to euthanasia. Some are likely euthanized prematurely due to inadequate pain relief and other treatments. By the time I arrive, they are already psychologically prepared to euthanize their pet and I feel that it would be unkind and unhealthy for me to broach the possibility of hospice at that point.

Additional assorted mentions

There is clear overlap among the above four themes and several others mentioned by respondents that did not fit neatly into the above categories but are indeed noteworthy. Two veterinarians mention that they wished their clients were aware of at-home euthanasia service and two would like their clients to be familiar with palliated natural death as an alternative to euthanasia. Four respondents expressed interest in their clients planning before the euthanasia what to do with their pet's body as well as after-care for themselves in terms of seeking support for their own grief.

Finally, five respondents wished their clients understood that there was no "right" or "perfect time" to end their pet's life. While this relates to the quality-of-life theme discussed above, we are speaking here more directly to assuaging the psychological discomfort of their human clients (i.e. as a protection against feelings of guilt) rather than the pet's suffering. For example, one veterinarian wrote,

> Providing end of life care is a team effort and there is no right or wrong way for owners to approach it. We practice so that all owners feel comfortable with their choice and their pet is ALWAYS our priority throughout the entire process.

Another veterinarian wrote,

> I wish that all clients knew that there is no one magical, perfect 'right time' to euthanize their pet, and that guilt and sorrow are different emotions - while sorrow at a loss is normal, there is no need to feel guilt, shame, or blame at oneself for a decision to end another being's suffering.

As the latter quote shows, there is clear overlap among the information these veterinarians wish their clients knew before asking them to provide EOL care to their pets, demonstrating the many hats and roles veterinarians play in EOL care.

Most challenging aspects of providing EOL care

We asked veterinary professionals to describe the most challenging aspects of their work providing hospice and palliative care. Seventy-eight veterinarians responded, identifying one or more challenges they face. Given the nature of the IAAHPC membership, it is not surprising the most mentioned single theme revolves around the challenge of educating pet owners and veterinarians about the palliative and hospice care services they provide (mentioned by 19 respondents). This challenge is closely connected in veterinarians' comments to the challenge of being called too late to help suffering pets (mentioned by 13 respondents), not having enough time to spend with each client (mentioned by 13 respondents) and the challenge of operating a business (mentioned by 13 respondents), as exemplified by the following veterinarian's comment:

> The fact that it is a new, emerging field that is not well known or understood. Marketing and advertising must remain a strong focus for my business, rather than concentrating on the medicine. Also, the fact that I feel like an emergency ambulance driver many days as clients always wait until the last possible moment, when their pet is suffering and dying, and want me to come right away for euthanasia.

That veterinarians' challenges are multifaceted and thus transcend single classification are illustrated by the following which nicely exemplifies the dynamic and complex nature of veterinary care, particularly among those providing at-home EOL care:

> A lot of people who call me have been to another veterinarian who has told them that the animal is suffering and must be euthanized. Some are angry and want a second opinion, others are unsure what to do and some trust their vet. It is difficult to go to a house, have an animal meet you at the door and then have to euthanize it, because the vet said it was time. If the people are ready, it is different. Most people have not heard of hospice and I have to carefully educate them, some are understanding and wish more time, others have made the difficult decision and just want it to be over with.

Burnout and self-care were also mentioned frequently (17% of veterinarians who answered this question), typically as the only challenge identified by the respondent, using the fewest number of words: "the mental aspect"; "personal burn out"; "self-care"; "dealing with my sorrow"; "'isolating"; "draining"; "compassion fatigue"; and "dealing with my sorrow." For those who provided more than a couple of words to describe the challenge of self-care the veterinarian's personality (e.g. "working as a person with a highly sensitive personality and being able to separate these emotions from personal time off"), the bonds they share with clients and pets (e.g. "emotional bonds with owners and becoming too attached with pets/owners"), and the difficulty managing clients' grief ("it can be draining when you put so much effort into families and dealing with their emotional well-being while trying to maintain your own") affects their ability to cope.

A final challenge expressed by veterinarians (8 of the respondents) involves the cost of providing comprehensive EOL care and how that balances against the human clients' perception of EOL care and its financial value. This clearly relates to the issue of burnout that is common among veterinarians, in general, but perhaps more pronounced among those offering at-home EOL services. For example, one veterinarian writes,

> convincing owners and other vets that what we offer is different then [sic] what they might think and it's not all about keeping pets alive at all cost no matter what til they die naturally or unassisted. that the services have value and they should expect to pay for our time. they will receive much more then [sic] they pay for. i wish i could dedicate myself entirely to this work and not have to worry so much about getting paid, unfortunately this work does not yet pay.

The financial rewards of providing veterinary EOL care was not highlighted by a single veterinarian in our study, which is perhaps why running their own business was also mentioned by 13 respondents as a challenging aspect of their work. This is further illustrated by a veterinarian who writes:

> Once I do have hospice clients, it is also much more labor intensive in the management of cases compared to euthanasia. There can be a great deal of follow up and consultation as such owners are clearly extremely attached and worried for their pet's comfort. At present I do not charge a fee for unlimited access to me (text/ email) but am considering doing so.

The challenge of running your own business and managing the intensive labor required of EOL care is compounded by the general public's perception that veterinarians should be cheap or free because they love animals. One veterinarian counters this potential confusion with clients around cost by setting a fee structure beforehand so that "Finances are clear before I ever come to their house so I don't have to deal with the emotional drain of people telling me I should do things for free if I love animals."

Most rewarding aspects

Perhaps not surprising, relieving suffering and providing pets with a "good death" was the reward noted most frequently (38%) by the 80 veterinarians who answered this question, followed by the appreciation they are shown by the pets' families (29%). These two themes are illustrated by this veterinarian who wrote,

> By far the most personally rewarding is seeing the relief in the pet and when I come to help them transition. (Granted not every pet sees me this way!). This also transfers to the family. It is especially gratifying to hear owners say things like, "that was so much better than I expected' or 'that was so peaceful' or "thank you so much for making this so much easier for us."

A similar sentiment is articulated by the veterinarian who states, "The drain I take on is visible to my families. I have never been so respected or revered as I am by my families. I also know I have given the best death possible to my patients, who deserve nothing less." For most respondents, these themes overlapped and included references to enjoying seeing the human–animal bond, developing relationships with their clients and/or their clients' pets and providing palliative care that extends the quality time that pets and humans are able to spend together. The following veterinarian's comment best demonstrates the confluence of these myriad themes:

> The relationships formed with caretakers and pets. I leave each visit refreshed and excited about my life. I used to dislike being a vet and was constantly looking for other careers. I now like my job and my life. My clients all want me there, they haven't wandered into my clinic with a sick pet and no money. Finances are clear before I ever come to their house so I don't have to deal with the emotional drain of people telling me I should do things for free if I love animals.

Providing EOL care in their clients' homes was explicitly mentioned by six veterinarians in our study as a rewarding part for them but a critical part of providing their human clients and their pets with a stress-free EOL experience. One veterinarian wrote, "I can see the benefit to the pet and to the client by helping them in their home without the stresses of that trip to the veterinary clinic. The clients are most appreciative that someone is willing/able to visit them at home."

Discussion

Veterinarians in our study seemed concerned about their clients feeling guilty about the EOL care they chose for their pets. Our respondents also expressed a desire for their human clients to have thought through the aftercare options—both in terms of the disposal of their animals' remains but also support options to deal with grief—which is consistent with the suggestion that pet owners need to be made aware that support is available to them after death, in addition to making them aware of how to access it if necessary. If euthanasia is the EOL choice by the client and guilt is felt, the veterinarians in our study emphasize—as is consistent with previous research (Dickinson, 2014)—that euthanasia is the final gift the pet owner can give to the animal. And, as Paul notes (2019), euthanasia is the "last arrow" in the veterinarians' quiver.

Regarding Internet information being helpful or harmful for a client's knowledge regarding EOL issues, the respondents tended to feel that such information was usually helpful, though some misinformation exists. Some veterinarians note that their own websites helped to empower the clients before contacting them. A few veterinarians said their clients tended to not seek such information on the Internet. Certainly, Internet information for the most part would stimulate questions, if nothing else, for the client to ask the veterinarian when meeting.

What was it that veterinarians wish their clients understood regarding EOL issues before calling for an appointment? Grief was the largest concern expressed. As noted earlier, reactions to pet deaths do not differ significantly from human deaths, as pets are fictive kin, yet the veterinarians in our study seem to feel that their clients perceive their grief as abnormal. This is an area in which veterinary schools could include information in their curricula and/or offer workshops to deal with this topic. Our respondents report the most challenging aspects of providing palliative and hospice care is the lack of knowledge by clients regarding hospice and palliative care and the emotional needs of both the client and the veterinarian. Pet loss and grief management is a significant source of stress for veterinarians and contributes to compassion fatigue (Burfitt, 2019), necessitating additional training in this area.

Veterinary schools and veterinary tech programs could reduce this concern by providing more information regarding EOL issues. As previously noted, EOL issues are not a top priority in U.S. veterinary education. As palliative and hospice care with animals is relatively new, it simply is not common knowledge that such exists. The second author of this paper in researching veterinarians in England in 2013 learned that many of them had never heard of hospice with pets. Hopefully, they are better informed now. The IAAHPC in the United States has done an excellent job of broadcasting hospice and palliative care with animals.

Many of the issues identified in the literature and from these respondents can be addressed by the IAAHPC's certification program in animal hospice. The veterinarians and veterinary technicians in our study are very familiar with this certification and many have completed it. Overall, these respondents seem to feel rather positive and rewarded in their profession regarding palliative and hospice care with gratitude from their clients and a good feeling about helping to relieve suffering and helping pets to die peacefully. It should be noted that the decision to seek hospice care does not rule out euthanasia, as emphasis should be that a natural death is not necessarily the goal of animal hospice. Animal hospice offers and discusses all options openly, without judgement and with honesty to manage the reality with expectations (Gregersen, 2016).

Veterinary medicine is laden with practitioners who are passionate about science, nonhuman animals, and medicine. Being a good doctor, however, is not just about veterinary science, but it is also about understanding humans (Owens, 2015), a sentiment revealed in the responses of the veterinarians in our study. The strong association between pet owner's burden and measures of psychosocial function align closely with work in human caregiver relationships, and understanding the affective states motivating animal behavior is important to the clinician's effective case management (Spitznagel *et al.*, 2017). To manage potential discomfort in interactions with clients, veterinarians must develop specific impression management strategies such as body language, spoken language, eye contact, and emotion labor (Hochschild, 1983). Veterinarians want to show their competence and make clients feel like they care about their animals; they do not want to be too emotional or not emotional enough when giving bad news, as giving bad news is one of the more complicated aspects of their interaction with clients.

Performing for clients is an interactional tool used to protect the professional self from potential threats toward a positively valued professional self (Hochschild, 1983).

Veterinarians use numerous strategies when interacting with clients who decide to euthanize companion animals, one of which is to protect the self by distancing through humor (Owens, 2015). The symbolic interactionist approach can be utilized when analyzing the interpretive processes veterinarians use when discussing with clients and situations in which the professional self is threatened. Veterinarians must learn how to protect their professional selves to cooperate with difficult people and can address this issue by building trusting relationships and providing performances to clients through verbal and nonverbal communication and becoming more comfortable (Goffman,

1959). The veterinarians in our sample of IAAHPC members seem to realize the importance of developing trust, showing concern about what it is their clients know before coming to them with an ill or dying pet. They want their clients to understand that grief is normal, whether following the death of a *Homo sapien* or fictive kin with their pet. They want to know what their client knows about gauging the quality of life of their companion animal and they wish that pet owners would seek help regarding EOL issues sooner rather than later.

Conclusion

While we do not have the answers to the concerns of the veterinarians in this study, studies involving veterinary education reveal 75% of U.S. veterinarians surveyed agreed that veterinary schools should place more emphasis on communication skills with owners of terminally ill animals and only 33% of respondents felt well prepared by their veterinary training to deal with EOL issues (Dickinson *et al.*, 2011). If such an orientation were emphasized more in veterinary schools, perhaps veterinarians would be equipped to better educate the public about their services and what knowledge they should strive to have prior to contacting their veterinarian about an EOL issue. Public relations with consumers might in the end assist clients of veterinarians to better handle the very emotional aspects of EOL issues with their pet. The websites of the veterinarians can provide accurate Internet information which could help to answer many of the queries the client might have and state information such as it is okay to grieve over the death of a beloved animal. The webpage could help the client to better understand how to gauge a pet's quality of life and how animals display pain. Additionally, the euthanasia process could be explained. Such sharing of information with the client could go a long way towards making this whole process more tolerable and less traumatic for both the client and the veterinarian (as well as the animal).

The generalizability of the findings reported here is limited given that the IAAHPC is a unique organization focused exclusively on EOL issues, education, and advocacy. On a personal note, the co-authors of this paper, being sociologists and not veterinarians, have been very favorably impressed with the compassion of veterinarians and veterinary tech professionals after attending the IAAHPC conferences in recent years. These professionals obviously love what they do, though the job is challenging and stress producing. There is information in the media citing various studies which show a high suicide rate among veterinarians in the U.S. Part of these findings are contributed to the fact that veterinarians must deal with EOL issues.

Though our sample is small, these reporting veterinary professionals seemingly receive much praise and gratitude from their work on EOL issues and find their profession to be most rewarding. Perhaps their knowledge gained and participation in the IAAHPC Conferences and workshops gives them needed support, though we have no data to support this. A future study comparing IAAHPC members with veterinary professionals not so affiliated would be worthwhile.

References

Bartram, D.J. and Baldwin, D.S. (2008) Veterinary surgeons and suicide: Influences, opportunities and research directions. *Veterinary Record* 162, 36–40. DOI: 10.1136/vr.162.2.36.

Bartram, D.J., Yadegarfar, G. and Baldwin, D.S. (2009) Psychosocial working conditions and work-related stressors among UK veterinary surgeons. *Occupational. Medicine* 59, 334–41. DOI: 10.1093/occmed/kqp072.

Bartram, D.J. and Baldwin, D.S. (2010) Veterinary surgeons and suicide: A structured review of the possible influences on increased risk. *Veterinary Record* 166, 388–397. DOI: 10.1136/vr.b4794.

Burfitt, J. (2019) The emotional toll of euthanasia on vets. *Vet Practice* 1–3. Available at: https://vetpracticemag.com.au/the-emotional-toll-of-euthanansia-on-vets/

Dickinson, G.E. (2014) Household pet euthanasia and companion animal last rites. *Phi Kappa Phi Forum* 94, 4–6.

Dickinson, G.E. and Hoffmann, H.C. (2019) Animal hospice and palliative care: Veterinarians' experiences and preferred practices. *Journal of Veterinary. Behavior* 32, 57–61. DOI: 10.1016/j.jveb.2019.04.008.

Dickinson, G.E., Roof, P.D. and Roof, K.W. (2011) A survey of veterinarians in the US: Euthanasia and other end-of-life issues. *Anthrozoos* 24, 167–174. DOI: 10.2752/175303711X12998632257666.

Gardner, D.H. and Hini, D. (2006) Work-related stress in the veterinary profession in New Zealand. *New Zealand Veterinary Journal* 54, 119–124. DOI: 10.1080/00480169.2006.36623.

Goffman, E. (1959) *The Presentation of Self in Everyday Life.* Doubleday, Garden City, NY.

Goldberg, K.J. (2016) Veterinary hospice and palliative care: A comprehensive review of the literature. *Veterinary. Record* 178, 369–374. DOI: 10.1136/vr.103459.

Gregersen, S. (2016) Getting the best result at the end using animal hospice. *Veterinary Nursing Journal* 31, 271–275. DOI: 10.1080/17415349.2016.1208335.

Hart, L.A. and Yamamoto, M. (2017) Euthanasia, pet loss, and grief for owners and veterinarians. *Merck Veterinary Manual*. Available at: https://www.mreckvetmanual.com/behavior/the-human-animal-bond/euthanasia-pet-loss

Hochschild, A.R. (1983) *The Managed Heart: The Commercialization of Human Feeling*. University of California Press, Berkeley, CA.

Huggard, P.K. and Huggard, E.J. (2008) When the caring gets tough: Compassion fatigue and veterinary care. *Veterinary Script* May, 14–16. Available at: http://compassionfatigue.org/pages/HuggardVetScript.pdf

Jones-Fairnie, H., Ferroni, P., Silburn, S. and Lawrence, D. (2008) Suicide in Australian veterinarians. *Australian Veterinary Journal* 86, 114–116. DOI: 10.1111/j.1751-0813.2008.00277.x.

Mellanby, R.J. (2005) Incidence of suicide in the veterinary profession in England and Wales. *Veterinary Record* 157, 415–417. DOI: 10.1136/vr.157.14.415.

Milner, A.J., Niven, H., Page, K. and LaMontagne, A.D. (2015) Suicide in veterinarians and veterinary nurses in Australia: 2001–2012. *Australian Veterinary Journal* 93, 308–310. DOI: 10.1111/avj.12358.

Mitchener, K.L. and Ogilvie, G.K. (2002) Understanding compassion fatigue: Keys for the caring veterinary healthcare team. *Journal of the American Animal Hospital Association* 38, 307–310. DOI: 10.5326/0380307.

Nowell, L.S., Norris, J.M., White, D.E. and Moules, N.J. (2017) Thematic analysis: Striving to meet the trustworthiness criteria. *International Journal of Qualitative Methods* 16, 1–13. DOI: 10.1177/1609406917733847.

O'Dair, H. (2015) Euthanasia of pets: Strengthening end-of-life-care. *In Practice* 37, 143–145. DOI: 10.1136/inp.h805.

Owens, N. (2015) Protecting the self: Veterinarians' perspectives on dealing with people. *Society & Animals* 23, 105–127. DOI: 10.1163/15685306-12341362.

Paul, M. (2019) Veterinary euthanasia: The last act of love. *The MJH Life Sciences* 50, 1–8. Available at: https://www.dvm360.com/view/veterinary-euthanasia-last-act-love

Platt, B., Hawton, K., Simkin, S. and Mellanby, R.J. (2012) Suicidal behaviour and psychosocial problems in veterinary surgeons: A systematic review. *Social Psychiatry Epidemiology* 47, 223–240. DOI: 10.1007/s00127-010-0328-6.

Spitznagel, M.B., Jacobson, D.M., Cox, M.D. and Carlson, M.D. (2017) Caregiver burden in owners of a sick companion animal: A cross-sectional observational study. *Veterinary. Record* 181, 321. DOI: 10.1136/vr.10429.

Tomasi, S.E., Fechter-Leggett, E.D., Edwards, N.T., Reddish, A.D., Crosby, A.E. *et al*. (2019) Suicide among veterinarians in the United States from 1979 through 2015. *Journal of the American Veterinary Medical Association* 254, 104–112. DOI: 10.2460/javma.254.1.104.

Tran, L., Crane, M.F. and Phillips, J.K. (2014) The distinct role of performing euthanasia on depression and suicide in veterinarians. *Journal of Occupational Health Psychology* 19, 123–132. DOI: 10.1037/a0035837.

3 One Owner's Perspective After a Pet Hospice Journey

Allison C. Hudock*
Independent Researcher, 189 N. Marengo Ave., Apt 210 Pasadena, CA, USA

Abstract
I was the sole pet parent to my beloved cat, Peaches, who received a devastating advanced cancer diagnosis in June 2023. Upon my decision not to pursue chemotherapy for Peaches, I became her sole hospice caregiver in the subsequent months until her death in November 2023. This commentary provides my perspective as a pet parent and caregiver during the time of a traumatic life-limiting diagnosis, my decision to pursue hospice care over treatment, the challenges of navigating hospice care as a sole caregiver without adequate support, and my hindsight and takeaways since her passing.

Keywords: hospice, lymphoma, caregiver, human–animal bond

Commentary

Peaches was diagnosed with advanced small cell gastrointestinal lymphoma in June 2023 following diagnostics and emergency surgery. I knew she was sick but never expected to hear the "C" word, and I had no experience with cancer in all my years as a cat mom. Once she recovered enough to travel, we had her first oncologist appointment where I learned about lymphoma, chemotherapy protocols and life expectancy with and without treatment. I left that appointment with 3 pieces of paper – 2 chemo protocols and the pamphlet for a euthanasia/aftercare service I was directed to pick up in the lobby. I was in an absolute state of shock.

We had just moved to a new state far away from home and brought each other comfort. I had to rely on veterinarians we had just met to help make critical decisions for Peaches. My anger that the cancer wasn't found earlier even after proactive vet care and diagnostics morphed into sadness. Yes, she was 12, but we had only been together for 2 years, and that was not enough time.

The decision for hospice in lieu of treatment was mine alone, and while it was a heavy weight to carry, I did so without regret. I had just put Peaches through a huge life-saving operation in lieu of immediate euthanasia. Unfortunately, this resulted in a difficult recovery despite her excellent medical care. I wanted more time with Peaches, but treatment was another huge ask, and I had met my quota. The reality was the odds of remission were not in her favor. My commitment was to her quality of life, knowing full well that she would pass away sooner this way.

I didn't know what our hospice journey would look like, but I assumed the hospital

*Corresponding author: allison.hudock@gmail.com

would offer support and guidance, just like for humans. I agreed to the few in-person oncologist check-ins out of desperation. I had so many questions. I felt abandoned. Near the end of Peaches' life, I found tele-hospice services via internet research, but it seemed pointless to engage them. Peaches' oncology vet tech would ask me at each checkup how I was doing and how much sleep was I getting. She could see my physical toll. I'll always remember her kindness. Her compassion should not be the exception.

I initially looked at Peaches post-diagnosis through the emotional lens of "she's dying of cancer", which triggered the dreaded anticipatory grief. After the hospice decision, there was a sense of peace within me, and I now looked at her as "she's living with cancer". We then went along each day with gratitude and rolled with the changes, of which there were many. I focused less on when the last day would arrive.

Peaches was the recipient of my "on the fly" hospice care. Her supportive care routine included limited prescription meds and some supplements, with adjustments as needed. Every day I was making decisions based on "is this is in Peaches' best interest?" I felt immense pressure to figure it all out, consumed with helpless thoughts, and a constant fear I wasn't doing enough. Was I missing her signs and signals – is she in pain or has the jaundice emerged? How can I comfort her?

I spent my non-working time on internet research and chatting with other pet cancer parents on social media. I should have been resting during Peaches' now 2 h sleeping spans. But my life revolved around Peaches, her before me. I watched her like a hawk, recording notes in the quality-of-life calendar I found online. It gave me a sense of control that I was desperate for and ultimately revealed her decline.

Peaches crossed the rainbow bridge in my loving arms on November 6, 2023, via euthanasia at the hospital, after a new sudden symptom that morning forced me to make this rapid decision. I have never made a euthanasia decision so quickly, but I couldn't bear to see her suffering. I left the hospital in a state of shock with an empty carrier. It felt like I had just fallen off a treadmill going 1000 miles per hour. I had to physically let go of her, and it broke me.

Hindsight is always 20/20. I believe veterinarians need to meet the caregiver/pet parent where they are and make them feel seen and heard when delivering a life-limiting diagnosis, be compassionate and supportive as they navigate this new unknown, engage in compassionate end-of-life conversations with clients and recognize if/when a referral to a hospice vet may be more appropriate, and understand that because the human–animal bond runs so deep, caregiver burnout is real in providing hospice care and needs to be addressed.

I look back and recognize what could have helped Peaches' hospice be "better". Knowing about and preparing a hospice care plan would have been ideal, in part for me to feel some control over very uncharted territory. Awareness and education on the use of the quality-of-life scale and pain scale would have eased some of my fears of not being able to read Peaches' signs. More frequent checkups via phone or video would have been helpful to communicate Peaches' status in real time and provide much-needed caregiver support. The hospice journey with Peaches was life-changing, and I know these lessons and her spirit will guide me as I share her story and provide care for future cats.

Conflict of Interest

The author declares there are no conflicts of interest.

Funding

The author declares that no funding was received in the preparation of this commentary. IAAHPC is sponsoring Article Processing Charges (APC) for this special issue.

Author Contributions

The author declares that AI was not used in the preparation of this commentary.

Ethics Statement

The author confirms that all relevant guidelines were followed in the preparation and submission of this commentary.

Data Availability

Research data was not used.

4 Compassionate End-of-Life Care: Development, Implementation, and Evaluation of a Comprehensive Euthanasia Course in Veterinary Education From 2019–2024

Virginia K. Corrigan[1]*, Kathleen Cooney[2] and Raeann Foster[3]
[1]University of Tennessee College of Veterinary Medicine, Departments of Academic Affairs and Small Animal Clinical Sciences, University of Tennessee Institute of Agriculture, Knoxville, TN, USA; [2]Companion Animal Euthanasia Training Academy (CAETA), Lutz, FL, USA; [3]Virginia Maryland College of Veterinary Medicine, Department of Small Animal Clinical Sciences, Virginia Tech, Blacksburg, VA, USA

Abstract

Background: End-of-life (EOL) and euthanasia best practices are vital but underrepresented areas in veterinary education. The Compassionate End-of-Life Care course at the Virginia-Maryland College of Veterinary Medicine (VMCVM) was developed to address this gap by offering third year veterinary students specialized training in EOL care with emphasis on euthanasia for a variety of species. Methods: The course was created as an in-person elective course and evolved into a hybrid model during the COVID-19 pandemic. The course was presented by the Companion Animal Euthanasia Training Academy (CAETA) and included certification and micro-credentialing as a Certified Peaceful Euthanasia Veterinarian (CPEV). This chapter evaluates the course as an elective within the third year of the Doctor of Veterinary Medicine curriculum at the VMCVM using two surveys with both quantitative and qualitative data collection methods. The first survey obtained data on the course between 2019 and 2021. Additional data using Student Perceptions of Teaching (SPOT) surveys from 2022, 2023, and 2024 were incorporated to provide longitudinal feedback on course effectiveness, instructor performance, and overall course satisfaction. Results: College integration was effective because of strong and consistent collaborative efforts between the passionate VMCVM faculty and CAETA administrators. Student feedback from course evaluations highlighted improved human–animal interaction skills, enhanced confidence in euthanasia techniques, and increased preparedness for EOL care in clinical practice for a variety of species. The hybrid format increases flexibility while maintaining high student satisfaction. Longitudinal student surveys (2022–2024) indicated consistently high ratings for instructor effectiveness, course relevance, and overall satisfaction, demonstrating sustained course value with minor fluctuations and highlighting areas for ongoing refinement. Conclusions: This chapter presents the development, implementation, and evaluation of a novel hybrid euthanasia course in veterinary medicine that offers a replicable model for other institutions to integrate EOL education into their

---

*Corresponding author: vkiefer@utk.edu

curricula. Future opportunities exist for deeper exploration of EOL competencies in veterinary professional education, including those around hospice and palliative care, team-based veterinary healthcare, and inter professional collaboration.

Keywords: veterinary education, hospice care, palliative care, euthanasia, hybrid curriculum, human–animal bond, micro-credentialing, CAETA, communication, ethics

Introduction

Veterinarians and veterinary healthcare team members frequently guide end-of-life (EOL) decisions and play an essential role in ensuring a "good death" for animal patients by navigating complex technical, emotional, and ethical challenges (Persson *et al.*, 2020; Bubeck, 2023). Despite the increasing recognition of the importance of EOL care for animals, veterinary education has historically not kept pace with clinical advancements in this area (Goldberg, 2016).

Comprehensive education in animal hospice, palliative care, and euthanasia remains variable across veterinary curricula globally, highlighting the need for structured educational approaches that effectively prepare veterinarians and veterinary healthcare team members for the complexities of EOL care (Littlewood *et al.*, 2020; Cooney *et al.*, 2021). Because euthanasia represents one of the most emotionally charged and morally complex moments in veterinary practice, ensuring a positive human–animal bond experience throughout the EOL process is essential. Structured education in euthanasia techniques and communication strategies strengthens the veterinarian and veterinary health care team's ability to preserve trust, compassion, and dignity in the human–animal relationship during these pivotal moments.

The ability to deliver compassionate and effective EOL care is recognized as a fundamental competency of veterinarians (Cooney *et al.*, 2021). However, structured EOL training in veterinary curricula often inadequately addresses the critical elements. Veterinarians report feeling underprepared for euthanasia work and a desire for more training during schooling (Kogan and Cooney, 2023). This is significant, given the prevalence of euthanasia as one of the most common procedures in veterinary medicine (Pegram *et al.*, 2021; Cooney and Kipperman, 2023). Competency in this domain requires both technical proficiency and strong communication and emotional intelligence skills to adequately support pet owners during difficult decisions (Persson *et al.*, 2020).

Surveys of veterinary curricula in the United States in 2020 illustrated limited but essential training in euthanasia, averaging only about 2.8 instructional hours on euthanasia methods, despite unanimous acknowledgment of its importance as a core competency (Cooney *et al.*, 2021). Many schools emphasize euthanasia pharmacology and clinical signs of death; however, direct hands-on training may not be consistently provided (Cooney *et al.*, 2021). Veterinarians' level of confidence in performing the medical procedure and managing communication components appears to increase during clinical practice years, through direct experience. As of 2024, more than 12 new veterinary colleges are in development (AVMA, 2024), with unknown numbers of euthanasia and EOL-related content and its effects on the human–animal interactions.

Australian and New Zealand veterinary schools similarly demonstrate variability in EOL training, predominantly incorporating euthanasia education within clinical rotations during students' final years, often relying on opportunistic rather than structured learning (Littlewood *et al.*, 2020). Decision making education in these contexts focuses on animal welfare, quality of life, client preferences, and financial considerations, yet lacks consistent structured delivery (Littlewood *et al.*, 2021). Similarly, a survey of veterinary schools in the United Kingdom indicated growing inclusion of EOL issues, yet training depth and approach remained uneven, frequently limited to elective modules or single lectures (Dickinson *et al.*, 2014). Cornell University's College of Veterinary Medicine successfully developed an elective communication course focused on euthanasia for 4th-year veterinary students (Schultz *et al.*, 2022).

Post-graduate training programs are available for EOL care. The International Association for Animal Hospice and Palliative Care (IAAHPC) offers a professional certification program for veterinarians and credentialed veterinary technicians, and is also approved by the Registry of Approved Continuing Education (RACE) (IAAHPC, 2025). This program includes approximately 100h of coursework available to veterinarians, veterinary students, and veterinary technicians covering various aspects of EOL care, including pain management, euthanasia, and advanced approaches in animal hospice care (IAAHPC, 2025). Currently, both the University of Pennsylvania and Midwestern University offer part of the IAAHPC's certification program to veterinary students as an elective, but it does not include euthanasia-related content. The Companion Animal Euthanasia Training Academy (CAETA) provides detailed training to veterinary professionals in all aspects of companion animal euthanasia (Cooney, 2024). This program is designed for veterinary professionals to demonstrate mastery of technical euthanasia skills, client communication, ethical decision making, adequate recordkeeping and controlled substance handling, and to provide tangible proof of competency in these areas for immediate use in practice (Cooney *et al.*, 2021; Cooney, 2024). Veterinarians without such training run the risk of animal harm and client dissatisfaction, and may be ill-equipped to meet professional standards (Gray and Radford, 2022; Cooney, 2023; Kogan and Cooney, 2023). As of 2025, the CAETA 10h certification program is being taught at six veterinary colleges, with VMCVM being the first to include up to 20 additional hours of euthanasia-related content (CAETA, 2022).

Embedded micro-credentialing and certificate programs have emerged as innovative approaches to address gaps in veterinary education by formally recognizing specialized knowledge and competencies that are also valued in the workplace. Such programs, increasingly integrated into higher education, offer structured, competency-based pathways to certification, enhancing learner confidence, marketability, and workplace readiness (Brown *et al.*, 2021; Thi Ngoc Ha *et al.*, 2023).

Beyond formal education, the "hidden curriculum," which is embedded in learning opportunities and interactions involved with the formal curriculum, also shapes veterinary professional students' learning experiences and professional development (Roder and May, 2017; Kunze and Seals, 2020). Extracurricular activities, such as pet loss support hotlines and specialized student organizations, can supplement formal training by providing experiential learning in grief support, communication strategies, and ethical decision making (Alves and Scorsolini-Comin, 2025). Clinical rotation provides numerous informal and opportunistic learning environments. Structured debriefings post-euthanasia procedures have been proposed as additional strategies to enhance experiential learning in the informal curriculum (Littlewood *et al.*, 2021), and carried into private practice settings for euthanasia protocol improvements (Cooney, 2024). An analysis of 22 studies published between 1989 and 2023 revealed that veterinary training in EOL care predominantly focused on euthanasia techniques and client communication but often lacked structured content on managing veterinarian grief and emotional support (Alves and Scorsolini-Comin, 2025).

This article presents an overview of the development, implementation, and evaluation of an elective EOL care course developed collaboratively by the VMCVM and CAETA from 2019 to 2024. This hybrid-format two-credit, 30h course, incorporating CAETA's Certified Peaceful Euthanasia Veterinarian certification (CAETA, 2025), was designed to comprehensively address identified gaps in veterinary EOL education by combining formal instruction, hands-on training, structured ethical discussions, and focused client communication training. The course aimed to equip veterinary students with essential knowledge, technical skills, and emotional competencies necessary to navigate real-world euthanasia cases effectively and compassionately.

Methods

The EOL care course was initially introduced in 2019 as a one-credit elective at the VMCVM to provide third-year veterinary students with structured training in technical competencies, communication strategies, and ethical considerations around euthanasia. Initially, conducted in a hybrid online and in-person format in 2019, the course transitioned to a fully online format in 2020 because of the COVID-19 pandemic. By 2021, the course evolved into a two-credit (30 h) hybrid model integrating asynchronous online lectures with in-person practical sessions to maximize flexibility and enhance hands-on learning opportunities, based on student feedback and course evaluations.

The curriculum for the two-credit elective course encompasses holistic EOL care content (Table 4.1). The original one-credit course comprised 15 h of content, including 10 asynchronous online modules, complemented by a weekend of synchronous sessions taught in person. This evolved into 20 h of asynchronous content taken ideally before the synchronous weekend. Students also had access to optional synchronous office hours hosted via Zoom for additional interaction and clarification of the course material.

The specific learning objectives established for this course were:

1. Debate ethical implications and communication nuances regarding euthanasia.
2. Evaluate the pros and cons of different euthanasia techniques and drugs to select appropriate agents and techniques for specific species and situations.
3. Apply species-specific pre-euthanasia sedation and anesthesia protocols.
4. Administer euthanasia solution via the five main routes.
5. Apply appropriate regulations for the use of controlled substances.
6. Integrate client bereavement support, pet memorialization, and aftercare services where appropriate.
7. Evaluate compassion fatigue and its implications.
8. Appraise the American Veterinary Medical Association (AVMA) Guidelines for the Euthanasia of Animals.

The course aligns with competency-based curricular frameworks in veterinary education. The American Association of Veterinary Medical Colleges (AAVMC) has developed a framework for competency-based veterinary education (CBVE) (Matthew *et al.*, 2020). As previously described, two of the nine domains of competence have sub-competencies that specifically address euthanasia (Schultz *et al.*, 2022). These competencies are clinical reasoning and decision making, and communication. The specific sub-competencies that are addressed in this course include (1) considers euthanasia as a management option when appropriate and (2) engages clients in difficult conversations such as financial decisions and

Table 4.1. Integrated CAETA content for two-credit EOL care course.

Asynchronous content	Synchronous content
Pet loss support	Overview of companion animal euthanasia
Euthanasia around the world	Emotionally intelligent euthanasia
Home euthanasia	Caregiver and pet considerations
Behavioral and convenience euthanasia	Physiology and pharmacology
Modern pet aftercare	Pre-euthanasia sedation and anesthesia
Exotic euthanasia	Euthanasia techniques
Livestock euthanasia (non-companion)	Challenging situations
Companion livestock and equine euthanasia	Euthanasia case review
Compassion fatigue	Technique laboratory
Meaningful client communication	
Controlled substance handling	
Recorded appointment viewings	

EOL care (e.g. palliative care and euthanasia) (Matthew *et al.*, 2020).

Content delivery was structured such that the first ten contact hours were delivered synchronously during an intensive weekend session, and these sessions were recorded and asynchronously accessible. This content included a synchronous in-person 2 h cadaver euthanasia technique laboratory. The remaining 20 contact hours were exclusively online and asynchronous. For the online portion, students were assigned to complete interactive discussions and peer interactions on a discussion board, and final case-based project. Students had to complete modules one through ten to obtain CAETA certification and micro-credentials as part of the course. The contents provided by the CAETA are summarized in Table 4.1.

The student assessments included a mix of quizzes, discussion board activities, and a final essay-based case project. Assessments were numerically scored and translated into a Pass/Fail grade, with an overall passing threshold set at 64%. Students were also graded based on their attendance at in-person lectures and labs. Obtaining CAETA certification micro-credentials is required.

The original course evaluation presented in this study was conducted using structured surveys completed by students who participated in the one-credit 2019 (hybrid) and 2020 (fully online) iterations of the course (n = 46). These evaluations were administered in October 2020, gathering both quantitative and qualitative feedback to inform the ongoing course development.

Student Perceptions of Teaching (SPOT) surveys were conducted annually from 2022 to 2024 for the two-credit hour version of the course, providing structured feedback on course quality, instructor effectiveness, organization, relevance to students' degree programs, and responsiveness of course leadership to student concerns. The SPOT survey utilized Likert-scale items allowing students to rate their agreement or satisfaction levels across multiple domains, alongside qualitative opportunities to elaborate on their experiences. The surveys were administered anonymously via an online platform toward the end of each course offering, ensuring voluntary and confidential participation. Response rates ranged from approximately 18 to 63% across the 3 years, offering longitudinal insights into the trends in course delivery and effectiveness.

Qualitative feedback from the SPOT surveys conducted between 2022 and 2024 were analyzed thematically. Students provided narrative responses highlighting aspects of the course that they found particularly beneficial and areas for potential improvement. Qualitative responses were reviewed and summarized to identify recurring themes related to course structure, content delivery, hands-on components, and overall effectiveness.

The evaluation data were systematically analyzed to identify key areas for improvement, guiding subsequent enhancements in course content, delivery methods, and assessment practices. All data were collected anonymously through routine course and institutional evaluation processes designed for internal program improvement. These activities were under the category of program evaluation and not human subjects research. As such, no IRB review or determination was obtained prior to data analysis.

Results

The original course evaluation survey was completed in October 2020, with a total of n = 46 student responses. The students were asked to respond to the survey if they had participated in the 2019 and 2020 course offerings. Participation was voluntary and all responses were collected anonymously. Qualitative and quantitative data were also obtained. The 2019–2020 course evaluation survey questions can be viewed in Appendix 1.

Participants reported significantly increased confidence in euthanasia techniques, particularly in methods beyond the traditional intravenous (IV) injection. Qualitative responses highlighted intra-organ methods such as intrahepatic and intrarenal injections as particularly informative, with many students reporting that exposure to these techniques was entirely new and valuable. Among the survey respondents, the hands-on cadaver laboratory was identified as the most informative aspect of the course (49.4%), followed by live lectures and modules

(42.2%). Only a small proportion (6%) found online modules to be the most beneficial.

The qualitative feedback from the 2019–2020 survey emphasized that students appreciated the instructor's detailed instructions and demonstration of euthanasia techniques, particularly valuing the guidance on subtle handling of syringes and needles, and effective client communication strategies during sensitive euthanasia discussions. The laboratory sessions provided essential practical experience, allowing students to practice diverse euthanasia methods first, significantly enhancing their confidence and technical skills. Quantitatively, the online modules were viewed positively, with 60.9% of the students rating them as moderately to extremely useful. Specifically, the "Livestock and Equine Euthanasia" module ranked as the most useful online module, selected by 32.6% of students as their top choice. Conversely, "Euthanasia Around the World" was rated the least useful by 54.3% of the respondents.

Despite the positive feedback, students identified areas for improvement. Approximately 46.4% of students felt that online lectures could be enhanced, requesting more succinct content and clearer supplemental resources. Feedback also indicated a preference for additional time dedicated to hands-on practice in the cadaver lab, suggesting that less time was spent on lecture demonstrations during lab sessions. The course format was generally well-received, although a significant majority (71.7%) preferred the original hybrid structure with substantial in-person interaction rather than a fully online format. Qualitative responses revealed that the students found the hybrid approach conducive to learning, balancing flexibility and direct engagement. Additionally, students suggested additional topics for future course iterations, requesting more extensive coverage of bereavement support, client communication in challenging situations, and ethical considerations surrounding convenience euthanasia. There was a strong interest (86.9%) in an expanded elective course incorporating animal hospice and palliative care, indicating a broader desire for comprehensive training in EOL veterinary care. Overall, the EOL care elective course significantly enhanced students' practical euthanasia competencies, client communication skills, and appreciation for the broader scope of EOL care, including hospice and palliative approaches. The CAETA certification and micro-credential components were also highly valued, providing students with the perception of enhanced confidence and marketability upon entering the veterinary workforce.

2022–2024 SPOT Course course evaluation survey questions can be viewed in Appendix 2. Quantitative SPOT survey results from 2022 to 2024 revealed positive and relatively stable perceptions of the Compassionate End-of-Life Care course across three consecutive years (Table 4.2). Instructor effectiveness ratings demonstrated a notable upward trend, increasing from an average rating of 4.67 (out of six) in 2022 to 5.87 in 2023, before moderating slightly to 5.40 in 2024. Students consistently rated the course as highly relevant to their degree, with mean scores ranging from 4.41 to 6.90 (out of seven). The overall course ratings improved significantly from 3.98 (out of 5) in 2022 to 4.52 in 2023, with a slight decrease to 3.81 in 2024. Course organization ratings followed a similar pattern, increasing notably from 5.08 in 2022 to a peak of 6.62 in 2023, and then adjusting downward to 4.37 in 2024. These results collectively reflect sustained student appreciation for the course's value and instructional quality while highlighting

Table 4.2. Quantitative data from SPOT course evaluation surveys 2022–2024.

Metric	2022	2023	2024
Instructor effectiveness (Mean/6)	4.67	5.87	5.4
Overall course rating (Mean/5)	3.98	4.52	3.81
Course organization (Mean/7 in 2022–2023; Mean/5 in 2024)	5.08	6.62	4.37
Course relevance (Mean/7 in 2022–2023; Mean/5 in 2024)	6.73	6.9	4.41
Leadership responsiveness (Mean/7 in 2022–2023; Mean/5 in 2024)	6.24	6.43	4.19

Table 4.3. Qualitative data from SPOT course evaluation surveys 2022–2024.

Year	Key positive themes	Suggested improvements	General student sentiment
2022	Self-paced learning appreciated, comprehensive module content, valuable weekend in-person lectures and cadaver labs	Maintain comprehensive content, consider enhancing clarity in module presentation	Strongly positive; course recommended as a requirement for all students
2023	High praise for asynchronous format, valuable cadaver labs, excellent overall course design and practical demonstrations	Increase interactive elements online, additional hands-on practice requested	Highly positive; significant value seen in practical lab sessions
2024	Strong appreciation for lab components, practical euthanasia techniques, structured and engaging in-person sessions	Maintain or expand practical hands-on experiences; continue clear and structured delivery	Consistently positive; emphasis on practical applicability and course organization

opportunities for continued improvement in course delivery and organization.

Qualitative feedback from the 2022–2024 SPOT surveys revealed additional evaluation data (Table 4.3). Students reported consistent appreciation for hands-on laboratory experiences, particularly cadaver labs, which they found invaluable for practicing euthanasia techniques. Students positively noted the comprehensive and practical nature of the course content, emphasizing its relevance and applicability in clinical practice. The asynchronous format introduced in 2022 has been praised to enhance flexibility and self-paced learning. Across all years, students consistently highlighted the structured organization and engaging delivery of course materials, with suggestions for maintaining and expanding practical in-person experiences. The feedback underscored strong support for the continued inclusion of the course within the veterinary curriculum, with several students recommending it become mandatory for all veterinary students. Qualitative SPOT survey feedback also revealed that students frequently described the Certified Peaceful Euthanasia Veterinarian (CPEV) credential as an asset that would differentiate them in the job market and boost their confidence when discussing euthanasia care with clients. Several students remarked that having a formal certification increased their sense of professionalism and readiness to provide compassionate EOL care.

Discussion

The implementation of the EOL care elective course enhanced veterinary education at this institution by filling the gap in euthanasia training. The course evaluations revealed enhanced self-reported confidence in navigating complex EOL technical and non-technical competencies. The hybrid model provides a balance between flexibility and experiential learning, making it a potentially viable option for integration into other veterinary programs worldwide.

A key strength of the course was its emphasis on real-world applications, with students gaining valuable hands-on experience. Students particularly valued the hands-on laboratory and the ability to learn new techniques and protocols for sedation, anesthesia, and euthanasia. Ethical considerations were also integrated into the curriculum, helping students learn to navigate and reflect on the moral complexities of decision making around euthanasia. Another strength was the incorporation of a micro-credential. CAETA certification provided students with a credential that they perceived would be valuable in their future careers.

In addition to these strengths, areas of improvement were elucidated. The hybrid model, while beneficial in many respects, presents challenges in ensuring uniform student engagement across both the online and in-person components. Future iterations of the course could benefit from additional interactive elements in online modules, such as live discussion sessions and virtual case simulations. Additionally, expanding access to live euthanasia cases could further enhance the hands-on learning experience.

The addition of longitudinal SPOT survey data from 2022 to 2024 underscored the consistent improvements and sustained strengths of the Compassionate End-of-Life Care course. The improvements noted in instructor effectiveness and course organization between 2022 and 2023 could reflect specific changes in instructional strategies, course management, and responsiveness to student feedback. The slight moderation of these ratings in 2024 could be due to cohort-specific dynamics or changes in course execution, suggesting that ongoing evaluations and adaptive instructional methods are crucial for maintaining high course standards. Overall, the longitudinal data supported the course's continuing effectiveness and relevance, while highlighting areas for ongoing vigilance and responsiveness to student needs.

Future directions for the course could include longitudinal tracking of student competencies and outcomes after graduation, along with expanded inter professional collaboration and education opportunities incorporating veterinary technicians, veterinary social workers, and other veterinary healthcare professionals. These enhancements would further refine the curriculum and ensure that veterinary graduates are fully prepared to provide compassionate, team-based, and high-quality EOL care to their patients and clients.

This study has several limitations that should be acknowledged. First, the evaluation relied exclusively on post-course analysis and lacked pre-course baseline data to objectively quantify students' actual knowledge and skill growth. Consequently, the observed improvements are based on students' self-reported perceptions of competency and confidence rather than the direct measurement of clinical proficiency or communication skills. Self-report data inherently carry the potential for response bias, with students possibly overstating positive outcomes or satisfaction due to social desirability. Additionally, the absence of a control group limits the ability to conclusively attribute improvements solely to course content and format. Lastly, as the survey data were collected anonymously and retrospectively, there was a limited ability to clarify ambiguous responses or explore individual experiences in depth, potentially reducing the richness of the qualitative data.

Conclusion

The development and implementation of the Compassionate End-of-Life Care elective course represents a potentially valuable curricular innovation in veterinary education. The hybrid model and micro-credentialing approach could offer an adaptable and scalable solution for other professional veterinary education institutions. Embedding these topics into the core curriculum would help ensure that future veterinary healthcare professionals and veterinary teams are equipped to competently and confidently support both animal patients and their human caregivers in some of the most challenging moments of veterinary practice.

Furthermore, enhancing veterinary professional students' skills in compassionate euthanasia practices has a meaningful impact on preserving the human–animal bond. Sensitive and competent management of EOL care ensures that the bond between client and animal is honored, even at its most vulnerable stage. Training veterinary professional students to prioritize emotional support, effective communication, and humane procedures helps mitigate the grief associated with loss and reinforces client trust in the veterinary profession. By equipping future veterinarians with these competencies, the course supports not only technical proficiency, but also relational care essential to high-quality veterinary practice. Effective veterinary hospice and euthanasia education ultimately benefits all stakeholders: animals receive more humane and compassionate care at the EOL; clients are better supported through difficult decisions and grief, and veterinary healthcare professionals enter the profession more confident and better prepared for the moral, ethical, and emotional complexities of the field.

Conflict of Interest

Kathleen Cooney is the founder and has a financial interest in CAETA, which delivered the Certified Peaceful Euthanasia Veterinarian (CPEV) training referenced in this course. His involvement in the project was focused on course delivery and content expertise and was not involved in the design of the evaluation instruments or in the analysis of results. The remaining authors declare no conflicts of interest.

Ethics Statement

This project involved program evaluation activities and did not constitute human subjects research. Therefore, Institutional Review Board (IRB) approval was not required or obtained. All data were collected anonymously through standard course evaluation mechanisms for internal quality improvement.

Acknowledgments

The authors would like to acknowledge Dr Jennifer Hodgson for her instrumental contributions and support for the development and implementation of this new course. The authors would also like to acknowledge the faculty and staff at the VMCVM for their support of the course and the laboratory, and to the students who took the course and spent their time to provide feedback to inform future iterations of the course.

Author Contributions

VKC contributed in conceptualization, methodology, formal analysis, investigation, data curation, writing (original draft, review and editing), and project administration; KC performed in writing (review and editing), and resources; and RF contributed in writing (review and editing), investigation, and resources.

Funding Statement

No external funding sources were used in the preparation of this study.

Data Availability

All relevant data are within the article and its supporting information files.

Acronyms and Definitions

AAVMC	American Association of Veterinary Medical Colleges
AVMA	American Veterinary Medical Association
CAETA	Companion Animal Euthanasia Training Academy

CBVE	Competency-Based Veterinary Education
CPEV	Certified Peaceful Euthanasia Veterinarian
EOL	End-of-Life
IAAHPC	International Association for Animal Hospice and Palliative Care
IRB	Institutional Review Board
IV	Intravenous
RACE	Registry of Approved Continuing Education
SPOT	Student Perceptions of Teaching
VMCVM	Virginia-Maryland College of Veterinary Medicine

Supplementary Content

Refer to supplementary material on the CABI Digital Library: https://www.cabidigitallibrary.org/doi/book/10.1079/9781836994046.0000. See p.vii for details.

References

Alves, A. and Scorsolini-Comin, F. (2025) Training veterinarians to deal with death and the dying process: A scoping review. *New Zealand Veterinary Journal* (2), 67–76. DOI: 10.1080/00480169.2024.2424189.

AVMA (2024) More Veterinary Colleges in Line for Accreditation Evaluations. Available at: https://www.avma.org/news/more-veterinary-colleges-line-accreditation-evaluations (accessed 10 March 2025).

Brown, M., Mhichíl, M.N.G., Beirne, E. and Lochlainn, C.M. (2021) The global micro-credential landscape: Charting a new credential ecology for lifelong learning. *Journal of Learning for Development* 8(2), 228–254. DOI: 10.56059/jl4d.v8i2.525.

Bubeck, M.J. (2023) Justifying euthanasia: A qualitative study of veterinarians' ethical boundary work of 'good' killing. *Animals* 13(15), 2515. DOI: 10.3390/ani13152515.

CAETA (2022) Virginia-Maryland Veterinary College Takes the Lead in Euthanasia Training. CAETA Newsletter (blog). Available at: https://caetainternational.com/virginia-marylandveterinary-college-takes-the-lead-in-euthanasia-training/ (accessed 13 March 2025).

Cooney, K. (2024) "How I approach a meaningful euthanasia appointment." Royal Canin Vet Focus (blog). Available at: https://vetfocus.royalcanin.com/en/practice-management/how-iapproach-a-meaningful-euthanasia-appointment (accessed 13 March 2025).

Cooney, K. and Kipperman, B. (2023) Ethical and practical considerations associated with companion animal euthanasia. *Animals* 13(3), 430. DOI: 10.3390/ani13030430.

CAETA (2025) The CAETA Peaceful Euthanasia Certification. Companion Animal Euthanasia Training Academy (blog). Available at: https://learn.caetainternational.com/ (accessed 13 March 2025).

Cooney, K., Dickinson, G.E. and Hoffmann, H. (2021) Euthanasia education in veterinary schools in the United States. *Journal of Veterinary Medical Education* 48(6), 706–709. DOI: 10.3138/jvme-2020-0050.

Cooney, K. (2023) *Euthanasia in animal end-of-life care*. In: Shanan, A., Pierce, J. and Shearer, T. (eds) *Hospice and Palliative Care for Companion Animals*, 2nd edn. John Wiley & Sons, Inc, Hoboken, NJ, pp. 318–331. DOI: 10.1002/9781119808817.ch24.

Dickinson, G.E., Roof, K.W., Roof, P.D. and Paul, E.S. (2014) UK veterinarians' experiences with euthanasia. *Veterinary Record* 175(7), 174–174. DOI: 10.1136/vr.102636.

Goldberg, K.J. (2016) Veterinary hospice and palliative care: A comprehensive review of the literature. *Veterinary Record* 178(15), 369–374. DOI: 10.1136/vr.103459.

Gray, C. and Radford, A. (2022) Using electronic health records to explore negotiations around euthanasia decision making for dogs and cats in the UK. *Veterinary Record* 190(9), e1379. DOI: 10.1002/vetr.1379.

IAAHPC (2025) Veterinary PCertification in Pet Hospice and Palliative Care. Available at: https://iaahpc.org/veterinary-certification/ (accessed 13 March 2025).

Kogan, L.R. and Cooney, K.A. (2023) Defining a 'good death': Exploring veterinarians' perceptions of companion animal euthanasia. *Animals* 13(13), 2117. DOI: 10.3390/ani13132117.

Kunze, A.J. and Seals, C. (2020) Exploring fourth-year students' perceptions of the hidden curriculum of a doctor of veterinary medicine program through written reflections. *Education in the Health Professions* 3(3), 121. DOI: 10.4103/EHP.EHP_23_20.

Littlewood, K., Beausoleil, N., Kj Stafford, C., Stephens, T.C., Fawcett, A. *et al.* (2020) How management of grief associated with ending the life of an animal is taught to Australasian veterinary students. *Australian Veterinary Journal* 98(8), 356–363. DOI: 10.1111/avj.12960.

Littlewood, K., Beausoleil, N., Kj Stafford, C., Stephens, T.C., Quain, A. *et al.* (2021) How decision-making about euthanasia for animals is taught to Australasian veterinary students. *Australian Veterinary Journal* 99(8), 334–343. DOI: 10.1111/avj.13077.

Matthew, S.M., Bok, H.G.J., Chaney, K.P., Read, E.K., Hodgson, J.L. *et al.* (2020) Collaborative development of a shared framework for competency-based veterinary education. *Journal of Veterinary Medical Education* 47(5), 578–593. DOI: 10.3138/jvme.2019-0082.

Pegram, C., Gray, C., Packer, R.M.A., Richards, Y., Church, D.B. *et al.* (2021) Proportion and risk factors for death by euthanasia in dogs in the UK. *Scientific Reports* 11(1), 9145. DOI: 10.1038/s41598-021-88342-0.

Persson, K., Selter, F., Neitzke, G. and Kunzmann, P. (2020) Philosophy of a 'good death' in small animals and consequences for euthanasia in animal law and veterinary practice. *Animals* 10(1), 124. DOI: 10.3390/ani10010124.

Roder, C.A. and May, S.A. (2017) The hidden curriculum of veterinary education: Mediators and moderators of its effects. *Journal of Veterinary Medical Education* 44(3), 542–551. DOI: 10.3138/jvme.0416-082.

Schultz, M.A., Morrisey, J.K., Kaplan, L.K., Colón, J.L., McVety-Leinen, D.G. *et al.* (2022) A scalable and effective course design for teaching competency-based euthanasia communication skills in veterinary curricula. *Journal of Veterinary Medical Education* 49(4), 484–491. DOI: 10.3138/jvme2020-0133.

Thi Ngoc Ha, N., Spittle, M., Watt, A. and Dyke, N. (2023) A systematic literature review of micro-credentials in higher education: A non-zero-sum game. *Higher Education Research & Development* 42(6), 1527–1548. DOI: 10.1080/07294360.2022.2146061.

5 The Untapped Potential of Registered Veterinary Technicians in Hospice Care

Emily Piche*

The Art of Goodbye – Hospice and Euthanasia Training Institute, Tiny Township, Ontario, Canada

Abstract

Background: As veterinary medicine evolves to include more comprehensive hospice and end-of-life care, Registered Veterinary Technicians remain an underutilized resource in hospice and palliative care programs. This systematic review investigates the barriers and opportunities for Registered Veterinary Technicians to assume leadership roles in veterinary hospice care. Methods: A systematic review of peer-reviewed veterinary literature from 2000 to 2024 was conducted using PubMed, CAB Abstracts, and Google Scholar. Search terms included "veterinary hospice," "palliative care," "Registered Veterinary Technician," "veterinary nurse," "hospice and end-of-life care," and "access to care." Inclusion criteria were English-language studies focused on veterinary medicine, with emphasis on Registered Veterinary Technician roles, training, clinic economics, and accessibility of care. Human health and non-hospice veterinary studies were excluded except where explicitly used for comparative context. A total of 86 articles were screened; 21 met all inclusion criteria and were analyzed thematically. Results: Thematic analysis revealed six recurring themes: (1) underutilization of Registered Veterinary Technicians; (2) misunderstandings around Registered Veterinary Technician abilities; (3) nurse-led hospice care; (4) lack of dedicated hospice training; (5) Registered Veterinary Technicians can help increase access to care; and (6) high veterinarian workload limits hospice capacity. Despite the potential of Registered Veterinary Technicians to support compassionate hospice and end-of-life care, training gaps, cultural resistance, economic oversight, and regulatory ambiguity persist. Conclusions: Registered Veterinary Technicians are well-positioned to lead and enhance veterinary hospice services. Addressing training deficiencies, expanding scope-of-practice clarity, and promoting technician-led care models may help veterinary practices better serve animals and families during the most vulnerable life stage.

Keywords: registered veterinary technician, veterinary nurse, palliative care, veterinary hospice, access to care, hospice and end of life care

Introduction

Veterinary hospice and end-of-life care are emerging disciplines designed to support quality of life for companion animals with life-limiting conditions. Despite increasing client demand for compassionate hospice and end-of-life options, many veterinary practices struggle to provide timely, continuous, and accessible services. Registered Veterinary Technicians represent an

*Corresponding author: info@theartofgoodbye.ca

untapped resource in this space. This review systematically examines the current literature to understand how Registered Veterinary Technicians can be more effectively integrated into veterinary hospice programs.

Methods

A systematic review was conducted in alignment with Preferred Reporting Items for Systematic Reviews and Meta-Analyses guidelines. Searches were performed across PubMed, CAB Abstracts, and Google Scholar using combinations of keywords: "Registered Veterinary Technician," "veterinary nurse," "palliative care," "veterinary hospice," "access to care," and "hospice and end-of-life care." Articles were included if they:

- were published between 2000 and 2024;
- focused on veterinary medicine (not human medicine, except where noted);
- explored technician or nurse roles in hospice or palliative contexts;
- included discussion of training, scope of practice, access to care, economic impacts, or client perspectives

Articles focusing solely on human health care, theoretical ethics, or unrelated areas of veterinary medicine were excluded, with one exception used for comparative discussion. Of 86 screened articles, 21 met all inclusion criteria.

Results

Thematic analysis of the 21 included studies revealed six primary themes concerning Registered Veterinary Technicians in veterinary hospice care:

Theme 1: Underutilization of registered veterinary technicians

Registered Veterinary Technicians are often underused despite their training and capabilities, resulting in reduced job satisfaction and increased turnover. Studies highlight that maximizing Registered Veterinary Technician contributions could enhance both staff retention and quality of care (Larkin, 2018).

Theme 2: Misunderstandings around registered veterinary technician abilities

There are prevalent misconceptions among veterinary teams regarding the full scope of Registered Veterinary Technician skills. This misunderstanding limits their integration into hospice care and impedes optimal clinic workflow and patient outcomes (American Animal Hospital Association, 2023a; American Association of Veterinary State Boards (AAVSB), 2024).

Theme 3: Nurse led hospice care

Technician-led hospice care models demonstrate improved patient comfort and enhanced communication with clients. Empowering Registered Veterinary Technicians in these roles fosters compassionate end-of-life care and increases client satisfaction (Carter, 2020; Hall and Richards, 2020).

Theme 4: Lack of dedicated hospice training

A consistent lack of formal hospice training among veterinary professionals causes discomfort and variability in care delivery. This gap highlights the need for dedicated hospice and palliative education in veterinary curricula and continuing education (Dickinson and Sullivan, 2011; Hunt *et al.*, 2016).

Theme 5: Registered veterinary technicians can help increase access to care

Expanding the roles of Registered Veterinary Technicians improves clinic efficiency, enabling veterinary practices to offer more accessible hospice and palliative services. Studies show that effective utilization of Registered Veterinary Technicians can reduce barriers to care for clients and patients (Ontario Veterinary Medical Association, 2020; American Animal Hospital Association, 2023b).

Theme 6: High veterinarian workload limits hospice capacity

High workloads and burnout among veterinarians reduce the time available for hospice discussions and follow-up care. This limits the overall capacity of veterinary practices to provide comprehensive hospice services (Fritschi *et al.*, 2023; Steffey *et al.*, 2023).

Discussion

This review demonstrates that Registered Veterinary Technicians remain consistently underutilized in hospice and end-of-life care. Despite growing client demand, regulatory progress, and demonstrated competencies, many veterinary practices fail to leverage the skills of Registered Veterinary Technicians in this sensitive domain.

Veterinarians experience overwhelming caseloads that limit their ability to provide extended time and support required during hospice discussions and follow-up care. Delegating these responsibilities to trained Registered Veterinary Technicians has been shown to improve both client experience and clinical workflow.

These findings align with broader workforce utilization trends seen in human healthcare, where expanding the roles of nurses and allied professionals has improved patient satisfaction and access. Within veterinary medicine, increased reliance on Registered Veterinary Technicians may not only improve the quality of care but also alleviate workforce burnout and financial inefficiencies.

However, this review also reveals critical limitations: the veterinary literature lacks in-depth data on Registered Veterinary Technician-led hospice outcomes, and few studies investigate client perspectives directly. Furthermore, there is insufficient training infrastructure for Registered Veterinary Technicians in hospice and end-of-life specialties, reflecting a need for educational reform.

Strengths of this review include a robust, multi-database literature search, adherence to Preferred Reporting Items for Systematic Reviews and Meta-Analyses methodology, and thematic organization rooted in both clinical and operational contexts. Limitations include potential language bias and underrepresentation of unpublished or regional models of care.

Future research should focus on outcomes of Registered Veterinary Technician-led hospice models, development of standardized training curricula, and cross-country comparisons in scope-of-practice utilization. Engaging with clients, educators, and policy makers will be crucial to elevate and integrate the contributions of Registered Veterinary Technicians across all stages of veterinary care.

Conclusion

Registered Veterinary Technicians have the training, empathy, and proximity to clients necessary to lead compassionate and effective hospice programs. Their strategic deployment could resolve critical access and continuity gaps in veterinary hospice and end-of-life care. To get there, educational reforms, clinic-level restructuring, and cultural shifts within the profession must occur.

Conflict of Interests

The author is the owner of a hospice and end of life care training company. This affiliation may present a potential conflict of interest, as the author's business may benefit from the promotion and integration of hospice care programs in veterinary practice. Additionally, the author's role as a

Registered Veterinary Technician may present a further potential conflict of interest. However, the author affirms that the research and conclusions presented in this paper were conducted impartially and with the intent to advance knowledge in the field of veterinary hospice care.

Funding

International Association of Animal Hospice and Palliative Care (Grant/Award Number: No grant number).

Data Availability

Data available upon request.

Ethics Statement

The author confirms that the research meets any required ethical guidelines, including adherence to the legal requirements of the study country.

References

American Animal Hospital Association (2023a) Technician utilization guidelines. Available at: https://www.aaha.org/trends-magazine/january-2023/

American Animal Hospital Association (2023b) Proper Team Utilization. AAHA Trends. Available at: https://www.aaha.org/trends-magazine/january-2023/f2-tech-utilization/

American Association of Veterinary State Boards (AAVSB) (2024) AAVSB Releases Conclusions of the North American Veterinary Team Delegation Survey. AAVSB. Available at: https://www.aavsb.org/news/aavsb-releases-conclusions-of-the-north-american-veterinary-team-delegation-survey/ (accessed 9 August 2025).

Carter, K. (2020) The role of the veterinary technician in end-of-life care. *Veterinary Clinics of North America: Small Animal Practice* 50(3), 639–645. DOI: 10.1016/j.cvsm.2019.12.012.

Dickinson, G.E. and Sullivan, M. (2011) A survey of veterinarians in the U.S.: Euthanasia and other end-of-life issues. *Journal of Veterinary Medical Education* 38(4), 365–373. DOI: 10.3138/jvme.38.4.365.

Fritschi, L. *et al* (2023) Burnout and work-life balance in veterinarians: A cross-sectional survey. *Journal of Veterinary Internal Medicine* 37(4), 1234–1242. DOI: 10.1111/jvim.16839.

Hall, M.R. and Richards, J.C. (2020) Evaluating the role of veterinary nurses in animal hospice and palliative care. *Veterinary Nursing Journal* 35(4), 212–219. DOI: 10.1002/vnj3.2020.35.4.212.

Hunt, G., Shaw, J.R., Adams, C.L. and Dolan, E.D. (2016) Veterinary students' attitudes toward end-of-life decisions and communication in companion animal practice. *Journal of Veterinary Medical Education* 43(4), 293–302. DOI: 10.3138/jvme.0716-075R.

Larkin, M. (2018) Prime issue for veterinary technicians: Underutilization. *JAVMA News*, Available at: https://www.avma.org/javma-news/2018-11-15/prime-issue-veterinary-technicians-underutilization

Ontario Veterinary Medical Association (2020) Optimizing Veterinary Technician Roles to Improve Practice Efficiency and Access to Care. Available at: https://www.veterinarypracticenews.com/better-utilize-vet-techs/

Steffey, M.A., Griffon, D.J., Risselada, M., Scharf, J., Buote, M. *et al.* (2023) Veterinarian burnout demographics and organizational impacts. *Frontiers in Veterinary Science* 10, 1184526. DOI: 10.3389/fvets.2023.1184526.

6 Veterinary End-of-Life Mobile Practitioners: Motivators, Challenges, Job Fulfillment, and Burnout

Lori R. Kogan[1]*, Jennifer Currin-McCulloch[2], Kellie Littrell[3] and Emma Brown[4]
[1]Department of Clinical Sciences, Colorado State University, Fort Collins, CO, USA; [2]School of Social Work, Colorado State University, Fort Collins, CO, USA; [3]Texas Tech University School of Veterinary Medicine, Lubbock, TX, USA; [4]Department of Sociomedical Sciences, Columbia University, New York, NY, USA

Abstract
A growing specialty within veterinary medicine is end-of-life (EOL) care, including EOL mobile practice. EOL care is a broad term referring to euthanasia services, as well as hospice and palliative care for terminally-ill patients. This study was designed to better understand how EOL mobile veterinarians feel about their work, including the benefits and challenges, their reasons for choosing this career, and their levels of professional fulfillment and burnout compared to other veterinary professionals. To this end, an online, anonymous, cross-sectional survey was developed using Qualtrics, and adult EOL mobile practitioners were recruited for the study. A total of 162 veterinarians responded to the survey. Results suggest that the primary reasons why veterinarians are drawn to mobile EOL work include the ability to make a positive impact and provide personalized care to pets and families, and enjoy a better work environment. When participants were asked to indicate how challenging they found 16 EOL mobile practitioner work-related factors, the factors reported as "very challenging" by the largest number of participants included a lack of health benefits (24/99, 24%), followed by the hassle of the business side (e.g., taxes, recordkeeping, etc.) (21/122, 17.2%). When assessing burnout and professional fulfillment, a total of 21/142 (14.80%) indicated they felt burned out and 99/142 (69.72%) participants' scores fell above the cutoff for professional fulfillment, suggesting that mobile EOL practitioners have higher job fulfillment and lower burnout than other veterinary professionals. These results suggest that engagement in euthanasia, per se, does not necessarily lead to a negative impact on mental health. While not for everyone, mobile EOL practice appears to be a viable career path for some veterinarians.

Keywords: euthanasia, end-of-life, palliative care, veterinarian, mobile, in-home, job fulfillment, job satisfaction, burnout

*Corresponding author: lori.kogan@colostate.edu

Introduction

Euthanasia, defined as "the use of humane techniques to induce the most rapid, painless and distress-free death possible to induce death in a manner that is in accord with an animal's interest and/or because it is a matter of welfare' (Leary *et al.*, 2020) is a common cause of companion animal death (Pegram *et al.*, 2021; Cooney and Kipperman, 2023). Veterinarians play a unique role in the final stages of an animal's life, empowered to deliver euthanasia in a compassionate manner with the overarching goal of providing a peaceful and meaningful experience for both pets and pet owners alike (Morris, 2012; Gates *et al.*, 2017; Kollias *et al.*, 2023).

An increasing number of people view their pets as family members (Rowan and Kartal, 2018; Volsche, 2019; Kogan *et al.*, 2022a, b), with studies consistently reporting that the depth of attachment and connection humans feel toward their pets is similar to bonds between people (DeGroot, 1984; Carmack, 1985; Archer, 1997; Field *et al.*, 2009; Sable, 2013; Messam *et al.*, 2019; Behler, 2020; Cowling *et al.*, 2020). One consequence of this human–animal attachment is significant grief and loss when the life of a companion animal ends (Chur-Hansen, 2010; Kogan *et al.*, 2022a). As a result of the close bond owners feel with their pets, and the move towards Fear Free/Low Stress Handling, euthanasia has evolved over time into much more than the medical procedure (Pierce, 2014), requiring not only technical competency to ensure a humane death for animals, but encompassing numerous ethical considerations and compassionate communication skills (Yeates, 2010; Batchelor and McKeegan, 2012a; Hernandez *et al.*, 2018; Kipperman *et al.*, 2018; Quain, 2021; Cooney and Kipperman, 2023; Gates *et al.*, 2023; Pepper *et al.*, 2023). To offer technical guidance, several guidelines pertaining to appropriate drug protocols and routes of administration have been published (Cooney, 2020; Leary *et al.*, 2020; Robertson, 2020). Several entities offer euthanasia-focused veterinary continuing professional development (e.g., The Companion Animal Euthanasia Training Academy (CAETA), Australian Veterinary Palliative Care Advisory Council, etc.), and recent publications highlight competencies required for facilitating humane euthanasia (Cooney and Kogan, 2022; Kogan and Cooney, 2023).

There is a growing body of literature that addresses important elements in creating a 'good death' from both a pet owner and veterinary professional viewpoint. Pet owners' definition of a good euthanasia experience includes a sense of compassion and confidence from their veterinarian, the creation of a low-stress environment, and the provision of adequate information and support (Matte *et al.*, 2020; Shearer, 2020; Cooney and Kogan, 2022). In a 2022 study, when pet owners were asked what differentiates a good from a bad death, results indicated that owners want their pet to experience little to no pain or anxiety throughout the entire process, with their pet in a state of sleep before the final injection is given (Cooney and Kogan, 2022). The ability to remain with their pet during the entire procedure was also a top priority for nearly all owners; not being allowed to be with their pet during the entire procedure was viewed negatively by over 90% of owners (Cooney and Kogan, 2022), sentiments found in several other studies (Wu *et al.*, 2021; Owczarczak-Garstecka *et al.*, 2022). In terms of location, pet owners preferred in-home euthanasia over other locations and were much more likely to report a positive experience in that setting (Kogan and Cooney, 2023).

Veterinary mobile practice, as opposed to traditional brick-and-mortar practice, is a viable career option for veterinarians considering alternative ways to practice veterinary medicine. While large animal mobile practices have long been the norm, small animal mobile practices have more recently increased in popularity (Koch, 2021). Most mobile veterinarians function as small businesses, providing many of the same services as brick-and-mortar hospitals, including physical exams, vaccinations, blood work, euthanasia, disease management and senior health (Drake, 2016; Barnette, 2020). Other mobile veterinarians contract to provide or refer specific services (e.g., radiography, surgery, dentistry, etc.) through brick-and-mortar hospitals or work for corporate mobile businesses.

A growing specialty within veterinary medicine is end-of-life (EOL) care (Bishop *et al.*,

2008; Paz *et al.*, 2024), including EOL mobile practice. EOL care is a broad term used in veterinary medicine most often to refer to euthanasia services but also encompassing hospice and palliative care for terminally-ill patients. Performing euthanasia has been described as emotionally challenging; a burden and stressor that can cause psychological distress (Bartram and Baldwin, 2008, 2010; Fink-Miller and Nestler, 2018; Stetina and Krouzecky, 2022). Several studies have found that veterinarians are at increased risk of suicide when compared to the general population (Nett *et al.*, 2015; Fink-Miller and Nestler, 2018). Some previous research has suggested that involvement with euthanasia can have a negative psychological impact (Owens *et al.*, 1981; Rollin, 1986; Fogle and Abrahamson, 1990) and could negatively influence the development of depression, suicidal ideation, and suicidal behaviors (Owens *et al.*, 1981; Fogle and Abrahamson, 1990; Arluke, 1994; Bartram and Baldwin, 2008, 2010; Rollin, 2011). Yet, other studies suggest the relationship between performing euthanasia, depression and suicide risk is more complex and the positive aspects of euthanasia may buffer any negative effects (Morris, 2012; Tran *et al.*, 2014). Despite the growing number of EOL veterinarians, including EOL mobile practitioners, there is a dearth of research about this population. It is unknown why these veterinarians choose to focus exclusively on EOL care and how they feel about their jobs, including their levels of professional fulfillment and burnout. Therefore, we designed this study to better understand how EOL mobile veterinarians feel about their work, including the benefits and drawbacks, their reasons for choosing this career, and their levels of professional fulfillment and burnout compared to other veterinary professionals. We also explored the potential predictive factor of job characteristics (e.g., length of shift, on-call duties, etc.) and personal demographics on both professional fulfillment and burnout.

Methods

An online, anonymous, cross-sectional survey was developed using Qualtrics (Qualtrics, Inc., Provo, UT, USA). The survey was designed, reviewed, and pilot tested by approximately 10 EOL practitioners for ambiguity and/or potentially missing or inappropriate response options, with appropriate revisions made. The final survey (see Supplementary Material) and study design were approved by the Colorado State University Institutional Review Board (IRB #6365). Survey participants were recruited between October 2024 and November 2024 via EOL practitioners social media (Facebook, Twitter, Instagram).

Adult (ages 18 and older) EOL mobile practitioners were recruited for the study. Participant demographics were collected (age, gender, LGBTQ + identity, relationship status, children, length of time in veterinary medicine, length of time as mobile EOL practitioner). Participants were asked about their role before becoming an EOL mobile practitioner, how many hours and shifts they work per week, how many hours they work per shift, and to rank the months of the year in terms of busiest to slowest. They were asked how many days per month they are on call, if they hold any other jobs, to describe their current position (e.g., owner/part owner, work for small business, etc.) and how they learned about the field of EOL mobile practitioners.

Participants were asked to rate several potential factors in terms of importance in becoming an EOL mobile practitioner (e.g., "Escape an unhealthy work environment"', "Desire to help pets die peacefully in familiar surroundings", "Ability to receive heartfelt appreciation for the service provided") using a 4-point scale with 1 = does not apply, 2 = not at all/minimally important, 3 = moderately important, and 4 = very important.

Participants were also asked to indicate how challenging they find several aspects of EOL mobile practitioner work (e.g., "unpredictable schedule", "travel time and fuel costs", "need to be on-call") using a 3-point scale with 1 = not at all/minimally challenging, 2 = moderately challenging, and 3 = very challenging.

The Stanford Professional Fulfillment Index (PFI) (Trockel *et al.*, 2018) was used to assess self-reported professional fulfillment and professional burnout. The PFI includes a 6-item Professional Fulfillment subscale (e.g., "I feel happy at work", "I feel in control when dealing with difficult problems at work"), a 6-item Interpersonal Disengagement subscale (e.g., "Less empathetic with my colleagues", "Less connected with patients"), and a 4-item Work Exhaustion subscale (e.g., "A sense of dread when I think about the work I have to do", "Lacking in enthusiasm at work"). For all items, participants were instructed to reflect on their past 2 weeks and indicate how well the items described their experience using a 5-point scale ranging from 0 (not at all) to 4 (extremely). An average score was created for the Professional Fulfillment sub-scale; the initial validation study of the PFI reported evidence of the utility of a cut-point (cut point = 3.0) to identify dichotomous groupings that distinguish participants who were experiencing professional fulfillment and those who were not (Trockel *et al.*, 2018). Scores for the Work Exhaustion and Interpersonal Disengagement sub-scales were combined to assess burnout (score 0–10) with higher scores indicating more burnout symptoms. A cut-point of 1.33 was used to identify dichotomous groupings that distinguished participants experiencing burnout from those who were not (Trockel *et al.*, 2018). Prior studies indicate that the PFI is a valid and reliable assessment of professional fulfillment and burnout (Trockel *et al.*, 2018; Kogan *et al.*, 2020; Kogan and Rishniw, 2023a).

In the last part of the survey, participants were asked to indicate their perception of adequate emotional support resources using a 5-point Likert scale with 1 = strongly disagree to 5 = strongly agree. They were also asked how often they connect (in person or virtually) with other EOL practitioners using a 5-point Likert scale with 1 = never to 5 = daily. Interspersed throughout the survey, we included four qualitative open-ended questions to ascertain what mobile EOL veterinarians found to be (1) the benefits of EOL work, (2) the challenges of EOL practice, (3) the impact of their work on their children (if applicable), (4) and other feedback they wished to share about their work as a mobile EOL veterinarian.

Descriptive and inferential statistics were performed with SPSS, version 28. Linear regression was used to determine if personal demographics (relationship status (single/married or partnered), length of time in veterinary field, length of time as EOL practitioner, shifts per week, length of shifts, hours worked per week, on call duty, number of children (yes/no), age, and other jobs (yes/ no) could predict levels of professional fulfillment or burnout. Significance level was set at .05.

Qualitative analysis

We integrated Guest *et al.*'s (Guest *et al.*, 2011) applied thematic analysis methods to analyze participants' responses to the four-open ended survey items. Participants' responses to questions varied from one word to several sentences. The two coders (JCM and EB) are a doctoral trained palliative care social worker and a graduate student in a dual MSW/MPH program. The coding process included an individual reading of the dataset and an initial individual coding of a sample of responses from each open-ended item. JCM and EB then met to review coding terms and general themes that were interpreted from the data. Next, we coded the remaining data from all open-ended items independently and then met to discuss differences. We then determined main themes from the data and selected salient quotes to represent the themes.

Results

A total of 162 participants responded to the survey, all of whom reported being veterinarians. The majority were married/partnered (136/161, 84.5%) women (150/162, 92.6%), with an average age of 44.1 years (SD = 9.53; range 28 to 73). When asked about children (n = 159), 61 (38.4%) reported having no children, 28 (17.6%) having one child, 41 (25.8%) having two children, and 28 (17.6%) having three children or more. The majority of participants reported being in the veterinary field for 10 years or more (126/162, 77.8%), and being a mobile EOL practitioner for 1–5 years (84/162, 51.9%). Most participants reported that their previous role was within private practice (134/162, 82.7%). When asked how many hours they work per week (n = 162), the most common response was 30–40 h per week (41, 25.3%), followed by 21–30 h per week (31, 19.1%). The most common response when queried about the number of shifts worked per week was 5 (45/154, 29.2%), and the number of hours per shift was 8 (32/154, 20.8%). When asked about on call duties (n = 159), 76 (47.8%) reported not ever being on call, and 43 (27.0%) reported always being on call. When participants were asked if they held any other jobs (n = 160), 77 (48.1%) reported they also held a veterinary-related job and 75 (46.9%) reported not holding any other type of job. The majority of participants reported being the owner or part-owner of their business (120/162, 74.1%) (see Table 6.1 for demographics). When asked how they learned about mobile EOL practice as a career (n = 162), the most common response was from friends/ colleagues (86, 53.1%), followed by personal experience using the service (35, 21.6%) (Table 6.2). Participants were asked to rank order the 12 months from busiest (1) to slowest (12). The busiest months were January (X=4.88, SD=3.55) and June (X=5.61, SD=3.07); the slowest months were October (X=7.75, SD=3.49) and September (X=8.07, SD=3.05). (Table 6.3).

Reasons to become an EOL mobile practitioner

Participants were asked to indicate the importance of 28 potential reasons for choosing to be an veterinary EOL mobile practitioner. The items selected as very important by the largest number of participants included a desire to help pets die peacefully in familiar surroundings (135/154, 87.7%), the feeling of making a difference in a pet's final moments (128/154, 83.1%), flexible schedule (124/162, 76.5%) and control over appointment times and workload (123/162, 75.9%). The factors seen as least important/ applicable included the ability to perform small rituals or ceremonies if desired (30/154, 19.5%), less physical demands (30/162, 18.5%), personal growth from regularly confronting mortality and grief (26/161, 16.1%), and sold their hospital but wanted to stay in veterinary medicine (5/162, 3.1%) (Table 6.4).

Challenges as an EOL mobile practitioner

Participants were asked to indicate how challenging they find 16 EOL mobile practitioner work-related factors. None of the factors were rated as "very challenging" by more than 25% of the participants. The factor reported as "very challenging" by the largest number of participants was a lack of health benefits (24/99, 24%), followed by the hassle of the business side (e.g., taxes, recordkeeping, etc.) (21/122, 17.2%). The factors rated as moderately challenging by most participants included unpredictable income (63/125, 50.4%) and hassle of the business side (60/122, 49.2%) (Table 6.5).

Professional fulfillment and burnout

In the current sample, reliability of the professional fulfillment ($\alpha=.903$; $\Omega=.903$) and burnout scales ($\alpha=.902$; $\Omega=.900$) were excellent. The mean total scores for each of the PFI scales were calculated: Work Exhaustion scale: X=.95 (SD=.75); Interpersonal Disengagement scale: X=.42 (SD=.54); and Professional Fulfillment scale: X=3.19 (SD=.71). The mean total Burnout score (Work Exhaustion and Interpersonal Disengagement) was X=.65 (SD=.57). Using the suggested dichotomous burnout cutoff score of 1.33, the overall participant mean of .65 suggests that this population falls beneath the cutoff for burnout. A total of 21/142 (14.80%) scored above the cutoff for burnout, indicating they feel burned out.

Linear regression was used to determine if personal demographics (relationship status (single/married or partnered), length of time in veterinary field, length of time as EOL practitioner, shifts per week, length of shifts, hours worked per week, on call duty, number of children (yes/no), age, and other jobs (yes/no) could predict levels of burnout. The regression model was not significant ($p = .077$).

For the Professional Fulfillment scale, the mean score of 3.19 of this total sample fell above the suggested cutoff point of >3.0 for professional fulfillment. A total of 99/142 (69.72%) participants scored above the cutoff for professional fulfillment. Linear regression was used to determine if personal demographics relationship status (single/married or partnered), length of time in veterinary field, length of time as EOL practitioner, shifts per week, length of shifts,

Table 6.1. Demographics of EOL mobile veterinarians.

Gender (n = 162)		LGBTQ+ (n = 162)		Relationship status (n = 161)		Children (n = 159)	
Woman	150 (92.6%)	Yes	8 (4.9%)	Married/partnered	136 (84.5%)	None	61 (38.4%)
Man	8 (4.9%)	No	147 (90.7%)	Not married/partnered	25 (15.5%)	1	28 (17.6%)
Prefer not to answer	4 (2.5%)	Prefer not to answer	7 (4.3%)			2	41 (25.8%)
						3	23 (14.5%)
						4 or more	5 (3.1%)
						Prefer not to answer	1 (0.6%)
Length of time in veterinary medicine (n = 162)		Length of time as mobile EOL practitioner (n = 162)		Role before mobile EOL practitioner (n = 162)			
0–3 years	–	Less than 1 year	20 (12.3%)	Was not working outside the home (e.g., stay at home)	5 (3.1%)		
3–<5 years	8 (4.9%)	1–<3 years	44 (27.2%)	Straight from veterinary school/internship	11 (6.8%)		
5–<10 years	28 (17.3%)	3–<5 years	40 (24.7%)	Private practice	134 (82.7%)		
10 years or more	126 (77.8%)	5–<10 years	27 (16.7%)	Academia	1 (0.6%)		
		10 years or more	31 (19.1%)	Non-veterinary related job	1 (0.6%)		
				Other	10 (6.2%)		
Hours work per week (n = 162)		Shifts work per week (n = 154)		Hours work per shift (n = 154)			
1–5 hour	21 (13.0%)	1 or less	15 (9.7%)	1	6 (3.9%)		
6–10 hour	27 (16.7%)	2	17 (11.0%)	2	16 (10.4%)		
11–20 hour	24 (14.8%)	3	32 (20.8%)	3	15 (9.7%)		
21–30 hour	31 (19.1%)	4	25 (16.2%)	4	14 (9.1%)		
30–40 hour	41 (25.3%)	5	45 (29.2%)	5	12 (7.8%)		

>40 hour	18 (11.1%)	6	10 (6.5%)	6	23 (14.9%)
		7 or more	10 (6.5%)	7	5 (3.2%)
				8	32 (20.8%)
				9	5 (3.2%)
				10	20 (13.0%)
				11	2 (1.3%)
				12 or more	4 (2.6%)
Days on call per month (n = 162)		Hold any other jobs (n = 160)		Current position (n = 162)	
I am not on call	76 (47.8%)	Yes, veterinary related job	77 (48.1%)	Owner or part owner	120 (74.1%)
1–5	7 (4.4%)	Yes, non-veterinary related job	5 (3.1%)	Work for a small business	19 (11.7%)
6–10	5 (3.1%)	Yes, both veterinary and non-veterinary jobs	3 (1.9%)	Work for a corporation	18 (11.1%)
10–20	11 (6.9%)	No	75 (46.9%)	Other	5 (3.1%)
21 or more	17 (10.7%)				
I am always on call	43 (27.0%)				

Table 6.2. How EOL mobile practitioners learned about the field (n = 162).

	N	Percent (%)
Veterinary school	33	20.4
Friends/colleagues	86	53.1
Personal experience using the service	35	21.6
Online/educational presentation	21	13.0

Note: More than one answer was possible.

Table 6.3. Busiest and slowest months ranked by practitioners (N = 157).

	Rank	Mean	Standard Deviation
January	1	4.88	3.55
June	2	5.61	3.07
December	3	5.88	4.53
February	4	6.10	3.19
July	5	6.13	3.27
March	6	6.32	2.90
May	7	6.53	2.75
April	8	6.66	2.62
November	9	6.99	4.10
August	10	7.09	3.26
October	11	7.75	3.49
September	12	8.07	3.05

hours worked per week, on call duty, number of children (yes/no), age, and other jobs (yes/no) could predict levels of professional fulfillment. The regression model was significant ($p = .010$, $r^2 = .168$). The only variable that was significant ($p = 0.017$) was on call-duties. Those who reported having on-call duties had lower fulfillment than those who did not.

Emotional support

Participants were asked to indicate their perception of access to adequate emotional support services. The majority agreed or strongly agreed that they had adequate access (100/136, 73.5%), 26/136 (19.1%) were neutral, and 10/136 (7.4%) disagreed or strongly disagreed. When asked how often they connect (in person or virtually) with other EOL veterinarians, the most common response was weekly (36/136, 26.5%). A total of 29/136 (21.3%) reported never and 23/136 (16.9%) reported daily connecting with other EOL veterinarians (Table 6.6).

Qualitative findings

Benefits

One of the primary benefits of EOL work centered around the ability to offer care in clients' homes, often times a more peaceful setting for both the pet and the family than a veterinary hospital. Conducting the euthanasia process in the clients' homes offered more flexibility than a clinic setting, and gave practitioners time to connect with families, witness the human–animal bond, and fully listen to the families' needs. The home setting also allowed families to grieve in private. A practitioner summarized the benefits of working with families in their home:

> It's personable, private, peaceful and allows owners to spend final moments with their pet surrounded by family in comfort of their home. It's more convenient for owners so they don't have to bring their pets into a clinical or hospital setting which have proven to be more stressful on the pet. Owners appreciate the compassionate care provided.

Participants shared that being in the home was particularly impactful for the pets' final moments, as it was the least stressful environment for their physical and mental wellbeing.

Along with making a difference for families, participants also shared that being an EOL practitioner created fulfilling work experiences and offered meaning in their daily work. Practitioners elevated the meaning they find in their work such as "Providing a gift that I strongly feel every pet should receive (although not all can)."

EOL practitioners also highlighted the logistical benefits of their role, including being one's own boss, which enabled control and flexibility over their work schedule, freedom in their practice choices, and autonomy over income and pricing. One practitioner portrayed the

Table 6.4. Reported importance of 28 potential reasons for choosing to be a veterinary EOL mobile practitioner.

	Does not apply to me		Not at all/minimally Important		Moderately Important		Very Important	
Desire to help pets die peacefully in familiar surroundings (n = 154)	2	1.3%	1	0.6%	16	10.4%	135	87.7%
The feeling of making a difference in a pet's final moments (n = 154)	2	1.3%	6	3.9%	18	11.7%	128	83.1%
Flexible schedule (n = 162)	6	3.7%	7	4.3%	25	15.4%	124	76.5%
Control over appointment times and workload (n = 162)	6	3.7%	7	4.3%	26	16.0%	123	75.9%
Ability to make a significant emotional impact on families (n = 155)	1	0.6%	8	5.2%	40	25.8%	106	68.4%
Work life balance (n = 154)	7	4.5%	7	4.5%	35	22.7%	105	68.2%
Provide individualized client experience (n = 154)	1	0.6%	7	4.5%	43	27.9%	103	66.9%
Run your own business/be your own boss (n =162)	22	13.6%	17	10.5%	23	14.2%	100	61.7%
More time to counsel and comfort owners (n = 154)	7	4.5%	18	11.7%	42	27.3%	87	56.5%
Less stress (n = 162)	11	6.8%	19	11.7%	42	25.9%	90	55.6%
Increased connection with clients (n = 154)	7	4.5%	18	11.7%	47	30.5%	82	53.2%
Ability to receive heartfell appreciation for the service provided (n = 154)	8	5.2%	24	15.6%	51	33.1%	71	46.1%
Ability to help normalize discussions about EOL care (n = 154)	5	3.2%	19	12.3%	64	41.6%	66	42.9%
Ability to develop expertise in recognizing signs of suffering in animals (n = 153)	8	5.2%	26	17.0%	54	35.3%	65	42.5%
Ability to become an expert in end-of-ife care and pain management (n = 162)	9	5.6%	22	13.6%	65	40.1%	66	40.7%
Escape an unhealthy work environment (n = 161)	33	20.5%	20	12.4%	45	28.0%	63	39.1%
Ability to focus solely on end-of-life care rather than general practice (n = 155)	25	16.1%	26	16.8%	46	29.7%	58	37.4%

Continued

Table 6.4. Continued

	Does not apply to me		Not at all/minimally Important		Moderately Important		Very Important	
No need for a physical clinic space or expensive medical equipment (n = 162)	33	20.4%	27	16.7%	46	28.4%	56	34.6%
Bumed out and wanted something different than previous position (n = 161)	36	22.4%	28	17.4%	42	26.1%	55	34.2%
Different work environments and cultures (n = 161)	19	11.8%	27	16.8%	67	41.6%	48	29.8%
Lower staffing requirements (n = 161)	46	28.6%	34	21.1%	34	21.1%	47	29.2%
Fewer inventory and supply costs (n = 160)	31	19.4%	37	23.1%	46	28.8%	46	28.8%
Opportunity to educate other vets and pet owners about in-home euthanasia (n = 162)	16	9.9%	42	25.9%	58	35.8%	46	28.4%
Ability to travel (n = 154)	17	11.0%	64	41.6%	39	25.3%	34	22.1%
Ability to perform small rituals or ceremonies if desired (n = 154)	24	15.6%	55	35.7%	45	29.2%	30	19.5%
Less physical demands (e.g., long hours standing, handling large animals) (n = 162)	32	19.8%	62	38.3%	38	23.5%	30	18.5%
Personal growth from regularly confronting mortality and grief (n = 161)	30	18.6%	64	39.8%	41	25.5%	26	16.1%
Sold your hospital but want to stay in veterinary medicine (n = 162)	150	92.6%	5	3.1%	2	1.2%	5	3.1%

Table 6.5. Participants' reported challenge level of 16 EOL mobile practitioner job factors.

	Not at all/minimally challenging		Moderately challenging		Very challenging	
No health benefits (n = 99)	43	43.4%	32	32.3%	24	24.2%
Hassle of the business side (taxes, record keeping, inventory, etc.) (n = 122)	41	33.6%	60	49.2%	21	17.2%
Unpredictable income (n = 125)	43	34.4%	63	50.4%	19	15.2%
Potential safety risks in unfamiliar locations (n = 144)	70	48.6%	57	39.6%	17	11.8%
Unpredictable schedule (n = 131)	55	42.0%	61	46.6%	15	11.5%
Need to be on-call (n = 101)	47	46.5%	43	42.6%	11	10.9%
Lack of job security (n = 120)	71	59.2%	38	31.7%	11	9.2%
No vacation time (n = 99)	67	67.7%	24	24.2%	8	8.1%
Physical strain from lifting animals and equipment (n = 143)	68	47.6%	64	44.8%	11	7.7%
Need to create contract(s) (n = 93)	69	74.2%	17	18.3%	7	7.5%
Weather-related issues affecting travel (n = 139)	85	61.2%	44	31.7%	10	7.2%
Need to transport animals (n = 138)	82	59.4%	47	34.1%	9	6.5%
Need to hire and manage own technician (n = 51)	32	62.7%	16	31.4%	3	5.9%
Travel time and fuel costs (n = 140)	80	57.1%	52	37.1%	8	5.7%
Cost of liability insurance (n = 130)	96	73.8%	28	21.5%	6	4.6%
Minimal support from colleagues (n = 119)	91	76.5%	23	19.3%	5	4.2%

Table 6.6. Reported frequency of connecting with other EOL veterinarians for support (either in person or virtually) (n = 136).

	N	Percent (%)
Never	29	21.3
A few times a year	25	18.4
Monthly	23	16.9
Weekly	36	26.5
Daily	23	16.9

flexibility and independence afforded by their role as "schedule flexibility, total control over business, no need for employees, guaranteed outcome for clients, grateful clients, no worrying about patients, minimal multitasking." This role also is seen as an avenue for better work-life balance and a facilitator of family time outside of work. Additionally, EOL practitioners reported that their career had an overall positive impact on their children. It was conveyed that it helped their children to understand death and encouraged compassion, empathy, and maturity. A practitioner revealed the numerous positive impacts their work has had on their child:

> I think it has absolutely been positive for my daughter to see me more fulfilled at work, and have more flexibility in my schedule. Specifically speaking of end of life care, I think being able to talk about the difficult times and decisions pets and families go through helped when we were faced with losing our own dog – just that not being the first time we discussed death, euthanasia, grief, etc. gave us a foundation for discussions. She also sees that I allow myself to be emotional and keep some special stories with me, but not let the sadness overwhelm me.

Challenges

Despite the numerous benefits endorsed by EOL practitioners, some expressed challenges in their work. These challenges centered on the physical nature of the role, including bodily care and transportation of large animals, especially dogs. For example, a practitioner described the daily physical and emotional stressors of their role:

> There is certainly a big physical demand unless you have help with moving big patients. Also requires a certain level of agility and ability to get up and down from the ground as most patients are on the floor or their beds. Other challenges might be the various ways people grieve, you have to be good at reading a room. It truly goes beyond just normal good bedside manner. It's knowing what to say, when to say it and how. There is often a lot of patience that is involved with this job.

Many EOL practitioners reported working alone in their role, and desiring companionship with colleagues, the ability to problem solve with peers, and hands on assistance from support staff. Notably, when families experienced distressing grief responses, participants expressed the need for someone who could focus on the family's emotional needs while they cared for the animal. For example, a practitioner described their desire to have help with family dynamics: "They are there entirely as a bodyguard while I am focusing on the animal. I have never had a client be physically dangerous, but grief has made some clients say things that made me very uncomfortable."

Relatedly, participants reported experiencing an emotional toll from these difficult situations. Participants portrayed days which left them feeling "sad," "emotionally drained," or carrying the weight of "emotional wear and tear." Though most practitioners viewed the home environment as a positive aspect of the job, some noted concerns about the client's home being in an unfamiliar location, or feeling "unsafe" due to an "unpredictable" situation. A couple of practitioners mentioned the challenge in using their personal vehicle to transport deceased animals. Regarding this, a participant shared that "The negative, if any, is the regular smell of urine and feces in the vehicle we use for everyday life too."

Though many participants noted that they appreciate the independence of EOL work, being their own boss came with several temporal, travel, and logistical difficulties. This sense of adminstrative overwhelm was described by one practitioner as "Always kind of working as I am my own receptionist." While another participant summed up the stress of being a solo practioner as being a combination of the "inability of family members to agree, complex cases without colleague input, traffic and behind the scenes business management." There were concerns among participants about competition from larger corporations, difficulty in determining pricing, paying staff, and devising marketing strategies. Some also reported a lack of consistency with appointments, varying workload, scheduling dynamics, and inconsistent income. They described stress in balancing clients' urgent needs for euthanasia and not always being able to shift their schedule to be available. They lamented about "The unpredictability of when clients/patients will need me and the guilt of not being available all the time." Additionally, travel conditions, traffic, long distances, and weather presented barriers when getting to and from appointments. Finally, several participants reported financial concerns about retirement since they did not own physical property and would not have a space to sell upon retirement.

Discussion

This study aimed to explore the experiences, job fulfillment, and burnout levels of EOL mobile practitioners. The results of this study found that mobile EOL practitioners reported higher job fulfillment and lower burnout than veterinarians in traditional brick-and-mortar settings. Key factors motivating veterinarians to pursue EOL mobile practice include the ability to make a positive impact on pets and families, provide personalized care, and enjoy better work environments. Challenges identified in the study were primarily related to business aspects (e.g., lack of health benefits, unpredictable income, and scheduling) rather than an emotional toll.

A growing number of veterinarians are choosing to focus on EOL care (Bishop *et al.*, 2008; Kiselow, 2019; Paz *et al.*, 2024), including EOL mobile practice. While several studies have found that involvement with euthanasia can have a negative psychological impact and increase the likelihood of depression and suicidal behaviors (Owens *et al.*, 1981; Rollin, 1986; Fogle and Abrahamson, 1990; Arluke, 1994; Bartram and Baldwin, 2008, 2010; Rollin, 2011), other studies suggest the relationship between euthanasia and psychological distress is more nuanced (Tran *et al.*, 2014; Deacon and Brough, 2017; Crane *et al.*, 2023). Despite the growing number of EOL veterinarians, including mobile EOL practitioners, little research has been done to better understand this population and no studies are known to have assessed their job fulfillment and burnout.

A unique aspect of the veterinary profession that distinguishes it from other health professions is the constant exposure to euthanasia and grief of bereaved pet owners (Fernandez-Mehler *et al.*, 2013; Witte *et al.*, 2019). Euthanasia is a common means of death for companion animals; an important procedure that is critical not only for animal welfare (AVMA, 2020) but also the emotional well-being of the owner and owner-veterinarian relationship (Lagoni, 2011; Pierce, 2014). Yet, euthanasia is a frequently reported stressor in the veterinary profession, seen as placing substantial emotional demand on veterinary professionals (Bartram and Baldwin, 2008, 2010; Fink-Miller and Nestler, 2018; Marchitelli, 2019; Stetina and Krouzecky, 2022). Furthermore, some studies have linked it to psychological distress, higher work stress, and lower job satisfaction (Dickinson *et al.*, 2011; Morris, 2012; Fernandez-Mehler *et al.*, 2013; Scotney *et al.*, 2015).

A better understanding of the role euthanasia plays in veterinarians' well-being is critical given that veterinary practitioners are reported to be at higher risk of suicide, burnout, and depression when compared to other occupational groups (Fritschi *et al.*, 2009; Platt *et al.*, 2010; Hatch *et al.*, 2011; Witte *et al.*, 2019). It has been suggested that there are several ways that euthanasia may contribute to poor mental health, depression, and burnout (Tran *et al.*, 2014). Even in circumstances in which the veterinarian and client agree that euthanasia is appropriate, there are often intense emotional demands placed on the veterinarian by the grieving client (Adams *et al.*, 2000; Morris, 2012; Spitznagel *et al.*, 2022b). Veterinarians are often responsible for providing emotional support and comfort to pet owners (Morris, 2012; Spitznagel *et al.*, 2022a); in fact, many owners consider their veterinarian an important source of support in their grieving process (Fernandez-Mehler *et al.*, 2013; Dow *et al.*, 2019; Kogan and Cooney, 2023). This is despite the fact that only 55% of veterinarians report feeling very comfortable emotionally supporting clients with euthanasia and only 3% report feeling their veterinary school prepared them adequately for the communication aspects of euthanasia (Kogan and Cooney, 2023).

Conversely, other research suggests the negative impact of euthanasia for veterinarians and veterinary nurses is typically quite small (Tran *et al.*, 2014; Deacon and Brough, 2017; Quain, 2021; Kogan *et al.*, 2025). Results of our study, involving a population whose primary job is to provide euthanasia, would appear to support the premise that euthanasia, per se, does not negatively affect veterinarians' well-being (Tran *et al.*, 2014; Crane *et al.*, 2023). Instead, our results suggest that the relationship between euthanasia and poor mental health is nuanced and likely impacted by both professional competencies and the details of the euthanasia experience.

Most participants in our study reported previously working in private practice before transitioning their career into exclusively EOL care. In comparison to brick-and-mortar clinical practice, mobile positions are typically entrepreneurial positions with relatively low startup costs that offer the ability to provide personalized care to clients, set one's own schedule, and be one's own boss. The fact that 74% of participants reported being the owner or part-owner of their business suggests that many have the ability to control their workload and modify their work environment, elements identified as important for mental health and job satisfaction (Hilton *et al.*, 2023). These factors can improve work-life balance which has been found to positively impact well-being and retention in the field (Bell *et al.*, 2019; O'Connor, 2019; Barnette, 2020; Hagen *et al.*, 2020; VitusVet, 2020). Mobile practices also benefit pet owners by removing stressors associated with patient transport for a hospital visit and typically offering flexible hours to better accommodate owners' schedules (Drake, 2016; Koch, 2021).

In a recent study (Kogan and Rishniw, 2024), the most common reasons cited by mobile veterinarians for leaving their previous job (most often one in private practice) included hospital factors (e.g., administration, culture, leadership) personal empowerment factors (e.g., feeling their voice was heard, ability to practice the way they think most appropriate for each case), and schedule-related factors (e.g., ability to create a flexible personalized schedule, ability to leave work at scheduled time, and number of hours worked per week). Relatedly, in that same study the most common reasons given by mobile practitioners for choosing mobile work included wanting to be one's own boss, schedule flexibility, and the desire to escape an unhealthy work environment (Kogan and Rishniw, 2024). Similar sentiments have been expressed by veterinarians transitioning from private practice to laboratory work as well as studies exploring retention and recruitment challenges (Hatch *et al.*, 2011; Batchelor and McKeegan, 2012b; Kersebohm *et al.*, 2017; Arbe Montoya *et al.*, 2021; Anderson and Hobson-West, 2022; Li *et al.*, 2024).

Our study found that the most important factors in deciding to become an EOL mobile practitioner included having a positive impact on pets and families, the ability to provide personalized care to families and patients, and a better work environment. These sentiments can also be seen in responses to the open-ended question asking participants about the best part of being a mobile EOL practitioner. Frequent sentiments included providing the best possible experience for pets and their families and the ability to create a peaceful death in a home environment that allowed for grieving in private, similar to factors reported by Springer *et al.* (2024).

When asked about challenges encountered as a mobile EOL practitioner, only a minority of participants reported feeling very challenged by *any* job-related factors. For those experiencing challenges, the most commonly reported included a lack of health benefits, business-related tasks, unpredictable income, and an unpredictable schedule. Each of the remaining possible challenges were rated as very challenging by less than 12% of the participants. In a previous study exploring mobile practitioners, the work factors seen as bothersome included a lack of support from colleagues (cited by 61%) and a lack of job security (55%) (Kogan and Rishniw, 2024). However, we found that only 9% of respondents experienced lack of job security as very challenging while 59% reported it was not at all/minimally challenging. It should be noted, however, that this may have been influenced by the large number (53%) who reported having another job. We also found that only 4% of participants reported feeling a lack of support from colleagues was very challenging with 77% finding it not at all/minimally challenging. This is despite the fact that 40% of respondents reported they connect with other EOL veterinarians only a few times a year or less. Additionally, 74% of respondents noted feeling they have adequate emotional support, suggesting that a lack of support is not a significant challenge or detriment to most veterinarians pursuing this line of work. These findings suggest that many EOL mobile veterinarians do not appear to need frequent connection with other EOL practitioners, possibly because they are obtaining collegial support from other types of veterinary professionals. Responses to the open-ended question pertaining to the challenges associated with EOL mobile work found that practitioners reported strains from the physicality of the job, transporting large animals, inconsistent schedule and income. A small number referenced a lack of support from colleagues due to the isolation in the role and challenges with corporate competition and family grief dynamics.

In addition to the reasons for choosing EOL mobile work and its potential challenges, this study examined participants' job fulfillment and burnout. We found that the majority (70%) of respondents reported feeling fulfilled, and only

15% reported feeling burned out. In contrast, one recent study of veterinarians found that only 30% of the total sample scored above the cutoff for Professional Fulfillment (associates = 20%; owners = 34%) and 57% reported feeling burned out (associates = 63%; owners = 49%) (Kogan and Rishniw, 2023b). A study involving veterinary technicians found that 62% of respondents fell above the cutoff for burnout, and only 21% above the cutoff for fulfillment (Kogan *et al.*, 2025). These levels of fulfillment and burnout for EOL practitioners could be partly due to that fact that EOL mobile work appears to offer a satisfying work environment and job flexibility, both aspects found to predict job satisfaction (Kersebohm *et al.*, 2017; Li *et al.*, 2024).

These fulfillment and burnout scores counter the premise that involvement with euthanasia, per se, is associated with poorer mental health and burnout and support previous research suggesting the relationship and that when done under the right conditions, euthanasia can be a positive factor (Tran *et al.*, 2014; Crane *et al.*, 2023). Given that there appears to be a trend toward worse psychological health in more recent veterinary graduates (Fritschi *et al.*, 2009), and many veterinarians suffer from burnout (Hatch *et al.*, 2011; Mastenbroek *et al.*, 2014; Rhodes *et al.*, 2022; Steffey *et al.*, 2023; Varela and Correia, 2023), these results suggest that EOL veterinary care may be a specialty area that offers some professionals a viable career alternative to general practice.

The successful delivery of in-home euthanasia services requires EOL practitioners to master a specific set of client-centered approaches that differ significantly from traditional veterinary practice. Those who focus on EOL care understand that it is critical to conduct euthanasia in ways that best meet the needs of the patient and client. In one recent study, pet owners identified the most important elements of an at-home euthanasia in determining a good death experience as a veterinarian who comes adequately prepared, is friendly, provides a relaxed atmosphere, is willing to gather where the pet prefers, and provides private time before and after the euthanasia (Cooney and Kogan, 2022). These desires have been echoed in previous studies that find owners want to be allowed to witness the death of their pet (Dickinson *et al.*, 2011; Dickinson and Hoffmann, 2017; Adrian and Stitt, 2019; Quain *et al.*, 2022) and want reassurance that they are making the right choice (Adams *et al.*, 1999; Matte *et al.*, 2020). Most veterinarians also prefer having owners present during euthanasia, perhaps because they feel it reduces patient anxiety, increases patient comfort, and offers the opportunity to better understand the relationship between pet and owner (Kogan and Cooney, 2023). This personalized approach to euthanasia delivery aligns with the reported professional fulfillment of mobile EOL veterinarians, who value the ability to provide the type of EOL care that pet owners consistently identify as essential to their grief process.

The importance of communication surrounding EOL care cannot be overstated (Hamood *et al.*, 2014). Managing clients' emotions, validating clients' grief, and providing support, empathy, and reassurance are essential skills for EOL practitioners (Morris, 2012). Yet, most veterinarians do not receive adequate formal training in grief and bereavement management (Littlewood *et al.*, 2018, 2021; Gates *et al.*, 2023), and many veterinarians acknowledge that they experience difficulty communicating with grieving clients, a challenge that has been shown to correlate with higher levels of compassion fatigue and psychological distress (Dow *et al.*, 2019). Instead of training in veterinary school, the majority of veterinarians report that their skills for dealing with grieving clients are self-taught or received outside of their veterinary curriculum (Pilgram, 2010; Dickinson *et al.*, 2011; Morris, 2012; Dow *et al.*, 2019; Littlewood *et al.*, 2021; Gates *et al.*, 2023). One study, for example, found that 70% of veterinarians feel dissatisfied with the EOL training they received in veterinary school, with 42% reporting they received their EOL care training from The International Association of Animal Hospice and Palliative Care (IAAHPC) (Dickinson and Hoffmann, 2019). This lack of formal grief management training in veterinary education can be a barrier for some wishing to become EOL mobile practitioners, who routinely navigate intense emotional interactions with clients.

Equally important to the emotional and communication components of euthanasia are the technical aspects. One recent study found that only 4% of veterinarians report feeling their veterinary school training prepared them very well for the technical aspects of euthanasia (Kogan and Cooney, 2023). While more veterinarians report feeling very comfortable with the medical aspects of euthanasia compared to the emotional aspects (74% versus 55%), this still leaves approximately 25% of veterinarians who do not feel very comfortable with the procedure (Littlewood *et al.*, 2018; Kogan and Cooney, 2023). Yet, a reduction in adverse events could reduce potential stressors for both pet owners and veterinarians during the euthanasia process (Marchitelli, 2019; Kogan and Cooney, 2023). The technical proficiency in performing euthanasia procedures represents a crucial intersection between EOL mobile practice and the overall quality of EOL care. Creating a 'good death' experience necessitates minimizing the risk of adverse events (Cooney and Kogan, 2022). Despite the high percentage of veterinarians reporting comfort with medical aspects of euthanasia, adverse events do occur, and may negativly impact both practitioner confidence and client perceptions of the process. One pilot study on canine euthanasia found that 52% of investigated euthanasias included at least one adverse event, with 31% experiencing an increase in respiratory rate during euthanasia solution administration. Although changes in respiratory rate do not necessarily indicate patient discomfort or distress, rapid changes in respiratory rate may be perceived by pet owners as distressing (Marchitelli, 2019; Cooney and Kogan, 2022). When veterinarians were asked to rank a list of physiologic conditions and anatomical traits in order of euthanasia-related concerns, respiratory distress was ranked the highest (Kogan and Cooney, 2023). This technical dimension of euthanasia services is particularly relevant to understanding the professional experiences of EOL mobile practitioners, who must independently manage these procedures in varied home environments without the support infrastructure available in traditional clinical settings.

In addition to not being physically present during their pets' final moments, other elements reported by pet owners as negatively impacting the euthanasia experience included their pet appearing to be in pain, scared, or stressed in their final moments, thrashing or making sudden movements, or vocalizing when the euthanasia solution is injected (Cooney and Kogan, 2022). Trained, experienced veterinary professionals are essential in minimizing these types of adverse events, especially EOL mobile practitioners who often work alone and do not have immediate back up resources if something goes wrong. It is perhaps not surprising, therefore, that many comments from participants strongly recommended that this work should be performed by veterinarians. The chances of dysthanasia (i.e. bad death) (Kogan and Cooney, 2023) may be lessened by ensuring that only adequately trained and experienced veterinary professionals conduct the euthanasia procedure.

Conclusion

There are several limitations to our study, including a relatively small sample size. Given that the number of EOL mobile practitioners is unknown, it is not possible to determine what percentage of this population responded. As a result, caution is suggested when generalizing our findings to other EOL mobile veterinarians. Nevertheless, our survey, to our knowledge, is the first to survey mobile EOL practitioners. Another limitation is response bias. It is possible that individuals who feel strongly about EOL mobile work may have been more likely to respond to the survey (Springer *et al.*, 2024). Also, the majority of participants were likely regular users of social media for professional networking, which could have influenced their feelings of adequate support. It should also be noted that many participants held another job which may have impacted their levels of fulfillment and burnout. Additionally, it should be noted that this survey was released shortly after the Veterinary Professional Associate (VPA) Proposition 129 was voted into law within the state of Colorado (Colorado Government, 2024). This amendment creates the state-regulated profession of veterinary professional associate in the field of veterinary care. From the responses to the final open-ended question asking for any additional comments, it would appear that many respondents had concerns about the potential impact of VPAs on EOL care. It is possible that these concerns influenced their survey responses in unknown ways. Further research investigating potential barriers for veterinary professionals seeking EOL work and resources they need to be successful would be of value. In addition, exploring potential differences in the frequency of different types of euthanasia, including financial or convenience, could help elucidate differences in overall job fulfillment and burnout between mobile EOL practitioners and general practitioners in brick-and mortar settings.

In conclusion, this study found that mobile EOL practitioners have higher job fulfillment and lower burnout when compared to other veterinary professionals. This is despite the fact that their job focuses on euthanasia, suggesting that engagement in euthanasia, per se, does not necessarily lead to a negative impact on mental health. In addition, the primary reasons why veterinarians are drawn to EOL work are the ability to make a positive impact on pets and families, provide personalized care to families and patients, and enjoy a better work environment. Within this unique entrepreneurial pathway, it would appear that most veterinarians feel able to accomplish these goals, and in the process, create a positive death and dying experience for both their patients and clients. While not for everyone, mobile EOL practice appears to be a viable career path for some veterinarians.

Conflicts of Interest

The authors declare no conflicts of interest.

Funding

This research received no external funding.

Data Availability

Data are available upon request.

Author Contributions

All authors contributed to the conceptualization and writing of this manuscript. All authors have read and agreed to the published version of the manuscript.

Informed Consent Statement

Informed consent was obtained from all subjects involved in the study.

Supplementary Content

Refer to supplementary material on the CABI Digital Library: https://www.cabidigitallibrary.org/doi/book/10.1079/9781836994046.0000. See p.vii for details.

References

Adams, C.L., Bonnett, B.N. and Meek, A.H. (1999) Owner response to companion animal death: Development of a theory and practical implications. *The Canadian Veterinary Journal* 40(1), 33–39.

Adams, C.L., Bonnett, B.N. and Meek, A.H. (2000) Predictors of owner response to companion animal death in 177 clients from 14 practices in Ontario. *Journal of the American Veterinary Medical Association* 217(9), 1303–1309. DOI: 10.2460/javma.2000.217.1303.

Adrian, J.A.L. and Stitt, A. (2019) There for you: Attending pet euthanasia and whether this relates to complicated grief and post-traumatic stress disorder. *Anthrozoös* 32(5), 701–713. DOI: 10.1080/08927936.2019.1645515.

Anderson, A. and Hobson-West, P. (2022) "Refugees from practice"? Exploring why some vets move from the clinic to the laboratory. *Veterinary Record* 190(1), e773. DOI: 10.1002/vetr.773.

Arbe Montoya, A.I., Hazel, S.J., Matthew, S.M. and McArthur, M.L. (2021) Why do veterinarians leave clinical practice? A qualitative study using thematic analysis. *Veterinary Record* 188(1), e2. DOI: 10.1002/vetr.2.

Archer, J. (1997) Why do people love their pets? *Evolution and Human Behavior* 18(4), 237–259. DOI: 10.1016/S0162-3095(99)80001-4.

Arluke, A. (1994) Managing emotions in an animal shelter. In: *Animals and Human Society*. Routledge.

AVMA (2020) AVMA Guidelines for the Euthanasia of Animals. AVMA. Available at: https://www.avma.org/resources-tools/avma-policies/avma-guidelines-euthanasia-animals (accessed 15 January 2025).

Barnette, C. (2020) Mobile Veterinary Care: What You Need to Know Before Starting Your Own Practice on Wheels. Dispomed. Available at: https://www.dispomed.com/mobile-veterinary-care-what-you-need-to-know-before-starting-your-own-practice-on-wheels/ (accessed 15 January 2025).

Bartram, D.J. and Baldwin, D.S. (2008) Veterinary surgeons and suicide: Influences, opportunities and research directions. *Veterinary Record* 162(2), 36–40. DOI: 10.1136/vr.162.2.36.

Bartram, D.J. and Baldwin, D.S. (2010) Veterinary surgeons and suicide: A structured review of possible influences on increased risk. *The Veterinary Record* 166(13), 388–397. DOI: 10.1136/vr.b4794.

Batchelor, C.E.M. and McKeegan, D.E.F. (2012a) Survey of the frequency and perceived stressfulness of ethical dilemmas encountered in UK veterinary practice. *Veterinary Record* 170(1), 19–19. DOI: 10.1136/vr.100262.

Batchelor, C.E.M. and McKeegan, D.E.F. (2012b) Survey of the frequency and perceived stressfulness of ethical dilemmas encountered in UK veterinary practice. *The Veterinary Record* 170(1), 19. DOI: 10.1136/vr.100262.

Behler, A.M.C. (2020) "We lost a member of the family": Predictors of the grief experience surrounding the loss of a pet. *Human Animal Interaction Bulletin* 8(3), 18.

Bell, M., Cake, M. and Mansfield, C. (2019) Success in career transitions in veterinary practice: Perspectives of employers and their employees. *Veterinary Record* 185(8), 232–232. DOI: 10.1136/vr.105133.

Bishop, G.A., Long, C.C., Carlsten, K.S., Kennedy, K.C. and Shaw, J.R. (2008) The Colorado State University pet hospice program: End-of-life care for pets and their families. *Journal of Veterinary Medical Education* 35(4), 525–531. DOI: 10.3138/jvme.35.4.525.

Carmack, B.J. (1985) The effects on family members and functioning after the death of a pet. *Marriage & Family Review* 8(3–4), 149–161. DOI: 10.1300/J002v08n03_11.

Chur-Hansen, A. (2010) Grief and bereavement issues and the loss of a companion animal: People living with a companion animal, owners of livestock, and animal support workers. *Clinical Psychologist* 14(1), 14–21. DOI: 10.1080/13284201003662800.

Colorado Government (2024) Proposition 129: Establishing Veterinary Professional Associates. Available at: https://leg.colorado.gov/sites/default/files/images/2023-2024_145vbb.pdf (accessed 15 January 2025).

Cooney, K. (2020) Common and alternative routes of euthanasia solution administration. *Veterinary Clinics of North America: Small Animal Practice* 50. DOI: 10.1016/j.cvsm.2019.12.005.

Cooney, K. and Kogan, L. (2022) How pet owners define a "good death. *Dvm360* (8), 12–12.

Cooney, K. and Kipperman, B. (2023) Ethical and practical considerations associated with companion animal euthanasia. *Animals* 13(3). DOI: 10.3390/ani13030430.

Cowling, D.M., Isenstein, S.G.E. and Schneider, M.S. (2020) When the bond breaks: Variables associated with grief following companion animal loss. *Anthrozoös* 33(6), 693–708. DOI: 10.1080/08927936.2020.1824651.

Crane, M.F., Kho, M., Thomas, E.F., Decety, J., Molenberghs, P. *et al.* (2023) The moderating role of different forms of empathy on the association between performing animal euthanasia and career sustainability. *Journal of Applied Social Psychology* 53(11), 1088–1107. DOI: 10.1111/jasp.13000.

Deacon, R.E. and Brough, P. (2017) Veterinary nurses' psychological well-being: The impact of patient suffering and death. *Australian Journal of Psychology* 69(2), 77–85. DOI: 10.1111/ajpy.12119.

DeGroot, A. (1984) Preparing the veterinarian for dealing with the emotions of pet loss. In: Anderson, R.K., Hart, B.L. and Hart, L.A. (eds) *Pet Connection: Its Influence on Our Health and Quality of Life*, Vol. Available at. University of Minnesota. Available at: https://scholar.google.com/scholar_lookup?title=Preparing+the+veterinarian+for+dealing+with+the+emotions+of+pet+loss&author=DeGroot%2C+A.&publication_year=1984

Dickinson, G.E. and Hoffmann, H.C. (2017) Saying goodbye to family: Caretakers' experiences with euthanasia and honoring the legacy of companion animals. *Society & Animals* 25(5), 490–507. DOI: 10.1163/15685306-12341456.

Dickinson, G.E. and Hoffmann, H.C. (2019) Animal hospice and palliative care: Veterinarians' experiences and preferred practices. *Journal of Veterinary Behavior* 32, 57–61. DOI: 10.1016/j.jveb.2019.04.008.

Dickinson, G.E., Roof, P.D. and Roof, K.W. (2011) A survey of veterinarians in the US: euthanasia and other end-of-life issues. *Anthrozoös* 24(2), 167–174. DOI: 10.2752/175303711X12998632257666.

Dow, M.Q., Chur-Hansen, A., Hamood, W. and Edwards, S. (2019) Impact of dealing with bereaved clients on the psychological wellbeing of veterinarians. *Australian Veterinary Journal* 97(10), 382–389. DOI: 10.1111/avj.12842.

Drake, S. (2016) Mobile Vet Clinics: What Are They? Available at: https://www.petmd.com/dog/care/mobile-vet-clinics-what-are-they (accessed 15 January 2025).

Fernandez-Mehler, P., Gloor, P., Sager, E., Lewis, F.I. and Glaus, T.M. (2013) Veterinarians' role for pet owners facing pet loss. *Veterinary Record* 172(21), 555–555. DOI: 10.1136/vr.101154.

Field, N.P., Orsini, L., Gavish, R. and Packman, W. (2009) Role of attachment in response to pet loss. *Death Studies* 33(4), 334–355. DOI: 10.1080/07481180802705783.

Fink-Miller, E.L. and Nestler, L.M. (2018) Suicide in physicians and veterinarians: Risk factors and theories. *Current Opinion in Psychology* 22, 23–26. DOI: 10.1016/j.copsyc.2017.07.019.

Fogle, B. and Abrahamson, D. (1990) Pet loss: A survey of the attitudes and feelings of practicing veterinarians. *Anthrozoös* 3(3), 143–150. DOI: 10.2752/089279390787057568.

Fritschi, L., Morrison, D., Shirangi, A. and Day, L. (2009) Psychological well-being of Australian veterinarians. *Australian Veterinary Journal* 87(3), 76–81. DOI: 10.1111/j.1751-0813.2009.00391.x.

Gates, M., Hinds, H. and Dale, A. (2017) Preliminary description of aging cats and dogs presented to a New Zealand first-opinion veterinary clinic at end-of-life. *New Zealand Veterinary Journal* 65(6), 313–317. DOI: 10.1080/00480169.2017.1360161.

Gates, M., Kells, N., Kongara, K. and Littlewood, K. (2023) Euthanasia of dogs and cats by veterinarians in New Zealand: Protocols, procedures and experiences. *New Zealand Veterinary Journal* 71(4), 1–14. DOI: 10.1080/00480169.2023.2194687.

Guest, G., MacQueen, K.M. and Namey, E.E. (2011) *Applied Thematic Analysis*. SAGE Publications.

Hagen, J.R., Weller, R., Mair, T.S. and Kinnison, T. (2020) Investigation of factors affecting recruitment and retention in the UK veterinary profession. *Veterinary Record* 187(9), 354–354. DOI: 10.1136/vr.106044.

Hamood, W.J., Chur-Hansen, A. and McArthur, M.L. (2014) A qualitative study to explore communication skills in veterinary medical education. *International Journal of Medical Education* 5, 193–198. DOI: 10.5116/ijme.542a.975d.

Hatch, P.H., Winefield, H.R., Christie, B.A. and Lievaart, J.J. (2011) Workplace stress, mental health, and burnout of veterinarians in Australia. *Australian Veterinary Journal* 89(11), 460–468. DOI: 10.1111/j.1751-0813.2011.00833.x.

Hernandez, E., Fawcett, A., Brouwer, E., Rau, J. and Turner, P.V. (2018) Speaking up: Veterinary ethical responsibilities and animal welfare issues in everyday practice. *Animals* 8(1). DOI: 10.3390/ani8010015.

Hilton, K.R., Burke, K.J. and Signal, T. (2023) Mental health in the veterinary profession: An individual or organisational focus? *Australian Veterinary Journal* 101(1–2), 41–48. DOI: 10.1111/avj.13215.

Kersebohm, J.C., Lorenz, T., Becher, A. and Doherr, M.G. (2017) Factors related to work and life satisfaction of veterinary practitioners in Germany. *Veterinary Record Open* 4(1), e000229. DOI: 10.1136/vetreco-2017-000229.

Kipperman, B., Morris, P. and Rollin, B. (2018) Ethical dilemmas encountered by small animal veterinarians: Characterisation, responses, consequences and beliefs regarding euthanasia. *Veterinary Record* 182(19), 548–548. DOI: 10.1136/vr.104619.

Kiselow, M. (2019) Private practice oncology: Viewpoint on end-of-life decision-making. *The Veterinary Clinics of North America Small Animal Practice* 49(3), 519–527. DOI: 10.1016/j.cvsm.2019.01.010.

Koch, D. (2021) Mobile Veterinary Services: The Future of Veterinary Medicine. PetCoach. Available at: https://www.petcoach.co/article/

Kogan, L.R. and Cooney, K.A. (2023) Defining a "Good Death": Exploring veterinarians' perceptions of companion animal euthanasia. *Animals: An Open Access Journal from MDPI* 13(13), 2117. DOI: 10.3390/ani13132117.

Kogan, L.R. and Rishniw, M. (2023a) Relief and mobile veterinary careers may offer a path towards improved quality of life. *Journal of the American Veterinary Medical Association* 1(aop), 1–7. DOI: 10.2460/javma.23.07.0422.

Kogan, L.R. and Rishniw, M. (2023b) Veterinarians and moral distress. *Journal of the American Veterinary Medical Association* 261(5), 1–7. DOI: 10.2460/javma.22.12.0598.

Kogan, L.R. and Rishniw, M. (2024) Relief and mobile veterinary careers may offer a path towards improved quality of life. *Journal of the American Veterinary Medical Association* 262(2), 209–215. DOI: 10.2460/javma.23.07.0422.

Kogan, L.R., Wallace, J.E., Schoenfeld-Tacher, R., Hellyer, P.W. and Richards, M. (2020) Veterinary technicians and occupational burnout. *Frontiers in Veterinary Science* 7, 328. Available at: https://www.frontiersin.org/articles/10.3389/fvets.2020.00328

Kogan, L.R., Packman, W., Bussolari, C., Currin-McCulloch, J. and Erdman, P. (2022a) Pet death and owners' memorialization choices. *Illness, Crisis & Loss* 10541373221143046. DOI: 10.1177/10541373221143046.

Kogan, L.R., Carter, L. and Foltz, K. (2025) Perceptions and experiences of veterinary assistants, veterinary technicians/nurses, and veterinary technician specialists. *Journal of Veterinary Emergency and Critical Care* 35(5), 521–532. DOI: 10.1111/vec.70043.

Kogan, L.R., Wallace, J.E., Hellyer, P.W. and Carr, E.C.J. (2022b) Canine caregivers: Paradoxical challenges and rewards. *Animals* 12(9). DOI: 10.3390/ani12091074.

Kollias, N.S., Strand, E.B., Kogan, L.R., Houlihan, K.E., Thompson-Iritani, S. *et al.* (2023) Psychological implications of humane endings on the veterinary profession. *Journal of the American Veterinary Medical Association* 261(2), 185–192. DOI: 10.2460/javma.22.06.0234.

Lagoni, L. (2011) Family-present euthansia: Protocols for planning and preparing clients for the death of a pet. In: Blazina, C., Boyraz, G. and Shen-Miller, D. (eds) *Psychology of the Human–Animal Bond: A Resource for Clinicians and Researchers*. Springer Science + Business Media, Cham, Switzerland, pp. 181–202. DOI: 10.1007/978-1-4419-9761-6.

Leary, S., Pharmaceuticals, F., Underwood, W., Anthony, R., Cartner, S. *et al.* (2020) *AVMA Guidelines for the Euthanasia of Animals: 2020 Edition*.

Li, K., Mooney, E., McArthur, M., Hall, E. and Quain, A. (2024) A comparison between veterinary small animal general practitioners and emergency practitioners in Australia. Part 2: Client-related, work-related, and personal burnout. *Frontiers in Veterinary Science* 11. DOI: 10.3389/fvets.2024.1355511.

Littlewood, K.E., Beausoleil, N.J., Stafford, K.J., Stephens, C., Collins, T. *et al.* (2018) Exploring how end-of-life management is taught to australasian veterinary students. part 1: Technical euthanasia. *The Veterinary Record* 183(22), 691. DOI: 10.1136/vr.104775.

Littlewood, K.E., Beausoleil, N.J., Stafford, K.J., Stephens, C., Collins, T. *et al.* (2021) How decision-making about euthanasia for animals is taught to Australasian veterinary students. *Australian Veterinary Journal* 99(8), 334–343. DOI: 10.1111/avj.13077.

Marchitelli, B. (2019) An objective exploration of euthanasia and adverse events. *The Veterinary Clinics of North America. Small Animal Practice* 49(3), 553–563. DOI: 10.1016/j.cvsm.2019.01.016.

Mastenbroek, N.J.J.M., Jaarsma, A.D.C., Demerouti, E., Muijtjens, A.M.M., Scherpbier, A.J.J.A. *et al.* (2014) Burnout and engagement, and its predictors in young veterinary professionals: The influence of gender. *Veterinary Record* 174(6), 144–144. DOI: 10.1136/vr.101762.

Matte, A.R., Khosa, D.K., Coe, J.B., Meehan, M. and Niel, L. (2020) Exploring veterinarians' use of practices aimed at understanding and providing emotional support to clients during companion animal euthanasia in Ontario, Canada. *Veterinary Record* 187(9), e74–e74. DOI: 10.1136/vr.105659.

Messam, L.L., Mc, V. and Hart, L.A. (2019) Chapter 15—Persons experiencing prolonged grief after the loss of a pet. In: Kogan, L. and Blazina, C. (eds) *Clinician's Guide to Treating Companion Animal Issues*. Academic Press, Cambridge, MA, pp. 267–280. DOI: 10.1016/B978-0-12-812962-3.00015-0.

Morris, P. (2012) Managing pet owners' guilt and grief in veterinary euthanasia encounters. *Journal of Contemporary Ethnography* 41, 337–365.

Nett, R.J., Witte, T.K., Holzbauer, S.M., Elchos, B.L., Campagnolo, E.R. *et al.* (2015) Risk factors for suicide, attitudes toward mental illness, and practice-related stressors among US veterinarians. *Journal of the American Veterinary Medical Association* 247(8), 945–955.

O'Connor, E. (2019) Sources of work stress in veterinary practice in the UK. *Veterinary Record* 184(19), 588–588. DOI: 10.1136/vr.104662.

Owczarczak-Garstecka, S.C., Holland, K.E., Anderson, K.L., Casey, R.A., Christley, R.M. *et al.* (2022) Accessing veterinary healthcare during the COVID-19 pandemic: A mixed-methods analysis of UK and Republic of Ireland dog owners' concerns and experiences. *Veterinary Record* 191(3), e1681. DOI: 10.1002/vetr.1681.

Owens, C., Davis, R. and Smith, B. (1981) The psychology of euthanizing animals: the emotional components. *Human and Animal Bonding Collection*. Available at: https://www.wellbeingintlstudiesrepository.org/acwp_habr/4

Paz, B.F., Ferreira, M.G.P.A., Martins, K.R., Uccella, L. and Nardi, A. (2024) Practical principles of palliative care in veterinary oncology: Alleviating the suffering of the animal, owner, and veterinarian. *Veterinary Medicine International* 5565837. DOI: 10.1155/2024/5565837.

Pegram, C., Gray, C., Packer, R.M.A., Richards, Y., Church, D.B. *et al.* (2021) Proportion and risk factors for death by euthanasia in dogs in the UK. *Scientific Reports* 11(1), 9145. DOI: 10.1038/s41598-021-88342-0.

Pepper, B.M., Chan, H., Ward, M.P. and Quain, A. (2023) Euthanasia of dogs by Australian veterinarians: A survey of current practices. *Veterinary Sciences* 10(5). DOI: 10.3390/vetsci10050317.

Pierce, J. (2014) The Last Walk: Reflections on Our Pets at the End of Their Lives. University of Chicago Press. Available at: https://press.uchicago.edu/ucp/books/book/chicago/L/bo11097201.html

Pilgram, M.D. (2010) Communicating social support to grieving clients: The veterinarians' view. *Death Studies* 34(8), 699–714. DOI: 10.1080/07481181003761666.

Platt, B., Hawton, K., Simkin, S. and Mellanby, R.J. (2010) Systematic review of the prevalence of suicide in veterinary surgeons. *Occupational Medicine* 60(6), 436–446. DOI: 10.1093/occmed/kqq044.

Quain, A. (2021) The gift: Ethically indicated euthanasia in companion animal practice. *Veterinary Sciences* 8(8). DOI: 10.3390/vetsci8080141.

Quain, A., Mullan, S. and Ward, M.P. (2022) Low and no-contact euthanasia: Associated ethical challenges experienced by veterinary team members during the early months of the COVID-19 pandemic. *Animals* 12(5). DOI: 10.3390/ani12050560.

Rhodes, R.L., Noguchi, K. and Agler, L.-M.L. (2022) Female veterinarians' experiences with human clients: The link to burnout and depression. *International Journal of Workplace Health Management* 15(5), 572–589. DOI: 10.1108/IJWHM-01-2021-0007.

Robertson, S.A. (2020) Pharmacologic methods: An update on optimal presedation and euthanasia solution administration. *The Veterinary Clinics of North America. Small Animal Practice* 50(3), 525–543. DOI: 10.1016/j.cvsm.2019.12.004.

Rollin, B.E. (1986) Euthanasia and moral stress. *Loss, Grief & Care* 1(1–2), 115–126.

Rollin, B.E. (2011) Euthanasia, moral stress, and chronic illness in veterinary medicine. *Veterinary Clinics of North America: Small Animal Practice* 41(3), 651–659. DOI: 10.1016/j.cvsm.2011.03.005.

Rowan, A. and Kartal, T. (2018) Dog population & dog sheltering trends in the United States of America. *Animals* 8(5). DOI: 10.3390/ani8050068.

Sable, P. (2013) The pet connection: An attachment perspective. *Clinical Social Work Journal* 41(1), 93–99. DOI: 10.1007/s10615-012-0405-2.

Scotney, R.L., McLaughlin, D. and Keates, H.L. (2015) A systematic review of the effects of euthanasia and occupational stress in personnel working with animals in animal shelters, veterinary clinics, and biomedical research facilities. *Journal of the American Veterinary Medical Association* 247(10), 1121–1130.

Shearer, T. (2020) Nonpharmacologic methods to improve the euthanasia experience. *The Veterinary Clinics of North America. Small Animal Practice* 50(3), 627–638. DOI: 10.1016/j.cvsm.2019.12.011.

Spitznagel, M.B., Patrick, K., Gober, M.W., Carlson, M.D., Gardner, M. *et al.* (2022a) Relationships among owner consideration of euthanasia, caregiver burden, and treatment satisfaction in canine osteoarthritis. *The Veterinary Journal* 1997(286), 105868–105868. DOI: 10.1016/j.tvjl.2022.105868.

Spitznagel, M.B., Updegraff, A.S.G., Was, C., Martin, J.T., Sislak, M. *et al.* (2022b) An acceptance and commitment training program reduces burden transfer, stress, and burnout among veterinary healthcare teams. *Journal of the American Veterinary Medical Association* 260(12), 1554–1561. DOI: 10.2460/javma.22.05.0196.

Springer, S., Flammer, S.A. and Dürnberger, C. (2024) "Veterinary medicine is not finished when I have diagnosed an incurable disease, that's when it starts for me" – A qualitative interview study with small animal veterinarians on hospice and palliative care. *Frontiers in Veterinary Science* 11. DOI: 10.3389/fvets.2024.1440404.

Steffey, M.A., Griffon, D.J., Risselada, M., Buote, N.J., Scharf, V.F. *et al.* (2023) A narrative review of the physiology and health effects of burnout associated with veterinarian-pertinent occupational stressors. *Frontiers in Veterinary Science* 10. DOI: 10.3389/fvets.2023.1184525.

Stetina, B.U. and Krouzecky, C. (2022) Reviewing a decade of change for veterinarians: Past, present and gaps in researching stress, coping and mental health risks. *Animals* 12(22). DOI: 10.3390/ani12223199.

Tran, L., Crane, M.F. and Phillips, J.K. (2014) The distinct role of performing euthanasia on depression and suicide in veterinarians. *Journal of Occupational Health Psychology* 19(2), 123–132. DOI: 10.1037/a0035837.

Trockel, M., Boham, B., Lesure, E., Hamidi, M., Welle, D. *et al.* (2018) A brief instrument to assess both burnout and professional fulfillment in physicians: reliability and validity, including correlation with self-reported medical errors, in a sample of resident and practicing physicians. *US National Library of Medicine National Institutes of Health Search Database* 42(1), 11–24.

Varela, M. and Correia, I. (2023) Empathy and burnout in veterinarians and veterinary nurses: Identifying burnout protectors. *Anthrozoös* 36(1), 15–34. DOI: 10.1080/08927936.2022.2074189.

VitusVet (2020) Thinking of Starting a Mobile Vet Clinic? These 4 Benefits Might Surprise You. VitusVet. Available at: https://vitusvet.com/blog/thinking-of-starting-a-mobile-vet-clinic-these-4-benefits-might-surprise-you/ (accessed 15 January 2025).

Volsche, S. (2019) Pet parents and the loss of attachment. In: *Pet Loss, Grief, and Therapeutic Interventions*. Routledge, London.

Witte, T.K., Spitzer, E.G., Edwards, N., Fowler, K.A. and Nett, R.J. (2019) Suicides and deaths of undetermined intent among veterinary professionals from 2003 through 2014. *Journal of the American Veterinary Medical Association* 255(5), 595–608. DOI: 10.2460/javma.255.5.595.

Wu, H., Bains, R.S., Morris, A. and Morales, C. (2021) Affordability, feasibility, and accessibility: Companion animal guardians with (dis)abilities access to veterinary medical and behavioral services during COVID-19. *Animals* 11(8). DOI: 10.3390/ani11082359.

Yeates, J. (2010) Ethical aspects of euthanasia of owned animals. *Practice* 32(2), 70–73. DOI: 10.1136/inp.c516.

7 A Time to Say Goodbye: Empathy and Emotion Regulation Predict Timing of End-of-Life Decisions by Pet Owners

Jennifer Vonk[1]*, Esther Maria Corina Bouma[2] and Arie Dijkstra[2]
[1]Department of Psychology, Oakland University, MI, USA; [2]Department of Social Psychology, Faculty of Behavioral and Social Sciences, University of Groningen, Netherlands

Abstract
Little is known about how pet owners make end-of-life (EoL) decisions regarding their pets. We analyzed data from 1542 pet owners from North America and Europe that had made EoL decisions involving their dogs (n = 546) or cats (n=996). We measured participants' empathy towards animals, emotion regulation, and attitudes toward pets, and asked for demographic information about themselves and the most recent pet that they had euthanized. We asked them to indicate a preference for making a decision too early versus too late, the stage of an illness or injury at which they had made their decision to euthanize, and the amount of guilt they felt for making a decision too early and too late. We hypothesized that individuals with high levels of empathy would prioritize the reduction of their pet's suffering and would therefore make earlier decisions and feel greater guilt for having made decisions too late. This might be especially true for those with low emotion regulation as they might have more difficulty managing their own distress related to the pet's condition. In addition, we recognized that pet owners would also consider their desire to extend the pet's life - particularly when they had strong positive attitudes toward pets. Contrary to our predictions, those with higher reported empathy for animals were more likely to make decisions to euthanize at later stages compared to earlier stages. Cat owners made decisions later compared to dog owners. Higher levels of empathy and lower levels of emotion regulation predicted guilt for both early and late decisions. Further work is needed to explore how various owner characteristics impact EoL decisions. Our study makes a first attempt to understand this complex issue.

Keywords: euthanasia, dog, cat, empathy, emotion regulation, guilt

Introduction

It is widely believed that companion animals bestow many benefits for physical and mental health upon their caregivers (e.g., Kaufman and Kaufman, 2006; O'Haire, 2010; McConnell *et al.*, 2011; Marsa-Sambola *et al.*, 2017; Barker and Gee, 2021; Gee *et al.*, 2021) although results can be mixed (Barroso *et al.*, 2021; Albright *et al.*, 2022). Given the relatively shorter lifespans of pets compared to humans, one of the most difficult aspects of pet ownership can be the need to make end-of-life (EoL) decisions. Although caregivers are fortunate in being able to make EoL decisions to end the suffering of an elderly or diseased pet, which they typically

*Corresponding author: vonk@oakland.edu

cannot do for human companions (Sanders, 1995; Leary *et al.*, 2020), there is no guidebook for the optimal moment to make such decisions. Although researchers have actively explored the topic of grief following euthanasia (e.g., Thomas, 1982; McCutcheon and Fleming, 2002; Lagoni, 2011; Tzivian *et al.*, 2014; Testoni *et al.*, 2017; Adrian and Stitt, 2019; Littlewood *et al.*, 2020), and some studies have explored how veterinarians make euthanasia decisions (e.g., Sanders, 1995; Shaw and Lagoni, 2007), there is very little research regarding what factors influence pet owners' decisions regarding euthanasia. What sparse research does exist typically adopts a qualitative approach to identify environmental factors and attitudes underlying decisions to euthanize (Tzivian *et al.*, 2014; Niessen *et al.*, 2017; Bussolari *et al.*, 2018; Littlewood *et al.*, 2021b; Littlewood *et al.*, 2021a). Previous research has not examined pet owner characteristics specifically regarding how they influence the *timing* of EoL decisions regarding companion animals. This is particularly important because research has shown that the decision to euthanize is the strongest predictor of intense grief following the loss of a companion animal (Davis *et al.*, 2003). Furthermore, pet owners can experience significant guilt and self-blame after making such decisions (Hewson, 2014; Wong *et al.*, 2017).

Qualitative research has revealed a common theme of conflict between owner versus pet concerns when making EoL decisions (Sanders, 1995; Moore, 2011; Schuurman, 2017; Niessen *et al.*, 2017; Littlewood *et al.*, 2021a). Typically, this conflict is expressed in weighing concerns about pet health and suffering alongside concerns about the financial costs and emotional burden of caring for the pet on the owner (e.g., Spitznagel *et al.*, 2017). For example, Littlewood *et al.* (2021b) noted that a sample of 14 cat owners in New Zealand voiced human-centered and animal-centered concerns when interviewed about EoL decisions for their elderly and chronically ill cats. Human-centered concerns focused on the management of euthanasia, including the timing and finding a good veterinarian. Even within pet focused concerns, owners must weigh the suffering of the pet against the desire to extend the pet's life (Sanders, 1995; Tzivian *et al.*, 2014; Schuurman, 2017). Previous studies have not examined individual owner characteristics that might predict timing of euthanasia decisions. Although we recognize that there are many reasons that owners consider the euthanasia of pets other than illness or suffering, we were interested in individual traits that might predict differential weighing of the reduction of suffering and the extension of life as factors predicting the timing of EoL decisions. Therefore, our study focused on euthanasia in the context of degenerative disease or age.

We were particularly interested in how individual differences in traits like empathy and emotion regulation would interact to predict the weighing of the concerns and the preferred timing for EoL decisions. Researchers have acknowledged that emotion management is important both for veterinarians and pet owners during the process of making EoL decisions (Morris, 2012). We hypothesized that relatively higher levels of empathy would lead caregivers to make earlier decisions to euthanize because these individuals would want to reduce the suffering of their animal companions. Indeed, the difficulty in seeing their pet suffering was a primary reason for euthanasia given by Israeli pet owners (Tzivian *et al.*, 2014). The ability to recognize suffering might in itself require empathy. For example, empathy was the best predictor of perception of pain in dogs for Norwegian dog owners (Ellingsen *et al.*, 2010) and pain is one of the most important predictors of welfare (Broom, 2019). However, empathy leads to different outcomes depending on the individual's ability to cope with observing another in distress. Individuals can either direct affective responses to themselves, which results in anxiety and distress, or toward the distressed other, which leads to sympathy (Batson, 1998). We predicted that individuals with high empathy and poor emotion regulation would be inclined to make earlier decisions to reduce their own distress when dealing with an animal in declining health. Individuals high in empathy but also high in emotion regulation might be better able to cope with their own distress and place greater emphasis on extending the animal's life.

Recognizing the complexity of euthanasia decisions, we also considered how attitudes toward pets would potentially moderate these associations between empathy, emotion regulation, and EoL decisions. Ellingsen *et al.* (2010) identified attachment to pets, attitudes toward animals, and empathy for animals as among the five key factors for the human-dog relationship, along with anthropomorphism and belief in animal minds. Empathy is highly associated with attachment to pets (Melson, 1991; Poresky, 1996; Vizek Vidovi´c *et al.*, 1999), which is highly correlated with pet attitude scores (Brown *et al.*, 1996; Ellingsen *et al.*, 2010; Hawkins *et al.*, 2017). Greater attachment to pets is related to better care and welfare (Marsa-Sambola *et al.*, 2016; Muldoon *et al.*, 2016), as well as to feeling upset and wanting to assist an animal in distress (Ellingsen *et al.*, 2010). Positive attitudes toward animals are also associated with more humane treatment, more concern for animal welfare, and less cruelty (Taylor and Signal, 2005). In a Korean sample, positive pet attitudes were associated with several medical outcomes related to the welfare of pet dogs. Some of these outcomes were beneficial to the dogs' welfare, such as veterinarian visits and vaccinations, but some were detrimental, such as the frequency of obesity (Kim *et al.*, 2020). Stronger attachments to pets have been associated with more intense grief (e.g., Gosse and Barnes, 1994; Brown *et al.*, 1996; Field *et al.*, 2009; Schmidt *et al.*, 2018; Park and Jeong, 2022), which led us to predict that attachment could lead to later EoL decisions to stave off anticipatory grief (Shaw and Lagoni, 2007; Brockman *et al.*, 2008; Fernandez-Mehler *et al.*, 2013; Hewson, 2014). We predicted that more positive attitudes towards animals in general might mitigate against the inclination to euthanize earlier in the stage of illness because these traits would be linked to placing a higher value on the pet's life and a greater desire to extend that life. Better understanding the characteristics and factors that influence pet owner's decisions about when to euthanize pets may help facilitate effective communication between veterinary professionals and owners facing such decisions.

There is an absence of research explicitly examining cultural differences in attitudes toward pet euthanasia, although societal attitudes toward pet death are known to influence duration and intensity of grief (Gosse and Barnes, 1994; Planchon and Templer, 1996; Adams *et al.*, 1999). We thought that American and European (primarily Dutch and Flemish) respondents might differ in their decision making because of differing attitudes regarding euthanasia with Dutch and Flemish citizens tending to be stronger proponents of euthanasia, even for humans, compared to American citizens (van Tol *et al.*, 2012; Deak and Saroglou, 2017). Furthermore, Americans and Europeans differ about practices regarding the pets' freedom of movement with American pet owners being more likely to keep their cats exclusively indoors (e.g., Bouma *et al.*, 2021; Foreman-Worsley *et al.*, 2021). Therefore, we surveyed 1542 cat and dog owners in both North America (primarily the United States) and Europe (primarily the Netherlands and Belgium) regarding their attitudes toward their pets, empathy, emotion regulation, and decisions regarding EoL for their pets. We focused on cats and dogs rather than other types of pets because dogs and cats are the most common types of pet and more likely to be euthanized compared to some other types of pet. Although we gathered data from pet owners who had and had not had experience euthanizing pets, here we restricted our analyses to those who had made the difficult decision to euthanize at least one pet.

Method

Participants

A total of 2381 participants started the questionnaire. Participants who answered less than 75% of the questions (N = 390) and/or did not (strongly) agree with the statement 'I paid attention to the questions, and you should use my data' (N = 63) and/or failed at least two attention check questions (N = 99) were excluded. Significantly more men than women were excluded while significantly fewer participants of the Dutch cohort were excluded after data cleaning. The latter makes sense as they actively volunteered to be in the cohort and participate in research about cats. Of the sample of 1840, 1542 respondents had actually made the decision to euthanize their pet dog or pet cat (27% had to make this decision within the last year, 45% between one and 5 years ago, and 28% more than 5 years ago). The final sample for analysis consists of these 1542 participants of which 996 (63.6%) answered questions about the euthanasia of their cat and 546 (34.8%) about the euthanasia of their dog.

Measures

Emotion dysregulation

Emotion dysregulation was measured using the short version of the Difficulties in Emotion Regulation Scale (DERS-SF; Kaufman *et al.*, 2016). The DERS-SF consists of 18 items and contains six subscales including non-acceptance of emotional responses, difficulties engaging in goal-directed behavior, impulse control difficulties, lack of emotional awareness, limited access to emotion regulation strategies, and lack of emotional clarity. An example item is "When I'm upset, I have difficulty focusing on other things." Participants indicated their level of agreement with each statement using scales ranging from 1 (almost never) to 5 (almost always). It should be noted that higher scores indicate a greater difficulty regulating emotions. We included only the total score in analyses. Internal consistency as measured by Cronbach's alpha was high, $\alpha = .88$.

Empathy for animals

We adapted the Multi-Dimensional Emotional Empathy Scale (MDEES, Caruso and Mayer, 1998; Alloway *et al.*, 2016) for use with regard to empathy for animals. We asked participants to respond to 17 statements (from the original 30 statements) concerning the extent to which they are affected by the suffering of animals. For example, "The suffering of animals deeply disturbs me." They responded on a 7-point scale from 1 (strongly disagree) to 7 (strongly agree). Internal consistency was high, $\alpha = .82$.

Pet attitude scale

We used the Pet Attitude Scale (PAS, Templer *et al.*, 1981) to assess participants' attitudes toward pets generally[1]. This scale contains 18 items, such as "I love pets" and "I like to feed animals out of my hand." Internal consistency was adequate, $\alpha = .72$. Kennel workers scored higher on the PAS than social workers in the original study (Templer *et al.*, 1981), verifying that it could distinguish between those expected to have differing levels of interest and investment in pets. Scores on this measure are highly correlated with scores on measures of attachment to animals (e.g., Ellingsen *et al.*, 2010).

Outcome measures

TIMING. Using the matrix format, we asked respondents to respond to the following: "It is always difficult knowing what is the right time for euthanasia when trying to balance suffering and time left to live. Indicate whether you would prefer making the decision a little too early and avoiding suffering or making the decision a little too late and extending the amount of time left. Indicate your preference for deciding to euthanize your pet early versus late in their illness from 1 (strong preference for early decision) to 6 (strong preference for late decision)."

STAGE. Using a multiple choice format, we asked, "At what stage did you make the difficult decision to euthanize your pet?: 1 = As soon as I knew the pet was ill but before they showed any signs of suffering, 2 = As soon as they began to show signs of suffering, 3 = After they had shown some signs of suffering but while they were still eating and engaging in some of their usual activities, 4 = After they had shown some signs of suffering and as soon as they stopped eating or engaging in their usual activities, 5 = Once they stopped eating and had been inactive for several days, 6 = Once they were no longer responsive, 7 = I would not euthanize - I would allow the pet to die a natural death."

GUILT. We asked, "How much guilt did you feel about the following aspect surrounding the euthanasia of your latest pet. If an aspect is not applicable you can select n/a." For, guilt for making the decision too early, they responded to "Making the decision to euthanize too early." For guilt for making the decision too late, they responded to "Making the decision to euthanize too late." They responded on a Likert scale of 1 (not very much guilt) to 5 (a tremendous amount of guilt).

Procedure

Participants were asked to complete the measures at a secure website, Qualtrics.com. The questionnaire was available in Dutch and English and distributed by snowball sampling through several social media accounts (Facebook, Twitter, LinkedIn) asking people who own(ed) a pet cat or pet dog to participate. Authors shared the link to the survey on their own social media accounts and asked followers to participate and/or share the invitation with their own networks. Invitations to participate were also posted to two cat rescue group pages on Facebook. In addition, 648 Dutch cat owners were invited over e-mail. These cat owners previously participated in other cat research (Bouma *et al.*, 2021) and agreed to be invited for further research. The questionnaire was available between February 28 and April 1, 2022. The Dutch survey was reviewed and approved by the Institutional Review Board of the University of Groningen). The English survey was reviewed and approved by the Oakland University Institutional Review Board).

The introduction text in the survey mentioned that the topic of euthanasia might evoke negative feelings and that respondents could stop their participation any time if they felt uncomfortable. Furthermore, support websites were displayed at the end of the survey (depending on the country of residence specific websites for the United States, United Kingdom, The Netherlands and Belgium were shown). Respondents actively gave informed consent. The survey began with questions about the respondent (demographics including being a pet professional or not), the measures of empathy and emotion regulation described above, and questions about the experience with euthanasia of their own pet cat(s) or dog(s)[2]. If owners had experience euthanizing more than one pet, they were asked to answer the questions regarding their most recent experience and to indicate what type of pet this involved (dog or cat). They indicated how long ago they had made this decision and for how long they had had the pet they had to euthanize. They were asked whether they made the decision alone or with others, and if so, with whom. They could choose "by myself, with family members, with my vet, with close friends or other" and they could indicate all that applied. They were also asked to indicate the primary reason(s) for their decision to euthanize. They selected all that applied from "behavioral concerns, health-related concerns, age of pet, health of owner, high cost of pet care, busy work schedule, living arrangements or other." Respondents also answered questions concerning how they determined when it was time to euthanize their pet and the guilt that they felt as a result of this decision.

Statistical Analyses

Group differences between dog (coded as 1) and cat owners (coded as 2) and the Dutch (coded as 1) and English sample (coded as 0) were examined with independent sample t-tests and Pearson chi-square tests. The outcome variables, timing, stage, early guilt, late guilt were regressed on pet type (cat, dog), emotion dysregulation, empathy for animals, and attitudes toward pets. We entered pet type, emotion dysregulation, empathy, and attitudes on the first step of the models. On the second step, we entered all two-way interactions, but no three-way interactions as we did not have hypotheses about three-way interactions. Preliminary analyses revealed few effects of sample (Dutch, English) so, for the sake of parsimony, we did not include this variable in the final analyses. We applied a Bonferroni correction for multiple analyses and therefore set alpha to .0125 for results from the regression analyses. We considered that our variables may exhibit quadratic associations with our outcomes, so we also initially conducted analyses including quadratic terms but very few quadratic effects were significant, so we present the simpler models omitting quadratic terms. We used IBM SPSS (version 28) software package to analyze our data.

Results

Sample characteristics

The majority of the sample indicated that they made the decision to euthanize in consultation with their vet (59.9%) and/or family members (44.7%). A smaller proportion of the sample (23.4%) made the decision by themselves, and only 5% made the decision with close friends. No significant differences were present between cat and dog owners with regard to gender (comparing males to females only), age, ethnicity (Caucasian vs other) and child/marital status. Differences were present for education, animal professional and length of time with the pet: Cat owners were slightly more highly educated than dog owners ($\chi^2 = 12.78$, $p = .002$). The proportion of animal professionals was higher ($\chi^2 = 43.70$, $p < .001$) in dog owners compared to cat owners (39% vs. 23%). The time with the pet was longer for owners of cats compared to dogs ($\chi^2 = 22.85$, $p < .001$).

When comparing English to Dutch survey takers, Dutch owners were more likely to report on cats versus dogs, ($t_{649} = 9.13$, $p < .001$, 95%CI: −.31, −0.21). English speaking participants were slightly older on average ($t_{687} = 2.67$, $p = .01$, 95%CI: .53, 3.44), and slightly less highly educated ($\chi^2 = 43.70$, $p < .001$), but more likely to work as animal care professionals ($\chi^2 = 45.94$, $p < .001$). They were more likely to be non-Caucasian ($\chi^2 = 13.57$, $p < .001$). They also differed significantly in the time since euthanasia ($\chi^2 = 17.72$, $p < .001$), with more recent experience in general, and a tendency to have spent a longer period of time with the pet before the euthanasia ($\chi^2 = 16.95$, $p < .001$). In addition, English speakers reported higher levels of spirituality ($t_{685} = 7.46$, $p < .001$, 95%CI: .36, .61), and were more likely to believe that they would see their deceased pet again in an afterlife ($t_{685} = 2.45$, $p < .001$, 95%CI: .02, .22). Table 7.1 shows that most of our respondents, across samples, euthanized their pets as a result of injury, age, or illness.

Table 7.1. Primary reasons for deciding to euthanize by pet type.

	Pet type	
Reasons to euthanize	Cat	Dog
Behavioural problems	9	15
Health-related concerns of the pet	948	520
Age of the pet	292	212
Health-related concerns of humans	2	1
High costs of pet care	3	1
Busy work schedule	0	1
Moving/Living arrangements don't allow pets	0	0
Accident	10	3
Other reason	4	3
Total	996*	556*

Note. * Respondents could indicate more than one reason, so rows do not sum to the total number of participants.

Correlations Between Key Predictors and Outcomes

The bivariate zero-order correlations and descriptive statistics for all predictors and outcomes appear in Table 7.2. Emotion regulation was not related to the other predictors, but it was negatively related to the outcomes of timing and guilt. Empathy and attitudes toward animals were highly correlated and predicted stage and guilt (although attitudes did not predict guilt at making the decision too late). Interestingly, timing and stage were negatively associated, and, whereas timing was positively associated with both types of guilt, stage was not. Dog owners had higher levels of empathy for animals and more positive pet attitudes in general compared to cat owners.

Regressions

The results of the step-wise linear regressions for each of the four outcomes appear in Table 7.3.

Timing

There were no significant effects of timing with our adjusted alpha level.

Stage

There were significant main effects of pet type ($\beta = .072$, $t = 2.79$, $p = .005$, 95%CI: .045, .257) and empathy ($\beta = .083$, $t = 2.563$, $p = .010$, 95%CI: .020, .154). Respondents were more likely to make later decisions for cats than for

Table 7.2. Zero-order correlations and descriptive statistics for the key predictors and outcomes.

	1	2	3	4	5	6	7	8
1. Pet Type	–							
2. Emotion Dysregulation	.009	–						
3. Empathy for Animals	–.052*	–.001	–					
4. Pet Attitudes	–.108***	.041	.61***	–				
5. Timing	–.052*	.061*	–.002	–.007	–			
6. Stage	.063**	.020	.095***	.073**	–.23***	–		
7. Guilt Early	–.028	.109**	.179***	.124***	.254***	.062	–	
8. Guilt Late	.071*	.107***	.086**	.026	.327***	.013	.367***	–
Mean	1.646	1.962	6.164	6.215	2.850	3.330	2.270	3.010
Standard Deviation	0.478	0.538	0.587	0.426	1.140	1.012	1.454	1.480

Note. *p < .05; **p < .01; ***p < .001.

dogs. Respondents with higher levels of empathy for animals were also more likely to make later decisions.

Guilt for too early decisions

There were significant main effects of emotion dysregulation (β= .106, t=3.190, p = .001, 95%CI: .041, .172) and empathy (β = .159, t=3.780, p < .001, 95%CI: .082, .258). Respondents with greater difficulty regulating emotion and those with higher levels of empathy for animals experienced more guilt for having made decisions too early.

Guilt for too late decisions

There were significant main effects of emotion dysregulation (β = .104, t=3.207, p = .001, 95%CI: .040, .165) and empathy (β = .102, t=2.503, p = .012, 95%CI: .023, .194). Respondents with greater difficulty regulating emotion and those with higher levels of empathy for animals experienced more guilt for having made decisions too late. No significant interaction effects were present for any outcome with our adjusted alpha level.

Discussion

We surveyed 1542 dog and cat owners residing in North America and Europe with the goal of better understanding factors underlying decisions regarding the timing of euthanasia in these pets. Because of our interest in how owners balanced concern for suffering and their own desire to prolong time with their pets, we focused on euthanasia in the context of illness, injury or old age. We focused our analyses on pet owners that had previously been involved in at least one decision to euthanize a pet. Overall, there were no statistically significant effects of pet type, other than cat owners reporting making the decision at a later stage in disease compared to dog owners. Researchers have also found that, for pet dogs, but not cats, making the decision to euthanize compared to having a pet die without having euthanized was negatively correlated with extended grief (Planchon *et al.*, 2002). This might be related to dogs and cats behaving differently in response to pain (Hernandez-Avalos *et al.*, 2019). Whereas dogs will show pain or discomfort more openly (e.g. whining and pacing), cats are more likely to stay silent and out of sight, which might explain later recognition of their suffering by owners. Although it is possible that different decisions for cats compared to dogs reflected differences in the characteristics of cat versus dog owners, rather than attributes of the pets themselves, cat and dog owners did not significantly differ in age, gender, level of education, religious or spiritual beliefs, including their belief in the likelihood of being reunited with their pet in the afterlife, although the latter difference approached significance (t_{331} = 1.74, p = .08, 95%CI: −.01, .18): Dog owners were slightly more likely to think that they would

Table 7.3. Hierarchical linear regression results.

	Timing			*Stage*			*Guilt Too Early*			*Guilt Too Late*		
	R^2	ΔR^2	β	R^2	ΔR^2	β	R^2	ΔR^2	β	R^2	ΔR^2	β
Step 1	.007**	.004**		.015***	.012***		.044***	.039***		.024***	.020***	
Pet Type			.053*			.072**			–.019			.070*
Emotion Dysregulation			.061			.018			.106**			.104**
Empathy for Animals			–.004			.083**			.159**			.102**
Pet Attitudes			–.001			.026			.024			–.035
Step 2	.11	.004		.021***	.014***		.055***	.044***		.027**	.017**	
Pet × Dysregulation			.032			.186*			–.183			–.019
Pet × Empathy			–.019			–.139			–.158			–.157
Pet × Attitudes			.231*			.248*			.165			.170
Dysregulation × Empathy			.000			–.027			.046			–.019
Dysregulation × Attitudes			–.018			.024			–.053			–.002
Empathy × Attitudes			.005			–.019			.066			.031

Note. *p < .05; **p < .01; ***p < .001.

see their deceased pet again in an afterlife. Correlations between pet type and our predictors indicated that dog owners had somewhat higher levels of empathy for animals and more positive pet attitudes in general compared to cat owners. These differences may have led the dog owners to make earlier decisions to euthanize, although pet type did not significantly interact with empathy or attitudes to predict timing outcomes. A measure of attachment that captured specific attachment to the euthanized pet rather than general attitudes toward pets might be more likely to predict later decisions and we will include such a measure in future work.

We included the general measure of attitudes toward pets (Templer *et al.*, 1981) so that the questions were relevant for owners with multiple pets and those that had not euthanized a pet. Earlier research shows measures of attitudes toward pets to be highly correlated with measures of attachment (e.g., Brown *et al.*, 1996; Ellingsen *et al.*, 2010; Hawkins *et al.*, 2017) and empathy (Daly and Morton, 2006), and we also found a high correlation with empathy here. Bivariate correlations also indicated that attitude toward pets was associated with guilt related to making decisions too early and decisions being made at later stages of an illness or injury. Tzivian *et al.* (2014) found that Israeli pet owners often delayed the decision to euthanize because of their strong connections to their pets, as indicated in qualitative interviews about their euthanasia experiences. Despite these correlations, attitudes toward pets were not a significant predictor in our regression models. Perhaps this was due to shared variance with our other predictors; however, the predictors were not highly correlated and VIF factors indicated that there was no reason to be concerned about multicollinearity.

We had hypothesized that empathy for animals might predict either early decisions to reduce pet suffering or later decisions to extend the pet's life. However, we thought that the association between empathy and timing of decisions would be moderated by participants' ability to regulate their emotions such that those high in empathy but low in emotion regulation might be likely to make earlier decisions to euthanize to prevent dealing with the discomfort of seeing a beloved pet sick or in pain (Batson, 1998). Park and Jeong (2022) recently found that maladaptive emotion regulation strategies increased the effect of attachment on separation pain after pet loss. Contrary to our hypotheses, empathy and emotion regulation did not interact to predict the timing of euthanasia decisions. However, both factors independently predicted the amount of guilt that respondents felt; both for having made decisions too early as well as having made decisions too late. This might indicate that owners high in empathy and those low in emotion regulation feel greater guilt for making the decision to euthanize at all, regardless of the timing of the decision, compared to those lower in empathy and those with better emotion regulation.

Respondents high in empathy were more likely to make decisions further in the process when the pet's disease had begun to impact its activities. This was in contrast to our prediction that those high in empathy might be likely to make earlier decisions to reduce pet suffering. Our hypothesis was based on the expectation that owners high in empathy would have difficulties seeing their pets suffering – a primary reason cited by Israeli pet owners for euthanizing their pets (Tzivian *et al.*, 2014). Previous research found that empathy predicted opposition to euthanasia in human children (Deak and Saroglou, 2017) and adults (Portenoy *et al.*, 1997). Whereas opposition is not equivalent to delaying eventual euthanasia, it is possible that empathy is more strongly related to moral beliefs regarding the sanctity of life and not the reduction of suffering, which is what we had anticipated.

Interestingly though, this outcome variable (stage) was negatively correlated with respondent's self-reported preferences for making decisions early or later in the illness (timing). That is, respondents' self-reported preferences for making later decisions actually predicted having made decisions earlier in the progression of a pet's disease or condition. Given that respondents reported guilt for both too early and too late decisions, it is possible that the preference reported now in retrospect was adjusted based on the guilt felt for having made earlier decisions. Other studies have found only a small proportion of bereaved pet owners to display significant guilt following euthanasia, but these researchers did not focus on the specific timing of the decision to euthanize (Bussolari *et al.*, 2017;

McCutcheon and Fleming, 2002; Planchon *et al.*, 2002; Tzivian *et al.*, 2014). Previous research has shown that anticipatory grief can result in delaying euthanasia (Brockman *et al.*, 2008; Fernandez-Mehler *et al.*, 2013; Hewson, 2014), so we expected that greater attachment, which predicts greater grief, would lead to later decisions. However, the timing preference in our study was not significantly predicted by pet type, empathy or attitudes toward pets, or emotion regulation.

Limitations and Directions for Future Research

We omitted several potentially interesting variables in the current study in the interest of keeping the survey brief. It should be noted that our statistical models accounted for a very small portion of the variability in the timing of euthanasia decisions. Thus, we acknowledge there are many other important factors in EoL decisions that were not accounted for in our models but that should be considered. Although our sample was relatively large, future research would benefit from a more diverse sample. Our sample was predominantly white and, as is common in human–animal interaction research, our sample is not entirely representative for the general population as women and people with a relatively high educational level are over-represented. Women in particular are likely to have stronger attachments to pets compared to men (Brown *et al.*, 1996; Ellingsen *et al.*, 2010) whereas the results concerning the relationship between education and pet attachment is more mixed (Ellingsen *et al.*, 2010; Martens *et al.*, 2016; Taylor and Signal, 2006; Wong *et al.*, 2019). It is also highly likely that our sample was strongly biased toward individuals that heavily invested in their pets. Thus, we did not likely capture the attitudes or predictors of participants with less close relationships to their pets, but this is probably true of most relevant studies on human/pet relationships (see also Littlewood *et al.*, 2021a).

Sampling individuals with a diversity of religious beliefs would also be important given how ideas about an afterlife and whether animals have minds and souls likely influence EoL decisions as well (Sanders, 1995; Testoni *et al.*, 2017). However, previous research indicated that religious beliefs did not predict distress following euthanasia or the determination of euthanasia as appropriate (Davis *et al.*, 2003). We expected some differences between our North American and European samples given differing practices, such as the tendency for more Americans to restrict their pets to indoor only environments (Foreman-Worsley *et al.*, 2021), and differences in attitudes about euthanasia generally (van Tol *et al.*, 2012; Deak and Saroglou, 2017) might suggest differences in EoL practices as well. However, we did not find significant differences between our English speaking and Dutch speaking cohorts. Future research could further examine pet owners and euthanasia in various cultures.

In addition, although we asked some questions about the particular reasons for which the owner had to consider euthanasia, we did not analyze these factors here. The vast majority of our participants euthanized due to poor health or old age, so we did not have much variability in these factors. The underlying cause for the pet's suffering or the extent of their suffering may be more predictive than any of the factors we considered. Because these aspects were considered to some degree in our timing and stage outcome measures and not as predictors, we may have reduced some of the variability in responses. Furthermore, our survey was focused on pet owners who chose euthanasia because their pet was ill or suffering in some way. However, we did not explicitly ask questions about euthanasia following accidental injuries. We did not focus on decisions surrounding economic issues, behavioral issues, or decisions made solely for the convenience of the owner. This focus may have influenced the findings. We also did not account for the owners' desire for control concerning the timing of the death of their pets (Davis *et al.*, 2003), which future work should account for. Future work should also consider the owners' anticipatory grief and the extent to which this delays the euthanasia decision, as previous studies have found this to be an important factor (Shaw and Lagoni, 2007; Lagoni, 2011; Littlewood *et al.*, 2020; Littlewood *et al.*, 2021a). In addition, future work should also examine the role of behavioral concerns, age of pet, length of time with pet, and the extent to which other individuals (such as other pet caretakers and veterinarians) in the decision-making process.

Conclusions

Our study aimed to shed light on the process of making decisions surrounding euthanasia of a companion animal. We decided to focus on owner attributes such as empathy and emotion regulation and general attitudes toward pets, but we recognize that many other owner and pet attributes are important to making such difficult decisions. Contrary to our hypotheses, we found no evidence for an interaction between empathy and emotion regulation on the timing of euthanasia. However, both empathy and emotion regulation predicted guilt following euthanasia. Higher levels of empathy predicted later euthanasia decisions, in contrast to our predictions. Our results suggest that empathy may be related to the value of life, rather than reduction in suffering. Future work is needed to identify other factors underlying pet owners' decision-making processes regarding EoL care for their pets, and how these factors are weighed. This is an incredibly complex issue that is likely influenced by a myriad of factors not captured in the current survey. Although this is a difficult subject, it is an important one that deserves further research attention. It is our hope that a better understanding of how owner characteristics impact their decision-making will allow veterinary professionals to communicate options to an owner that address their concerns and reduce overwhelming feelings of guilt while allowing them to make the best decisions for their pets. Our results are one step in better understanding pet owner characteristics and their influence on EoL decisions.

Notes

[1] We did not use a measure of specific pet attachment or ask participants to respond with the most recently euthanized pet in mind specifically because some of the total respondents had multiple pets and some had not actually euthanized a pet and we wanted all respondents to respond to the same scale in the same way.

[2] If respondents had never had to make the decision to euthanize their own pet cat or dog, they were asked to imagine a situation where they had to do this. In the current study, we report data of only those respondents who had actually made the decision to euthanize a pet.

References

Adams, C.L., Bonnett, B.N. and Meek, A.H. (1999) Owners' response to companion animal death: Development of a theory and practical implications. *Canadian Veterinary Journal* 40, 33–39.

Adrian, J.A.L. and Stitt, A. (2019) There for you: Attending pet euthanasia and whether this relates to complicated grief and post-traumatic stress disorder. *Anthrozoös* 32(5), 701–713.

Albright, A.E., Cui, R. and Allen, R.S. (2022) Pet ownership and mental and physical health in older white and black males and females. *International Journal of Environmental Research and Public Health* 19(9), 5655.

Alloway, T.P., Copello, E., Loesch, M., Soares, C., Watkins, J. *et al.* (2016) Investigating the reliability and validity of the multidimensional emotional empathy scale. *Measurement* 90, 438–442.

Barker, S.B. and Gee, N.R. (2021) Canine-assisted interventions in hospitals: Best practices for maximizing human and canine safety. *Frontiers in Veterinary Science* 8, 615730.

Barroso, C.S., Brown, K.C., Laubach, D., Souza, M., Daugherty, L.M. *et al.* (2021) Cat and/or dog ownership, cardiovascular disease, and obesity: A systematic review. *Veterinary Sciences* 8(12), 333.

Batson, C.D. (1998) Altruism and prosocial behavior. In: Gilbert, D.T., Fiske, S.T. and Lindzey, G. (eds) *The Handbook of Social Psychology*. McGraw-Hill, pp. 282–316.

Bouma, E.M.C., Reijgwart, M.L. and Dijkstra, A. (2021) Family member, best friend, child or 'just' a pet, owners' relationship perceptions and consequences for their cats. *International Journal of Environmental Research and Public Health* 19(1), 193.
Brockman, B.K., Taylor, V.A. and Brockman, C.M. (2008) The price of unconditional love: Consumer decision making for high-dollar veterinary care. *Journal of Business Research* 61, 397–405.
Broom, D.M. (2019) In: Choe, C.J. (ed.) *Welfare Concepts*, 2nd edn. Elsevier Academic Press, San Diego, CA. Available at: https://doi.org/10.1016/B978-0-12-809633-8.01321-2
Brown, B.H., Richards, H.C. and Wilson, C.A. (1996) Pet bonding and pet bereavement among adolescents. *Journal of Counseling & Development* 74(5), 505–509.
Bussolari, C., Habarth, J., Kimpara, S., Katz, R., Carlos, F. *et al.* (2017) Posttraumatic growth following the loss of a pet: A cross-cultural comparison. *OMEGA - Journal of Death and Dying* 78(4), 348–368. DOI: 10.1177/0030222817690403.
Bussolari, C.J., Habarth, J., Katz, R., Phillips, S., Carmack, B. *et al.* (2018) The euthanasia decision-making process: A qualitative exploration of bereaved companion animal owners. *Bereavement Care* 37(3), 101–108.
Caruso, D.R. and Mayer, J.D. (1998) The multidimensional emotional empathy scale (MDEES). *UNH Personality Lab* 21.
Daly, B. and Morton, L.L. (2006) An investigation of human-animal interactions and empathy as related to pet preference, ownership, attachment, and attitudes in children. *Anthrozoös* 19(2), 113–127.
Davis, H., Irwin, P., Richardson, M. and O'Brien-Malone, A. (2003) When a pet dies: Religious issues, euthanasia and strategies for coping with bereavement. *Anthrozoös* 16(1), 57–74.
Deak, C. and Saroglou, V. (2017) Terminating a child's life? Religious, moral, cognitive, and emotional factors underlying non-acceptance of child euthanasia. *Psychologica Belgica* 57(1), 59–76.
Ellingsen, K., Zanella, A.J., Bjerkås, E. and Indrebø, A. (2010) The relationship between empathy, perception of pain and attitudes toward pets among Norwegian dog owners. *Anthrozoös* 23(3), 231–243.
Fernandez-Mehler, P., Gloor, P., Sager, E., Lewis, F.I. and Glaus, T.M. (2013) Veterinarians' role for pet owners facing pet loss. *Veterinary Record* 172(21), 555.
Field, N.P., Orsini, L., Gavish, R. and Packman, W. (2009) Role of attachment in response to pet loss. *Death Studies* 33(4), 334–355.
Foreman-Worsley, R., Finka, L.R., Ward, S.J. and Farnworth, M.J. (2021) Indoors or outdoors? An international exploration of owner demographics and decision making associated with lifestyle of pet cats. *Animals* 11(2), 253.
Gee, N.R., Rodriguez, K.E., Fine, A.H. and Trammell, J.P. (2021) Dogs supporting human health and well-being: A biopsychosocial approach. *Frontiers in Veterinary Science* 8, 630465.
Gosse, G.H. and Barnes, M.J. (1994) Human grief resulting from the death of a pet. *Anthrozoös* 7(2), 103–111.
Hawkins, R.D., Williams, J.M., Scottish Society, f. t and Prevention of, C. t (2017) Childhood attachment to pets: Associations between pet attachment, attitudes to animals, compassion, and humane behaviour. *International Journal of Environmental Research and Public Health* 14(5), 490.
Hernandez-Avalos, I., Mota-Rojas, D., Mora-Medina, P., Martínez-Burnes, J., Casas Alvarado, A. *et al.* (2019) Review of different methods used for clinical recognition and assessment of pain in dogs and cats. *International Journal of Veterinary Science and Medicine* 7(1), 43–54.
Hewson, C. (2014) Grief for pets–Part 1: Overview and some false assumptions. *Veterinary Nursing Journal* 29(9), 302–305.
Kaufman, K.R. and Kaufman, N.D. (2006) And then the dog died. *Death Studies* 30, 61–76.
Kaufman, E.A., Xia, M., Fosco, G., Yaptangco, M., Skidmore, C.R. *et al.* (2016) The difficulties in emotion regulation scale short form (DERS-SF): Validation and replication in adolescent and adult samples. *Journal of Psychopathology and Behavioral Assessment* 38(3), 443–455.
Kim, W.H., Min, K.D., Cho, S.I. and Cho, S. (2020) The relationship between dog-related factors and owners' attitudes toward pets: An exploratory cross-sectional study in Korea. *Frontiers in Veterinary Science* 493.
Lagoni, L. (2011) Family-present euthanasia: Protocols for planning and preparing clients for the death of a pet. In: Blazina, C., Boyraz, G. and Shen-Miller, D. (eds) *The Psychology of the Human-Animal Bond*. Springer, pp. 181–202.
Leary, S.U.W., Anthony, R., Cartner, S., Grandin, T., Greenacre, C. *et al.* (2020) AVMA Guidelines for the Euthanasia of Animals American Veterinary Medical Association. Schaumburg, IL, USA.

Littlewood, K., Beausoleil, N., Stafford, K. and Stephens, C. (2021a) "What would you do?": How cat owners make end-of-life decisions and implications for veterinary-client interactions. *Animals* 11(4), 1114.

Littlewood, K.E., Beausoleil, N.J., Stafford, K.J., Stephens, C., Collins, T. *et al.* (2021b) How decision-making about euthanasia for animals is taught to Australasian veterinary students. *Australian Veterinary Journal* 99(8), 334–343.

Littlewood, K.E., Beausoleil, N.J., Stafford, K.J., Stephens, C., Collins, T. *et al.* (2020) How management of grief associated with ending the life of an animal is taught to Australasian veterinary students. *Australian Veterinary Journal* 98(8), 356–363.

Marsa-Sambola, F., Williams, J., Muldoon, J., Lawrence, A., Connor, M. *et al.* (2016) Sociodemographics of pet ownership among adolescents in Great Britain: Findings from the HBSC Study in England, Scotland, and Wales. *Anthrozoös* 29(4), 559–580.

Marsa-Sambola, F., Williams, J., Muldoon, J., Lawrence, A., Connor, M. *et al.* (2017) Quality of life and adolescents' communication with their significant others (mother, father, and best friend): The mediating effect of attachment to pets. *Attachment and Human Development* 19(3), 278–297.

Martens, P., Enders-Slegers, M.J. and Walker, J.K. (2016) The emotional lives of companion animals: Attachment and subjective claims by owners of cats and dogs. *Anthrozoös* 29(1), 73–88.

McConnell, A.R., Brown, C.M., Shoda, T.M., Stayton, L.E. and Martin, C.E. (2011) Friends with benefits: On the positive consequences of pet ownership. *Journal of Personality and Social Psychology* 101(6), 1239–1252.

McCutcheon, K.A. and Fleming, S.J. (2002) Grief resulting from euthanasia and natural death of companion animals. *OMEGA-Journal of Death and Dying* 44(2), 169–188.

Melson, G.F. (1991) Studying children's attachment to their pets: A conceptual and methodological review. *Anthrozoös* 4, 91–99.

Moore, A.S. (2011) Managing cats with cancer: An examination of ethical perspectives. *Journal of Feline Medicine & Surgery* 13(9), 661–671.

Morris, P. (2012) Managing pet owners' guilt and grief in veterinary euthanasia encounters. *Journal of Contemporary Ethnography* 41(3), 337–365.

Muldoon, J.C., Williams, J.M. and Lawrence, A. (2016) Exploring children's perspectives on the welfare needs of pet animals. *Anthrozoös* 29(3), 357–375.

Niessen, S.J., Hazuchova, K., Powney, S.L., Guitian, J., Niessen, A.P. *et al.* (2017) The big pet diabetes survey: Perceived frequency and triggers for euthanasia. *Veterinary Sciences* 4(2), 27.

O'Haire, M. (2010) Companion animals and human health: Benefits, challenges, and the road ahead. *Journal of Veterinary Behavior* 5(5), 226–234.

Park, H.J. and Jeong, G.C. (2022) Relationship between attachment to pet and post-traumatic growth after pet loss: mediated moderating effect of cognitive emotion regulation strategy through separation pain. *Behavioral Sciences* 12(8), 291.

Planchon, L. and Templer, D. (1996) The correlates of grief after the death of a pet. *Anthrozoös* 9(2–3), 107–113.

Planchon, L.A., Templer, D.I., Stokes, S. and Keller, J. (2002) Death of a companion cat or dog and human bereavement: Psychosocial variables. *Anthrozoös* 10(1), 93–105.

Poresky, R.H. (1996) Companion animals and other factors affecting young children's development. *Anthrozoös* 9(4), 159–168.

Portenoy, R.K., Coyle, N., Kash, K.M., Brescia, F., Scanlon, C. *et al.* (1997) Determinants of the willingness to endorse assisted suicide: A survey of physicians, nurses, and social workers. *Psychosomatics* 38(3), 277–287.

Sanders, C.R. (1995, June) Killing with kindness: Veterinary euthanasia and the social construction of personhood. In: *Sociological Forum*, Vol. 2. pp. 195–214.

Schmidt, M., Naylor, P.E., Cohen, D., Gomez, R., Moses Jr, J.A. *et al.* (2018) Pet loss and continuing bonds in children and adolescents. *Death Studies* 44(5), 278–284.

Schuurman, N. (2017) Performing good death at the veterinary clinic: Experiences of pet euthanasia in Finland. *Area* 49(2), 208–214.

Shaw, J.R. and Lagoni, L. (2007) End-of-life communication in veterinary medicine: Delivering bad news and euthanasia decision making. *Veterinary Clinics: Small Animal Practice* 37(1), 95–108.

Spitznagel, M.B., Jacobson, D.M., Cox, M.D. and Carlson, M.D. (2017) Caregiver burden in owners of a sick companion animal: A cross-sectional observational study. *Veterinary Record* 181(12), 321–321.

Taylor, N. and Signal, T.D. (2005) Empathy and attitudes to animals. *Anthrozoös* 18(1), 18–27.

Taylor, N. and Signal, T. (2006) Attitudes to animals: Demographics within a community sample. *Society and Animals* 14(2), 147–157.
Templer, D.I., Salter, C.A., Dickey, S., Baldwin, R. and Veleber, D.M. (1981) The construction of a pet attitude scale. *The Psychological Record* 31(3), 343–348.
Testoni, I., Cataldo, L., Ronconi, L. and Zamperini, A. (2017) Pet loss and representations of death, attachment, depression, and euthanasia. *Anthrozoös* 30(1), 135–148.
Thomas, G.P. (1982) When a pet dies. *Modern Veterinary Practice* 63, 272–277.
Tzivian, L., Friger, M. and Kushnir, T. (2014) Grief and bereavement of Israeli dog owners: Exploring short-term phases pre- and post-euthanization. *Death Studies* 38(2), 109–117.
van Tol, D.G., Rietjens, J.A. and van der Heide, A. (2012) Empathy and the application of the 'unbearable suffering' criterion in Dutch euthanasia practice. *Health Policy* 105(2–3), 296–302.
Vizek Vidovi´c, V., Vlahovi´c ˇSteti´c, V. and Bratko, D. (1999) Pet ownership, type of pet, and socio-emotional development of school children. *Anthrozoös* 12(4), 211–217.
Wong, P.W., Yu, R.W. and Ngai, J.T. (2019) Companion animal ownership and human well-being in a metropolis—the case of Hong Kong. *International Journal of Environmental Research and Public Health* 16(10), 1729.
Wong, W.C., Lau, K.C.T., Liu, L.L., Yuen, G.S.N. and Wing-Lok, P. (2017) Beyond recovery: Understanding the post bereavement growth from companion animal loss. *OMEGA: Journal of Death and Dying* 75(2), 103–123.

8 Predictors of Opting for Advanced Medical Care versus Euthanasia for Companion Animals with Severe Cardiac Disease

Samantha Siess[1]*, George A. Kramer[2], Dar Ozer[2], Nikki Gaudette[2], Brienne Williams[2], Brittany Antal[2] and Anne Moyer[1]

[1]Department of Psychology, Stony Brook University, NY, USA; [2]Department of Cardiology, Atlantic Coast New York Veterinary Specialists Bohemia, NY, USA

Abstract

This study examined predictors of opting for advanced medical care versus euthanasia for a critically ill companion animal. These included holding an optimistic bias for poor prognostic information, level of attachment to one's companion animal, and satisfaction with one's veterinarian. Eighty owners of companion animals with a diagnosis of a severe cardiac disease were asked to indicate what they believed their companion animal's chance of survival and quality of life would be if they opted for intensive treatment. Participants showed an optimistic bias in their interpretation of the chance of survival (but not quality of life) of a companion animal with more severe prognoses, suggesting that this may serve as a self-protective strategy in the face of losing a beloved companion animal. Client satisfaction with communication and with the cost of care, but not attachment to one's companion animal, significantly increased the likelihood of approving the recommended course of hospitalization and intensive treatment. This is of particular importance in that, of those who did not approve the recommended treatment, the majority elected to take their companion animals home against medical advice, rather than opt for humane euthanasia, this likely resulted in undue suffering and an uncomfortable death. These findings support the need for training in communication in veterinary schools.

Keywords: veterinarian communication, decision-making, end-of-life, euthanasia, attachment, companion animals

Introduction

The relationship between companion animal owners and their pets represents a unique type of dyad, making critical care and end-of-life decisions complex. This type of surrogate decision making is stressful when done on behalf of human loved ones (Nelson *et al.*, 2017; Pignatiello *et al.*, 2018). This strain can be exacerbated in veterinary contexts because compnion animals cannot explicitly make their wishes known. Effective medical decision making by owners on behalf of companion animals and its psychological and social correlates are poorly understood and understudied,

*Corresponding author: ss3836@cornell.edu

providing little guidance for veterinary medical professionals in their interactions with clients.

In general, surrogate decision makers for human patients, on whom the majority of research has been conducted, may have impaired reasoning and information processing abilities (Majesko *et al.*, 2012; Netzer and Sullivan, 2014; Verceles *et al.*, 2014) and may be, at times, unrealistically optimistic. Even when not under the duress associated with a role such as surrogate decision maker, people's level of optimism has been found to be unrealistic, with a tendency to underestimate the probability of negative outcomes while overestimating the probability of positive outcomes (Weinstein, 1980; Rothman *et al.*, 1996; Waters *et al.*, 2011; Shepperd *et al.*, 2013, 2015). For instance, surrogate decision makers for critically-ill patients in the ICU showed an optimistic bias in interpreting hypothetical prognostic statements about a generic patient with a high but not a low risk of death (Zier *et al.*, 2012). Similarly, an optimistic bias in response to poor prognoses, but not for better prognoses, was replicated among a sample of undergraduates who made interpretations of hypothetical prognoses for a parent or generic patient (Siess *et al.*, 2014; Moyer *et al.*, 2017) and for their dogs (Siess *et al.*, 2018a, b) and who were not under the duress of actually serving as a surrogate decision maker.

In both veterinary and human medical settings, an overly optimistic appraisal of poor prognoses that results in a greater likelihood of intensive, life-sustaining measures, has the potential to result in undue, prolonged suffering among patients. In addition, intensive measures in the veterinary setting are often financially burdensome, as the majority of owners of companion animals in the US do not have pet health insurance (American Veterinary Medical Association, [AVMA], 2018, 2021a; North American Pet Health Insurance Association [NAPHIA], 2021). Thus, it is increasingly important for veterinarians to have a better understanding of the tendency for distraught owners of critically-ill companion animals to have an overly optimistic appraisal of prognoses, outcomes of treatments, and a greater likelihood of electing intensive measures that may result in an extended poor quality of life of the animal and may have significant, detrimental financial burdens for the owner.

Animals provide companionship and social support and foster psychological well-being (Zasloff and Kidd, 1994; McNicholas *et al.*, 2005; McConnell *et al.*, 2011; Peacock *et al.*, 2012). Owners of companion animals report seeking and benefiting from closeness to their pet (Hall *et al.*, 2004; Prato-Previde *et al.*, 2006; Kurdek, 2008) as well as receiving comfort, encouragement, support, and relief in stressful circumstances (Allen *et al.*, 2002; Odendaal and Meintjes, 2003; Geisler, 2004; Kurdek, 2008). Owners also report using their companion animal as a secure base from which to explore new activities (Cusack, 1988; McNicholas and Collis, 1995). Moreover, loss of a companion animal is a source of significant grief (Lagoni *et al.*, 1994; Eckerd *et al.*, 2016; Bussolari *et al.*, 2018; Uccheddu *et al.*, 2019; Lee, 2020; Park and Royal, 2020). Although among adults, romantic partners are often the main source of a secure base figure (Hazan and Shaver, 1987), owners of companion animals have been shown to be attached to their pets in a similar manner (Zilcha-Mano *et al.*, 2011).

Owners of companion animals are seeking more regular and advanced veterinary care (Lau, 2012). It is increasingly likely that owners of companion animals will find themselves serving as a surrogate decision maker under dire veterinary circumstances (Siess *et al.*, 2015). To date, little attention has been paid to decision making in the context of veterinary medicine (Bley, 2017; Siess *et al.*, 2018a, b; Matte *et al.*, 2019; Marchitelli *et al.*, 2020; Spitznagel *et al.*, 2020). As such, the way in which owners of companion animals interpret prognoses given by veterinarians, the way in which available treatment options are explained, and the subsequent influences on decision making is unknown. Veterinarians report having difficulty with delivering poor prognoses (Fogle and Abrahamson, 1990; Butler and Degraff, 1996; Ptacek *et al.*, 2004), which induces stress and anxiety (Ptacek and Eberhardt, 1996; Ptacek *et al.*, 1999). Understanding the way in which owners of companion animals navigate their role as a surrogate decision maker in times of critical illness, such as the effect of caregiver burden (Spitznagel *et al.*, 2019a, b, 2020; Spitznagel and Carlson, 2019), has the potential to improve veterinarians' communication with their clients and subsequently reduce the burden of delivering and receiving poor prognoses.

In the current study, we examined whether an optimistic bias specifically for poor prognostic information (less than a 50% chance of survival), previously found only in hypothetical scenarios, is also present in a real-life veterinary setting. We also examined whether one's level of optimistic bias, attachment to one's companion animal, and satisfaction with one's veterinarian relate to the likelihood of choosing a treatment plan that is more intensive in terms of attempting to extend the life of a critically-ill companion animal. We selected a diagnosis of severe cardiac disease as a clinical situation whereby decisions are potentially influenced by many contextual and psychosocial factors and multiple courses of action are considered medically and ethically appropriate.

Ten percent of dogs and 10–15% of cats presented to primary veterinarians are diagnosed with cardiac disease (Ferasin and DeFrancesco, 2015; Keene *et al.*, 2019). Over time, they develop congestive heart failure, and have a very poor prognosis, with 80% dying within 2 years (Häggström *et al.*, 2008; Uechi, 2012; Keene *et al.*, 2019). The treatment for congestive heart failure, or, alternatively, euthanasia when necessary, is fairly standardized. Although it has a terminal prognosis, with treatment, dogs can have a good quality of life for a period of time (Atkins and Häggström, 2012; Ettinger *et al.*, 2017; Keene *et al.*, 2019). Treatment requires a significant commitment from the owner involving multiple daily medications, frequent veterinary visits and tests, and at-home monitoring. During acute congestive heart failure, an animal's quality of life is poor with clinical signs including dyspnea, lethargy, and inappetence (Ettinger *et al.*, 2017; Keene *et al.*, 2019). Given this lack of a clear medically or ethically preferable treatment path, and because there is a well-established protocol for treatment of acute congestive heart failure, it serves as a disease model amenable to research involving challenging treatment decisions.

Although there are many reasons for electing to decline intensive treatment or to euthanize a companion animal, poor quality of life is one of the most frequent reasons (Rollin, 2011). If an owner is unable to imagine their companion animal with an improved quality of life, treatment may be perceived as simply a means of prolonging suffering and may lead them to be more likely to decide to decline intensive measures. It is reasonable to acknowledge that the level of commitment required to extend the companion animal's lifespan may be too burdensome for many owners, particularly those with long work hours or other caregiving responsibilities (Spitznagel and Carlson, 2019) in addition to the financial burden associated with chronic treatments.

Study Overview

Study hypotheses

Hypothesis 1: Participants' ratings of their companion animals' chance of survival 2 years after treatment for severe cardiac disease would be more optimistic than their veterinarian's.

Rationale: Surrogates evaluating prognoses for hypothetical canine patients described in a vignette displayed a tendency for an optimistic bias for poor prognostic information (less than a 50% chance of survival) but not for less severe prognostic information (greater than a 50% chance of survival) about their dog even when not under the duress of actually being in a clinical treatment decision-making situation (Siess *et al.*, 2018b). In the case of a diagnosis of severe cardiac disease, the prognosis is fatal without intensive treatment (Ettinger *et al.*, 2017; Keene *et al.*, 2019). Thus, it is likely that owners will have an even stronger tendency to employ an optimistic bias for poor prognostic information in the case when the threat of loss is imminent.

Hypothesis 2: Participants' ratings of their companion animals' perceived quality of life with treatment for severe cardiac disease would be more optimistic than their veterinarian's.

Rationale: Similar to the rationale for chance of survival, it is likely that the optimistic bias will also be reflected in perceived anticipated quality of life for their companion animal.

Hypothesis 3: The greater the amount of optimistic bias for poor prognostic information and quality of life (if identified in the analyses for hypotheses 1 and 2), greater levels of attachment indicated by the greater amount of comfort received from one's companion animal, and greater client satisfaction (general satisfaction, technical quality, interpersonal manner, communication, financial aspects, accessibility and convenience, and time spent with the veterinarian), the greater would be the likelihood of choosing a more intensive treatment plan for severe cardiac disease.

Rationale: Previous research has shown that a greater amount of optimistic bias for poor hypothetical prognoses predicts a greater likelihood of approving the continuation of life sustaining measures in the case of a hypothetical human patient (Siess *et al.*, 2014; Moyer *et al.*, 2017) and treatment for canine B-cell lymphoma in the case of a hypothetical canine patient (Siess *et al.*, 2018a, b). It is likely that the emotional gravity associated with the impending loss of their companion animal without immediate treatment will result in an optimistic bias for the chance of survival as well as for quality of life. Together, it is probable that a higher perceived chance for survival and quality of life will result in a higher rate of owners choosing to approve a treatment plan that is more intensive for their companion animal. Levels of attachment have been associated with levels of caregiving and attentiveness to pets (Coy and Green, 2018). In the seminal work in humans (Ainsworth *et al.*, 2015) which has been extended into companion animals (Zilcha-Mano *et al.*, 2011), one of the four main criteria for an attachment figure is the use of the attachment figure as a source of comfort, encouragement, support and stress relief. In our study we examined whether the more comfort an owner receives from their companion animal, the closer their relationship and attachment is and, the more likely it is that an owner will strive to extend their companion animal's life. Lower levels of owner satisfaction with communication and the overall experience with the veterinarian may be associated with a lower amount of trust in the veterinarian as well as willingness to adhere to a post-hospitalization medical management plan. Similarly, in human medicine, poor communication, low levels of trust, and unmet expectations have been associated with poor patient satisfaction and subsequent adherence (Spernak *et al.*, 2007; Miaoulis *et al.*, 2009; Hillen *et al.*, 2011; Jerant *et al.*, 2014; Schoenthaler *et al.*, 2014). Although little attention has been paid to the significance of communication in veterinary settings, communication has been implicated as an important factor in client satisfaction and adherence (Case, 1988; Coe *et al.*, 2008). It is likely that the quality of interactions with the veterinarian, in terms of overall communication, time spent with the veterinarian, and interpersonal manner, in addition to satisfaction with technical quality and accessibility and convenience, may influence the extent to which owners feel comfortable going to greater lengths for potentially more costly and more extensive treatment for severe cardiac disease and will be more willing to elect for treatment and post-hospitalization medical management of the disease. Additionally, financial satisfaction plays a significant role in veterinary medicine as, as mentioned above, the majority of pet owners do not have health insurance coverage for their pets (AVMA, 2018, 2021b; NAPHIA, 2021).

Method

Participants

An a-priori power analysis was conducted, using G*Power, to determine the sample size required to detect a moderate effect size (d) of .32, with an α error probability of .05, and a power ($1-\beta$) of .80 (Faul *et al.*, 2007). The total sample size required was 79 and as such, 80 owners of companion animals receiving a diagnosis of severe cardiac disease were recruited from an emergency and multi-specialty referral veterinary hospital, over the course of 18 months, and received a $25 coupon that could be redeemed for veterinary services. They were 51 females and 29 males with an average age of 53.00 years (SD = 13.55; range = 20.00 to 82.00). The companion animals comprised 65 dogs with a mean age of 9.89 years (SD = 3.65; range = .42 to 17.58) and 15 cats with a mean age of 9.77 years (SD = 5.84; range = .75 to 19.83). Although the age ranges include ages less than 1 year of age, it should be noted that only 2 dogs and 1 cat were under the age of 1 year and only 13 dogs and 4 cats were under the age of 7 years. The study was approved, to be in compliance with ethical guidelines, by the institutional review board (IRB) at Stony Brook University.

Measures

Optimistic bias for prognostic information

The participant and the veterinarian independently indicated what they believed would be the dog or cat's chance of surviving for 2 years after intensive treatment is on a scale from 0% to 100% chance of surviving. The level of optimistic bias for prognostic information in terms of chance of survival was calculated as the difference in the perceived likelihood of survival indicated by the participant and by the veterinarian (based on clinical expertise as board certified small animal cardiologists). Positive values indicated that participants showed an optimistic bias and negative values indicated that they showed a pessimistic bias.

Optimistic bias for perceived quality of life

The participant and the veterinarian independently indicated what they believed the dog or cat's expected quality of life with intensive treatment would be on a 5-point Likert-type scale ranging from *very poor* to *very good*. The level of optimistic bias in terms of quality of life was calculated as the difference in the perceived quality of life as a result of the proposed treatment indicated by the participant and by the veterinarian.

Treatment plan decision

The medical record was reviewed to determine the treatment decision, and for those owners who decided to treat, the days of hospitalization and the outcome (survival versus death) as well as the age, breed of the dog or cat, and any other relevant medical history. For participants deciding to euthanize their dog or cat, the reason expressed for doing so was recorded.

Attachment

In accordance with our conception of attachment as related to having a figure that serves as a secure-base (Zilcha-Mano *et al.*, 2011), attachment to one's dog or cat was measured with the Comfort from Companion Animals Scale (Zasloff, 1996). It consists of 11 items rated on a 4-point Likert-type scale ranging from *strongly disagree* to *strongly agree*. It includes items such as "My pet provides me with companionship," "My pet is a source of constancy in my life," "I get comfort from touching my pet," and "My pet makes me feel safe." The internal consistency in this sample was $\alpha = .98$.

Client satisfaction

Client satisfaction was measured by a veterinary adaptation of The Patient Satisfaction Questionnaire Short-Form that included an additional question about financial aspects (PSQ-18; Marshall and Hays, 1994). The scale consists of 18 items rated on a 5-point Likert-type scale ranging from *strongly agree* to *strongly disagree*. Subscales include general satisfaction, technical quality, interpersonal manner, communication, financial aspects, accessibility and convenience, and the time spent with the veterinarian. The internal consistency in this sample was $\alpha = .83$.

Procedures

Participants were invited to participate in a study to examine client-veterinarian communication and interactions with staff members. Upon gaining informed consent, the cardiology veterinary technician administered the survey packet after the cardiologist spoke with participants about their dog or cat's diagnosis and recommended treatment plan. After the consultation, the veterinarian indicated in the medical record what they believed the numerical likelihood of survival 2 years after treatment was as well as what the dog or cat's quality of life would be with the recommended treatment. After completion of the survey packet, the technician reviewed the financial estimate for treatment, and the participant made their treatment decision. There were no alterations made to the natural flow of the consultations or treatment decision making process, as such, there was no risk to the safety of the companion animals in the study. Participants were sent a thank you note with information about the purpose of the study after the completion of all data collection.

Analytic strategy

All analyses were conducted using IBM SPSS Statistics 24 for windows (IBM Corp, 2016). To test the first and second hypotheses, a univariate ANOVA was conducted to determine if there was a difference in the amount of optimistic bias for the chance of survival and quality of life reported by owners based on the severity of the veterinarians' prognoses. Based on the consistent results from prior studies, prognoses were split into two categories: more severe prognoses and less severe prognoses. More severe prognoses were considered to be less than a 50% chance of two-year survival with intensive treatment and less severe prognoses were considered to be a 50% or greater chance of two-year survival with intensive treatment. To test the third hypothesis, a hierarchical logistic regression yielding a Wald statistic was performed on the decision to approve versus not approve the recommended hospitalization treatment plan with ten predictors. The first step of the model included predictors involving client satisfaction, including general satisfaction, and satisfaction with the technical quality of care, the interpersonal manner of the veterinarian, communication with the veterinarian, time spent with the veterinarian, financial aspects of care, and clinic accessibility and convenience. The second step of the model included comfort received from the companion animal. The third step of the model included the level of optimistic bias for chance of 2 year survival and an interaction between the amount of optimistic bias for chance of 2 year survival and the severity of the prognoses indicated by the veterinarian.

Results

Descriptive statistics

Prior to conducting statistical analyses, data were cleaned, missing values were replaced by the sample mean (n=7 instances across 4 subjects), and variables were tested for skewness and kurtosis. The data were examined for outliers, defined by more than three standard deviations away from the mean. One outlier was detected for a subject's indication of their animal's chance of 2 year survival. It was retained in the data because it seemed like an authentic response, based on interactions with the technician who collected the data.

Descriptive statistics and correlations between variables can be found in Table 8.1. Overall, the sample was highly attached to their companion animals, with an average score (M) on the comfort from companion animals scale of 41.33 (SD = 6.77) for owners of dogs and 42.77 (SD = 1.82) for owners of cats, out of a possible 44.00. Satisfaction with the provider was high for the subscales of general satisfaction for owners of dogs and cats, respectively (M = 4.29; SD = .62; M = 4.35; SD = .46), technical quality satisfaction (M = 4.10; SD = .48; M = 4.32, SD = .32), interpersonal manner satisfaction (M = 4.42; SD = .51; M = 4.62; SD = .49), communication satisfaction (M = 4.36; SD = .44; M = 4.51; SD = .42), accessibility and convenience satisfaction (M = 4.31; SD = .56; M = 4.33; SD = .50), and time spent with the veterinarian satisfaction (M = 4.25; SD = .54; M = 4.01; SD = .54), out of a maximum value of 5.00. Average financial satisfaction was lower, at 2.61 (SD = .94) for owners of dogs and 2.46 (SD = .89) for owners of cats. Of the 80 owners, 56 approved the recommended treatment for hospitalization and 24 did not approve the recommended treatment. Of those who did not approve the recommended treatment, 5 elected euthanasia and 19 took their companion animal home against medical advice (AMA).

Table 8.1. Descriptive statistics and correlations among study variables (N = 80).

Variables	OCS	OQL	P	CCA	GS	TQS	IMS	CS	FS	ACS	TSV
Optimism Chance of Survival (OCS)	1	.54***	–.50***	.09	–.01	.10	.03	.09	.09	.03	.06
Optimism Quality of Life (OQL)		1	–.04	.20	.14	.45***	.25*	.20	.17	.24*	.11
Prognoses (P)			1	.01	.02	.00	.05	–.10	.10	–.04	–.13
Comfort from Companion Animals (CCA)				1	.07	.25*	.01	.17	–.03	–.01	–.01
General Satisfaction (GS)					1	.59***	.40***	.70***	.10	.47***	.50***
Technical Quality Satisfaction (TQS)						1	.47***	.54***	.13	.50***	.39***
Interpersonal Manner Satisfaction (IMS)							1	.51***	.07	.42***	.52***
Communication Satisfaction (CS)								1	.22*	.48***	.51***
Financial Satisfaction (FS)									1	.03	.27*
Accessibility/Convenience Satisfaction (ACS)										1	.50***
Time Spent with Veterinarian Satisfaction (TSV)											1
Means	5.35	.33	39.30	41.60	4.31	4.15	4.46	4.39	2.58	4.31	4.21
Standard Deviations	29.68	.90	28.06	6.17	.59	.46	.51	.44	.93	.55	.54
Range	–75–80	–2–2	0–90	11–44	2.5–5	3–5	3–5	3.5–5	1–4.67	2.5–5	3–5
Minimum and Maximum Possible Scores	–100–100	–4–4	0–100	1–44	1–5	1–5	1–5	1–5	1–5	1–5	1–5

Statistical Significance: $^{*}p < .05$; $^{**}p < .01$; $^{***}p < .001$

Hypothesis 1: Examining the presence of an optimistic bias for the chance of two-year survival for severe prognoses

The largest proportion of participants, 52.50%, interpreted their dog or cat's prognosis in terms of chance of two-year survival more optimistically than the veterinarian's interpretation; 36.25% of participants interpreted the prognosis less optimistically; and 11.25% interpreted it similarly. For more severe prognoses of less than a 50% chance of survival, participants rated the likelihood of two-year survival on average 16.92% (SD = 26.03) above the estimate that the veterinarian made, indicating an optimistic bias. This was significantly different, $F(1,78) = 25.05$, $p<.001$, for less severe prognoses of 50% or greater chance of survival, which were rated on average 12.94% (SD = 25.93) *below* the estimate that the veterinarian made.

Hypothesis 2: Examining the presence of an optimistic bias for perceived quality of life with intensive treatment for severe prognoses

The largest proportion of participants, 43.75%, perceived their dog or cat's quality of life to be the same as the veterinarians did; 42.50% perceived it more pessimistically and 13.75% perceived it more optimistically. For more severe prognoses of less than a 50% chance of survival, participants rated the expected quality of life −.34 (SD = .91) *below* the estimate the veterinarian made. This was not significantly different for less severe prognoses of a 50% or greater chance of survival, which were rated −0.31 (SD = .90) *below* the estimate the veterinarian made, $F(1, 78) = .02$, $p = .89$. Also, the average expected quality of life for owners and veterinarians was similar, 3.35 (SD = .74) and 3.67 (SD = .67), on a 5-point scale, respectively.

Hypothesis 3: Predictors of treatment decision

Table 8.2 shows regression coefficients, Wald statistics, odds ratios, and 95% confidence intervals for odds ratios for each of the ten predictors. According to the Wald criterion, client satisfaction with communication and financial aspects significantly predicted the decision to approve the recommended treatment plan, $\chi^2 (1, N=80) = 5.17$, $p=.02$, $\chi^2 (1, N=80) = 5.26$, $p=.02$, respectively. Optimistic bias for prognoses, the interactive effects of the optimistic bias for prognoses with severity of prognoses, comfort received from companion animals, general patient satisfaction, satisfaction with the technical quality of care, interpersonal manner of the veterinarian, time spent with the veterinarian, and clinic accessibility and convenience did not contribute significantly to the model. The odds of approving the recommended treatment plan increased 9.18 times for every 1 unit increase in satisfaction with communication with the veterinarian and increased 2.18 times for every 1 unit increase in satisfaction with financial aspects.

Discussion

This study aimed to first determine whether the previously found optimistic bias for poor prognostic information for companion animals in hypothetical surrogate decision making scenarios was also present in a real life clinical veterinary setting. As hypothesized, more severe prognoses were associated with higher levels of optimistic bias in interpreting companion animals' likelihood of two-year survival following intensive treatment, with less severe prognoses with a 50% or more likelihood showing a reversal of this effect. This pattern of bias in interpretation of prognoses is in line with previous laboratory work on hypothetical surrogate decision makers for human patients (Siess *et al.*, 2014; Moyer *et al.*, 2017) and for canine patients (Siess *et al.*, 2018a, b). This is the first study to demonstrate this effect of an optimistic

Table 8.2. Hierarchical logistic regression analysis of owners of companion animals with severe cardiac disease's decision to approve the recommended treatment for intensive hospitalization as a function of patient satisfaction, comfort received from the companion animal, optimistic bias for the chance of two year survival, and the interactive effects of the optimistic bias for the chance of two-year survival with severity of prognoses.

				95% Confidence Interval for Odds Ratio	
Variables	B	Wald Chi-Square	Odds Ratio	Lower	Upper
Step 1					
General Satisfaction	−.25	.14	.78	.21	2.87
Technical Quality	−.15	.04	.86	.18	4.19
Interpersonal Manner	.01	.00	1.01	.25	4.14
Communication	2.21	5.17*	9.11	1.36	61.19
Financial Aspects	.82	5.26*	2.28	1.13	4.60
Time Spent with Veterinarian	−.10	.02	.91	.23	3.67
Accessibility/Convenience	−.07	.01	.93	.24	3.67
Step 2					
Comfort from Companion Animals	−.02	.17	.98	.89	1.08
Step 3					
Optimism Chance of Survival	−.00	.00	1.00	.97	1.03
Optimism Chance of Survival X	.00	.07	1.00	1.00	1.00
Severity of Prognoses					
Model		17.84			
(Constant)	−7.95	3.78			

*$p<.05$

appraisal of more severe prognoses in a clinical setting with actual decisions.

For human patients, in response to hypothetical numerical prognostic statements about either a parent or a generic patient, participants demonstrated an optimistic bias for those indicating a high risk of death (less than a 50% chance of survival) but not a low risk of death (greater than a 50% chance of survival; Siess *et al.*, 2014). Participants also demonstrated this pattern in response to hypothetical non-numerical prognostic statements such as "[They] probably will not survive" and "[They] probably will survive" (Moyer *et al.*, 2017). Additionally, the amount of optimistic bias for poor prognostic information was greater when the patient was described as a close other (parent) than a generic patient. Furthermore, when the prognoses were framed in a more threatening manner, that is, in terms of the chance of dying as opposed to the chance of surviving, the amount of optimistic bias increased. A follow-up study among a sample of owners of healthy dogs found the same pattern of an optimistic bias for poor quantitative prognoses with a high risk of death but not for prognoses with a lower risk of death (Siess *et al.*, 2018a) as well as for poor non-numerical prognoses (Siess *et al.*, 2018b).

Unrealistic optimism has been well documented in many situations, indicating that individuals have a tendency to be overly optimistic about the probability of negative outcomes happening to them (Weinstein, 1980;Shepperd *et al.*, 2013). Unrealistic absolute optimism is caused by a belief that one's personal outcomes will be more favourable than outcomes predicted by a quantitative standard.

Unrealistic comparative optimism is caused by a belief that one's personal outcomes will be more favourable than outcomes of others (Shepperd *et al.*, 2015). Reasons for unrealistic optimism have been theorized to be a result of motivation to believe the probability of an unfavorable outcome is less likely to occur (Tyler and Rosier, 2009), individuals having more information about themselves than others (Shepperd *et al.*, 2015), and the representative heuristic in which individuals consider how closely they match the stereotype of individuals who typically experience an unfavorable outcome when making predictions about their own likelihood (Tversky, 1977).

Unrealistic optimism has been implicated in predictions about outcomes for oneself and others, whereby individuals rated their own and others' risk of unfavorable outcomes lower than the actual risk. After making judgments about the likelihood of unfavorable outcomes occurring to themselves or others, individuals displayed an optimistic learning bias when told the actual likelihood of the event occurring was higher than expected, by discounting the additional risk optimistically (Kappes *et al.*, 2018). Given that individuals employ unrealistic optimism about the probability of unfavorable outcomes happening, it is not surprising that when faced with the distressing threat of loss of a beloved companion animal, the tendency to employ an optimistic bias occurs. This is supported by previous research in which individuals who reported a higher amount of comfort received from their dog, therefore a higher level of attachment, employed a greater amount of optimistic bias for hypothetical poor prognostic information (Siess *et al.*, 2018a, b), similar to the way biases were exacerbated in prior research when judgments were made regarding someone who was described as a close other (Siess *et al.*, 2014; Moyer *et al.*, 2017).

The reversal observed, which was also found in previous studies examining hypothetical scenarios involving a parent or generic patient (Siess *et al.*, 2014; Moyer *et al.*, 2017) or a dog (Siess *et al.*, 2018a, b) indicating a pessimistic bias for less severe prognoses, may be explained by defensive pessimism in which individuals cope by preparing for the worst (Norem and Cantor, 1986). By preparing for the possibility that, despite intensive treatment in the hospital and adherence with follow-up care, their animal may not survive, it is possible that owners may believe they are protecting themselves from disappointment and painful emotions should that occur. This speculation is supported by evidence that in preparation for negative outcomes, individuals may proactively attempt to reduce negative emotions if the event occurs (Sweeny and Shepperd, 2007).

Although it is not the veterinarian's responsibility to make difficult decisions on behalf of their clients, a greater understanding of the psychological processes influencing end-of-life decisions may allow for improved communication (Lummis *et al.*, 2020; Spitznagel *et al.*, 2020). This may result in clients having a better understanding of their animal's situation and feeling more comfortable with the difficult decision to euthanize when the odds of a successful procedure are low or the patient's quality of life may be poor. Many factors play a role in owners' end-of-life decision making, especially when quality of life with the recommended treatment is poor or uncertain (Siess *et al.*, 2015; Bley, 2017). Better communication from a veterinarian has the potential to help to alleviate these factors surrounding decisions (Marchitelli *et al.*, 2020).

The second aim of the study was to determine the extent to which an optimistic bias for poor prognostic information relates to an optimistically biased prediction of perceived quality of life for treatment of severe cardiac disease. It was hypothesized that participants' optimistic bias for severe prognoses would extend to an optimistic bias for the interpretation of perceived quality of life. In contrast to the hypothesis, the optimistic bias for the chance of two-year survival with the recommended treatment plan for intensive hospitalization did not appear to extend to an optimistic bias for perceived quality of life. Previous research has shown that the optimistic appraisal of poor prognostic statements is elevated when they are framed in a more threatening manner (in terms of likelihood of "dying" versus "surviving") and when one is emotionally closer to the patient for hypothetical human patients (Siess *et al.*, 2014) and for hypothetical canine patients (Siess *et al.*, 2018b). This defensive processing has been shown also in response to less precise, non-numerical prognostic statements such as,

"I think it is unlikely [he] will survive" is more likely to be interpreted in an optimistically-biased manner than "I think it is likely [he] will survive" (Moyer *et al.*, 2017; Siess *et al.*, 2018a). Perhaps the optimistic bias employed in the face of prognoses with a high threat of death is motivated primarily by self-protection from the threat of loss of the patient and is thus less likely to be activated in judgments related to quality of life. The sample of owners reported very high levels of attachment to their companion animal. Although the typical attachment figure for adults are family members, particularly spouses and parents, companion animals can serve as a secure attachment figure as well (Milberg and Friedrichsen, 2017). The four main criteria for an attachment figure are proximity maintenance during times of stress; use of the attachment figure as a source of comfort, encouragement, support and stress relief; use of the attachment figure as a secure base from which to explore; and finally, temporary or permanent separation from the attachment figure results in distress (Ainsworth *et al.*, 2015). It is not unlikely that among the sample of owners who reported very high levels of comfort received from their companion animal, many consider their animal to be an attachment figure. In that capacity, it is highly probable that owners who received a more severe prognosis for their companion animals' chance of survival experienced distress at the thought of being permanently separated from them, in line with the last criterion for an attachment figure (Ainsworth *et al.*, 2015). This may account for the optimistic bias employed for more severe prognoses about the chance of survival but not for the interpretation of quality of life as quality of life does not involve permanent separation from the attachment figure (companion animal). In a sample of family members of terminally-ill patients in palliative care, the threat of losing the attachment figure (patient) with the worsening of symptoms activated the attachment system, resulting in family members feeling less secure and seeking proximity to the patient (Milberg and Friedrichsen, 2017).

The third aim of the study was to determine whether one's level of optimistic bias related to the likelihood of approving a treatment plan for intensive hospitalization. It was hypothesized that the greater the amount of optimistic bias for poor prognostic information and quality of life, the greater the likelihood of choosing to approve a treatment plan with intensive hospitalization would be. The amount of optimistic bias did not significantly predict the decision to approve a treatment plan with intensive hospitalization. This result is not in line with previous findings in which the greater the amount of optimistic bias in interpreting prognoses about a hypothetical patient, the greater the likelihood was of approving more intensive life-sustaining measures over a transition to comfort care (Siess *et al.*, 2014; Moyer *et al.*, 2017). Similarly, individuals who employed a greater amount of optimistic bias for hypothetical poor prognostic information about their dog, the greater the likelihood was of the owners endorsing that they would approve life-prolonging treatments for canine B-cell lymphoma instead of euthanasia (Siess *et al.*, 2018a, b). This discrepancy is perhaps due to several factors. First, the sample of owners scored on average very high on the measure of attachment. Second, our sample was comprised of owners who were optimistic enough to agree to schedule a consultation with a board-certified veterinary cardiologist after referral from their primary veterinarian or by an emergency veterinarian. Based on the common prevalence of cardiac disease in dogs and cats in the population (Ferasin and DeFrancesco, 2015; Keene *et al.*, 2019), it is likely that there were a number of owners who received a referral and elected to euthanize, rather than have a consultation with a cardiologist, and thus would not have been captured in our sample. Certainly, some would have made a decision based on finances, however, it is possible that some elected euthanasia because they were either less attached to their companion animal or did not employ a strong optimistic bias. It is conceivable that the optimistic bias for severe prognoses was not a significant predictor of the decision to approve the recommended treatment plan for hospitalization as a result of this.

Further, it is important to note that of those who did not approve the recommended treatment, only 5 elected for euthanasia while 19 took their companion animal home AMA. This suggests that the majority of owners who declined the suggested treatment for intensive hospitalization may not have had a realistic understanding of their companion animal's condition in that their disease was so severe that they would likely not survive at home without treatment. When in congestive heart failure, animals exhibit distressing clinical signs that are visible and apparent to the non-professional's eye such as dyspnea (Ettinger *et al.*, 2017; Keene *et al.*, 2019). To decide to take such an animal home AMA is perhaps suggestive of an even stronger optimistic bias resulting in an unrealistically optimistic view of their companion animal's chance of survival. Individuals who are highly attached, have an optimistic bias for poor prognoses and approve the recommended treatment for intensive hospitalization, may in fact be the most realistic in recognizing that in the short term their animal will not survive or live comfortably without intensive treatment (Ettinger *et al.*, 2017; Keene *et al.*, 2019) as indicated by the veterinarian.

This issue is particularly important in terms of consequences for the animal, the owner, as well as for the veterinarian. First, the animal's recommended treatment plan for intensive hospitalization was given by the veterinarian because without it they would likely suffer and continue to decline without treatment. Therefore, it is the unfortunate reality that the majority, if not all, of the animals that went home AMA experienced some level of suffering and likely died a gruesome death at home. This decline in clinical state in the form of visible suffering, including gasping for air, likely caused significant distress for the owners who witnessed this (Ettinger *et al.*, 2017; Keene *et al.*, 2019). Further, owners who elected to take their animal home, are likely at a high risk of decisional regret and the development of psychiatric symptoms, that surrogate decision makers are already at risk for (Jones *et al.*, 2004; Corrigan *et al.*, 2007; Wendler and Rid, 2011; Kross *et al.*, 2011; Abou-Mrad *et al.*, 2012; Nelson *et al.*, 2017; Pignatiello *et al.*, 2018) because of the inevitable suffering and decline of their pet following their decision to leave the hospital against medical advice.

In addition to the impact that taking an animal home AMA has on the animal and for the owner, it is likely to have a negative impact on the veterinarian and veterinary staff involved. The veterinarian's goal is to treat patients when it is humane and can be beneficial and to end their suffering if that is not possible. Previous research has shown that when veterinarians believe they were able to achieve a 'good death' for patients, via humane euthanasia, they reported improved personal wellbeing. When unable to achieve a 'good death', they reported increased emotional strain, reduced wellbeing and job satisfaction, with detrimental effects on owners (Matte *et al.*, 2019). Ultimately, an owner's decision to take their animal home is something the veterinarian cannot do anything about other than attempt to change their mind. When these attempts fail, and the veterinarian observes an animal leaving the hospital to go home to suffer, this likely results in moral distress and contributes to the high rates of burnout in the veterinary profession (Siess *et al.*, 2015).

A further aim of the study was to determine whether attachment to the companion animal, as measured by the amount of comfort received from the companion animal, was related to the likelihood of approving a treatment plan for intensive hospitalization. It was hypothesized that the greater the attachment and therefore the greater the amount of comfort received from one's companion animal, the greater the likelihood of choosing to approve a treatment plan with intensive hospitalization would be. The amount of comfort received from the companion animal did not significantly predict the likelihood of approving the recommended treatment plan for hospitalization. This is likely due to the high skew in the scores ($M = 41.60$, Median $= 44.00$, $SD = 6.17$) towards the maximum possible score of 44. The owners in the sample were highly attached to their companion animal, therefore it is likely that the lack of variation in attachment resulted in the null result.

An additional aim of the study was to determine whether client satisfaction with the veterinary team is related to the likelihood of approving a treatment plan for intensive hospitalization. It was hypothesized that greater client satisfaction would result in a greater likelihood of choosing to approve a treatment plan with intensive hospitalization. As expected, greater client satisfaction with communication with the veterinarian significantly predicted a greater likelihood of approving the recommended treatment. Poor communication from health care providers has been reported as a common stressor among surrogate decision makers for human patients associated with low levels of confidence in the role (Butler and Degraff, 1996;

Hickman *et al.*, 2012; Majesko *et al.*, 2012; Torke *et al.*, 2012).

Results indicating that higher levels of satisfaction with communication from the veterinarian predicted a greater likelihood of approving the recommended treatment plan for hospitalization suggest that improved communication with the veterinarian may result in the owners feeling more confident in their role, specifically in their ability to make the "right" decision with regard to approving the recommended treatment plan, which many owners of companion animals with life threatening conditions struggle with (Bley, 2017). The significant majority of owners who did not approve the recommended treatment plan for hospitalization elected to take their animals home AMA and may have experienced distress decisional regret when their animal declined, placing them at higher risk for the development of negative psychological outcomes such as depression, anxiety, and PTSD (Jones *et al.*, 2004; Corrigan *et al.*, 2007; Wendler and Rid, 2011; Kross *et al.*, 2011; Abou-Mrad *et al.*, 2012; Nelson *et al.*, 2017; Pignatiello *et al.*, 2018). This finding is important in that poor communication from health care providers is a source of distress that surrogates report as a hindrance to their ability to make end-of-life decisions (Butler and Degraff, 1996; Hickman *et al.*, 2012; Majesko *et al.*, 2012; Torke *et al.*, 2012). This further suggests that interventions designed to improve communication by health care providers are worthwhile. Further supporting the need for greater training in communication in veterinary schools as veterinarians' abilities to have successful communications with owners of critically-ill companion animals will likely ease the burden of being a surrogate decision maker but may also result in better treatment of patients as well as reduced stressors on veterinarians.

Additionally, greater client satisfaction with their financial ability to pay for the recommended treatment significantly predicted a greater likelihood of approving the recommended treatment for intensive hospitalization. This result is not surprising as finances play a major role in veterinary medicine as the majority of pets are uninsured, requiring the vast majority of owners of companion animals to be able to pay a large amount of money on the spot (American Veterinary Medical Association, 2018; NAPHIA, 2021). In addition to the hurdle of being able to pay the large fee for hospitalization, all of the animals would need to be on several medications regularly and would need to have regular recheck examinations from the veterinary cardiologist. Additionally, the conditions experienced by the companion animals are chronic and terminal and, as such, the need for future hospitalization is inevitable (Keene *et al.*, 2019; Fuentes *et al.*, 2020). Recently, the American Veterinary Medical Association endorsed the active encouragement of owners of companion animals to obtain pet health insurance to help defray veterinary medical care costs in order to be able to provide high quality veterinary medical care (AVMA, 2021b).

General satisfaction, satisfaction with technical quality, interpersonal manner, time spent with the veterinarian, and accessibility and convenience did not significantly predict the decision to approve the recommended treatment. This is likely due to them all being highly rated with average scores of 4.31, 4.15, 4.46, 4.21, and 4.31 out of a maximum score of 5.00, respectively. The high ratings are not surprising as the hospital is a 24 hour multi-specialty and referral hospital and as such the equipment available is of high standard and the veterinarians were board-certified cardiologists with significant expertise. Consultations with the veterinary cardiologists are typically longer than a consultation with a primary veterinarian, it is likely that the consultations the owners had were longer than most appointments they have had with their primary veterinarians. The nature of the hospital being available 24-hours a day and 7 days a week likely explains the high rating for accessibility and convenience.

Limitations

The current study has potential limitations in that the sample consisted of owners of companion animals who were referred to see a veterinary cardiologist by their primary veterinarian, or by an emergency veterinarian, and agreed to a consultation. Owners of companion animals who declined to seek a consultation from a veterinary cardiologist or who euthanized prior to a consultation, were not captured. Additionally, the mean score for the Comfort from Companion Animals scale was very high, much higher than a previous sample of dog owners (Siess *et al.*, 2018b). This lack of variability likely affected its ability to serve as a predictor of the decision to treat the animal. Moreover, while our sample consisted of owners who reported nearly identical levels of attachment for dogs and cats, there may be differences in the typical levels of attachment to dogs and cats that would be captured in a more generalizable sample. Likewise, the age of companion animals may impact medical decisions, but was not a focus of the current study due to the nature of the disease processes in the sample. Additionally, the lack of variability in general satisfaction, technical quality, interpersonal manner, time spent with the veterinarian, and accessibility and convenience are likely why they were not significant predictors of decision to approve the recommended treatment. A replication of the study in a general veterinary practice setting may include more variability in the owners of companion animals in all respects and as such may result in significant differences in those components of patient satisfaction. Additionally, socioeconomic status and ethnicity were not included in the demographic variables measured limiting the generalizability of the results. Another potential limitation is that there was no data collected on past experiences with critically-ill companion animals which may impact the way in which owners of companion animals make end-of-life decisions for their current companion animals. Further, as this was the first study to examine these effects, we did not experimentally control for the ways in which prognoses and quality of life were presented to owners, which can have an impact on owners' perception of prognoses.

Conclusion

With the continued advancement of veterinary medicine and the inherent role of owners of companion animals as surrogate decision makers, more people will find themselves in the position of difficult decision making situations that are compounded with the threat of loss of a beloved companion animal. A more comprehensive understanding of the way in which owners of companion animals perceive high risk prognostic information about their companion animal, the role of attachment, and how factors such as optimism and quality of life factor into one's decision to pursue diagnostics, treat chronic diseases, or elect for euthanasia is crucial.

It is important to note that owners of companion animals, employ an optimistic bias for their animals' chance of survival when it is low as indicated by a veterinarian. This strongly supports findings that surrogates have a tendency to have an inaccurate understanding of their animals' risk of death when it is high. This is likely due to the strong attachment between an owner and a companion animal and likely arises as a form of self-protection from the threat of imminent loss. It is important to note that these individuals are likely at greater risk of experiencing high levels of distress in the event of the animals' death. Having established local referral locations for psychological counseling and support groups that can easily be provided at the time of diagnosis, may help to mitigate the distress that these individuals experience. The optimistic bias did not extend to the evaluation of the companion animals' quality of life, further suggesting the optimistic bias is likely in response to the threat of loss. The findings provide evidence for the notion that improved communication from veterinarians is necessary to reduce the burden on owners in their role as surrogate decision makers as well as for the treatment of their animals. Future research should be conducted to examine the specific aspects of communication that are most effective in improving owner satisfaction with communication.

References

Abou-Mrad, F., Mourad, C. and Najem, C. (2012) Depressive symptoms among surrogate decision makers in Lebanese ICUs. *Functional Neurology* 27(2), 95–99.

Ainsworth, M.D.S., Blehar, M.C., Waters, E. and Wall, S.N. (2015) *Patterns of Attachment: A Psychological Study of the Strange Situation*, 1st ed. Psychology Press. DOI: 10.4324/9780203758045.

Allen, K., Blascovich, J. and Mendes, W.B. (2002) Cardiovascular reactivity in the presence of pets, friends, and spouses: The truth about cats and dogs. *Psychosomatic Medicine* 64(5), 727–739. DOI: 10.1097/01.PSY.0000024236.11538.41.

American Veterinary Medical Association (2018) *2017-2018 Pet ownership and demographics sourcebook*. Available at: https://avma.org/resources-tools/reports-statistics

American Veterinary Medical Association (2021a) *Pet health insurance*. Available at: https://avma.org/resources-tools/avma-policies/pet-health-insurance

American Veterinary Medical Association (2021b) *Pet health insurance: Good for pets, good for practices*. Available at: https://avma.org/resources-tools/practice-management/pet-health-insurance-good-pets-good-practices

Atkins, C.E. and Häggström, J. (2012) Pharmacologic management of myxomatous mitral valve disease in dogs. *Journal of Veterinary Cardiology* 14(1), 165–184. DOI: 10.1016/j.jvc.2012.02.002.

Bley, C.R. (2017) Principles for ethical treatment decision-making in veterinary oncology. *Veterinary and Comparative Oncology* 16(2), 171–177. DOI: 10.111/vco.12347.

Bussolari, C.J., Habarth, J., Katz, R., Phillips, S., Carmack, B. *et al.* (2018) The euthanasia decision-making process: A qualitative exploration of bereaved companion animal owners. *Bereavement Care* 37(3), 101–108. DOI: 10.1080/02682621.2018.1542571.

Butler, C. and Degraff, P.S. (1996) Helping during pet loss and bereavement. *Veterinary Quarterly* 18(sup1), 58–60. DOI: 10.1080/01652176.1996.9694687.

Case, D. (1988) Survey of expectations among clients of three small animal clinics. *Journal of the American Veterinary Medical Association* 192(4), 498–502.

Coe, J.B., Adams, C.L. and Bonnett, B.N. (2008) A focus group study of veterinarians' and pet owners' perceptions of veterinarian-client communication in companion animal practice. *Journal of the American Veterinary Medical Association* 233(7), 1072–1080.

Corrigan, I., Samuelson, K.A., Fridlund, B. and Thome, B. (2007) The meaning of posttraumatic stress-reactions following critical illness or injury and intensive care treatment. *Intensive Critical Care Nursing* 23(4), 206–215. DOI: 10.1016/j.iccn.2007.01.004.

Coy, A.E. and Green, J.D. (2018) Treating pets well: The role of attachment anxiety and avoidance. *Human Animal Interaction Bulletin* 6(1), 14–31.

Cusack, O. (1988) *Pets and mental health*. Haworth Press, New York.

Eckerd, L.M., Barnett, J.E. and Jett-Dias, L. (2016) Grief following pet and human loss: Closeness is key. *Death Studies* 40(5), 275–282. DOI: 10.1080/07481187.2016.1139014.

Ettinger, S.L., Feldman, E.C. and Côté, E. (2017) *Textbook of Veterinary Internal Medicine: Diseases of the Dog and the Cat*. Elsevier.

Faul, F., Erdfelder, E., Lang, A.G. and Buchner, A. (2007) G*Power 3: A flexible statistical power analysis program for the social, behavioral, and biomedical sciences. *Behavior Research Methods* 39(2), 175–191. DOI: 10.3758/bf03193146.

Ferasin, L. and DeFrancesco, T. (2015) Management of acute heart failure in cats. *Journal of Veterinary Cardiology* 17(Suppl. 1), S173–189. DOI: 10.1016/j.jvc.2015.09.007.

Fogle, B. and Abrahamson, D. (1990) A survey of the attitudes and feelings of practicing veterinarians. *Anthrozoos* 3(3), 143–150. DOI: 10.2752/089279390787057568.

Fuentes, V.L., Abbott, J., Chetboul, V., Côté, E., Fox, P.R. *et al.* (2020) ACVIM consensus statement guidelines for the classification, diagnosis, and management of cardiomyopathies in cats. *Journal of Veterinary Internal Medicine* 34(3), 1062–1077. DOI: 10.1111/jvim.15745.

Geisler, A.M. (2004) Companion animals in palliative care: Stories from the bedside. *American Journal of Hospice & Palliative Medicine* 21(4), 285–288. DOI: 10.1177/104990910402100411.

Häggström, J., Boswood, A., O'Grady, M., Jöns, O., Smith, S. *et al.* (2008) Effect of pimobendan or benazepril hydrochloride on survival times in dogs with congestive heart failure caused by naturally occurring myxomatous mitral valve disease: The QUEST study. *Journal of Veterinary Internal Medicine* 22(5), 1124–1135. DOI: 10.1111/j.1939-1676.2008.0150.x.

Hall, M.J., Ng, A., Ursano, R.J., Holloway, H., Fullerton, C. *et al.* (2004) Psychological impact of the animal-human bond in disaster preparedness and response. *Journal of Psychiatric Practice* 10(6), 368–374. DOI: 10.1097/00131746-200411000-00005.

Hazan, C. and Shaver, P. (1987) Romantic love conceptualized as an attachment process. *Journal of Personality and Social Psychology* 52(3), 511–524. DOI: 10.1037/0022-3514.52.3.511.

Hickman, R.L., Jr, Daly, B.J. and Lee, E. (2012) Decisional conflict and regret: Consequences of surrogate decision making for the chronically critically ill. *Applied Nursing Research* 25(4), 271–275. DOI: 10.1016/j.apnr.2011.03.003.

Hillen, M.A., de Haes, H.C.J.M. and Smets, E.M.A. (2011) Cancer patients' trust in their physician-a review. *Psycho-Oncology* 20(3), 227–241. DOI: 10.1002/pon.1745.

Jerant, A., Fenton, J.J., Bertakis, K.D. and Franks, P. (2014) Satisfaction with health care providers and preventive care adherence: A national study. *Medical Care* 52(1), 78–85. DOI: 10.1097/MLR.0000000000000021.

Jones, C., Skirrow, P., Griffiths, R.D., Humphris, G., Ingleby, S. *et al.* (2004) Post-traumatic stress disorder-related symptoms in relatives of patients following intensive care. *Intensive Care Medicine* 30(3), 456–460. DOI: 10.1007/s00134-003-2149-5.

Kappes, A., Faber, N.S., Kahane, G., Savulescu, J. and Crockett, M.J. (2018) Concern for others leads to vicarious optimism. *Psychological Science* 29(3), 379–389. DOI: 10.1177/0956797617737129.

Keene, B.W., Atkins, C.E., Bonagura, J.D., Fox, P.R., Häggström, J. *et al.* (2019) ACVIM consensus guidelines for the diagnosis and treatment of myxomatous mitral valve disease in dogs. *Journal of Veterinary Internal Medicine* 33(3), 1127–1140. DOI: 10.1111/jvim.15488.

Kross, E.K., Engelberg, R.A., Gries, C.J., Nielsen, E.L., Zatzick, D. *et al.* (2011) ICU care associated with symptoms of depression and posttraumatic stress disorder among family members of patients who die in the ICU. *Chest* 139(4), 795–801. DOI: 10.1378/chest.10-0652.

Kurdek, L.A. (2008) Pet dogs as attachment figures. *Journal of Social and Personal Relationships* 25(2), 247–266. DOI: 10.1177/0265407507087958.

Lagoni, L., Butler, C. and Hetts, S. (1994) *The Human-Animal Bond and Grief*. Saunders.

Lau, E. (2012) *Veterinary visits up but pet ownership down*. Available at: http://news.vin.com/VINNews.aspx?articleId=24063

Lee, S.A. (2020) Does the DSM-5 grief disorder apply to owners of deceased pets? A psychometric study of impairment during pet loss. *Psychiatry Research* 285, 112800. DOI: 10.1016/j.psychres.2020.112800.

Lummis, M., Marchitelli, B. and Shearer, T. (2020) Difficult conversation in veterinary end-of-life care. *Veterinary Clinics of North America: Small Animal Practice* 50(3), 607–616. DOI: 10.1016/j.cvsm.2019.12.009.

Majesko, A., Hong, S.Y., Weissfeld, L. and White, D.B. (2012) Identifying family members who may struggle in the role of surrogate decision maker. *Critical Care Medicine* 40(8), 2281–2286. DOI: 10.1097/CCM.0b013e3182533317.

Marchitelli, B., Shearer, T. and Cook, C. (2020) Factors contributing to the decision to euthanize. *Veterinary Clinics of North America: Small Animal Practice* 50(3), 573–589. DOI: 10.1016/j.cvsm.2019.12.007.

Marshall, G.N. and Hays, R.D. (1994) *The Patient Satisfaction Questionnaire Short Form (PSQ-18)*. RAND.

Matte, A.R., Khosa, D.K., Coe, J.B. and Meehan, M.P. (2019) Impacts of the process and decision-making around companion animal euthanasia on veterinary wellbeing. *The Veterinary Record* 185(15), 480. DOI: 10.1136/vr.105540.

McConnell, A.R., Brown, C.M., Shoda, T.M., Stayton, L.E. and Martin, C.E. (2011) Friends with benefits: On the positive consequences of pet ownership. *Journal of Personality and Social Psychology* 101(6), 1239–1252. DOI: 10.1037/a0024506.

McNicholas, J. and Collis, G.M. (1995) The end of a relationship: Coping with pet loss. In: Robinson, I. (ed.) *The Waltham Book of Human-Animal Interaction: Benefits and Responsibilities of Pet Ownership*. Pergamon, pp. 127–143.

McNicholas, J., Gilbey, A., Rennie, A., Ahmedzai, S., Dono, J.-A. *et al.* (2005) Pet ownership and human health: A brief review of evidence and issues. *British Medical Journal* 331(7527), 1252–1254. DOI: 10.1136/bmj.331.7527.1252.

Miaoulis, G., Jr, Gutman, J. and Snow, M.M. (2009) Closing the gap: The patient-physician disconnect. *Health Marketing Quarterly* 26(1), 56–68. DOI: 10.1080/07359680802473547.

Milberg, A. and Friedrichsen, M. (2017) Attachment figures when death is approaching: A study applying attachment theory to adult patients' and family members' experiences during palliative home care. *Supportive Care in Cancer* 25(7), 2267–2274. DOI: 10.1007/s00520-017-3634-7.

Moyer, A., Siess, S. and Bhinder, S. (2017) How are non-numerical prognostic statements interpreted and are they subject to positive bias. *BMJ Supportive & Palliative Care* 7(4). DOI: 10.1136/bmjspcare-2017-001331.

Nelson, J.E., Hanson, L.C., Keller, K.L., Carson, S.S., Cox, C.E. *et al.* (2017) The voice of surrogate decision-makers: Family responses to prognostic information in chronic critical illness. *American Journal of Respiratory and Critical Care Medicine* 196(7), 864–872. DOI: 10.1164/rccm.201701-0201OC.

Netzer, G. and Sullivan, D.R. (2014) Recognizing, naming, and measuring a family intensive care unit syndrome. *Annals of the American Thoracic Society* 11(3), 435–441. DOI: 10.1513/AnnalsATS.201309-308OT.

Norem, J.K. and Cantor, N. (1986) Defensive pessimism: Harnessing anxiety as motivation. *Journal of Personality and Social Psychology* 51(6), 1208–1217. DOI: 10.1037/0022-3514.51.6.1208.

North American Pet Health Insurance Association (2021) *Pet Insurance in North America: State of the Industry*. Available at: https://naphia.org/industry-data

Odendaal, J.S. and Meintjes, R.A. (2003) Neurophysiological correlates of affiliative behaviour between humans and dogs. *Veterinary Journal* 165(3), 296–301. DOI: 10.1016/s1090-0233(02)00237-x.

Park, R. and Royal, K. (2020) A national survey of companion animal owners' self-reported methods of coping following euthanasia. *Veterinary Sciences* 7(3), 89. DOI: 10.3390/vetsci7030089.

Peacock, J., Chur-Hansen, A. and Winefield, H. (2012) Mental health implications of human attachment to companion animals. *Journal of Clinical Psychology* 68(3), 292–303. DOI: 10.1002/jclp.20866.

Pignatiello, G., Hickman, R.L., Jr and Hetland, B. (2018) End-of-life decision support in the ICU: Where are we now? *Western Journal of Nursing Research* 40(1), 84–120. DOI: 10.1177/0193945916676542.

Prato-Previde, E., Fallani, G. and Valsecchi, P. (2006) Gender differences in owners interacting with pet dogs: An observational study. *Ethology* 112(1), 64–73. DOI: 10.1111/j.1439-0310.2006.01123.x.

Ptacek, J.T. and Eberhardt, T.L. (1996) Breaking bad news. A review of the literature. *The Journal of the American Medical Association* 276(6), 496–502.

Ptacek, J.T., Leonard, K. and McKee, T.L. (2004) I've got some bad news...': Veterinarians' recollections of communicating bad news to clients. *Journal of Applied Social Psychology* 34(2), 366–390. DOI: 10.1111/j.1559-1816.2004.tb02552.x.

Ptacek, J.T., Fries, E.A., Eberhardt, T.L. and Ptacek, J.J. (1999) Breaking bad news to patients: physicians' perceptions of the process. *Supportive Care in Cancer* 7(3), 113–120. DOI: 10.1007/s005200050240.

Rollin, B.E. (2011) Euthanasia, moral stress, and chronic illness in veterinary medicine. *Veterinary Clinics of North America Small Animal Practice* 41(3), 651–659. DOI: 10.1016/j.cvsm.2011.03.005.

Rothman, A., Klein, W. and Weinstein, N. (1996) Absolute and relative biases in estimations of personal risk. *Journal of Applied Social Psychology* 26(14), 1213–1236. DOI: 10.1111/j.1559-1816.1996.tb01778.x.

Schoenthaler, A., Kalet, A., Nicholson, J. and Lipkin, M., Jr (2014) Does improving patient-practitioner communication improve clinical outcomes in patients with cardiovascular diseases? A systematic review of the evidence. *Patient Education and Counseling* 96(1), 3–12. DOI: 10.1016/j.pec.2014.04.006.

Shepperd, J.A., Klein, W.M.P., Waters, E.A. and Weinstein, N.D. (2013) Taking stock of unrealistic optimism. *Perspectives on Psychological Science* 8(4), 395–411. DOI: 10.1177/1745691613485247.

Shepperd, J.A., Waters, E., Weinstein, N.D. and Klein, W.M. (2015) A primer on unrealistic optimism. *Current Directions in Psychological Science* 24(3), 232–237. DOI: 10.1177/0963721414568341.

Siess, S., Marziliano, A., Maddaloni, J. and Moyer, A. (2014) Optimistic bias in interpreting poor prognoses predicts hypothetical end-of-life decision making. *Annals of Behavioral Medicine* 47, S283–S283.

Siess, S., Marziliano, A., Sarma, E.A., Sikorski, L.E. and Moyer, A. (2015) Why psychology matters in veterinary medicine. *Topics in Companion Animal Medicine* 30(2), 43–47. DOI: 10.1053/j.tcam.2015.05.001.

Siess, S., Paone, N. and Moyer, A. (2018a) The effect of severity of prognosis and framing on an optimistic bias for non-numerical prognoses in the veterinary setting. *Annals of Behavioral Medicine* 52, S55.

Siess, S., Sikorski, L. and Moyer, A. (2018b) Optimistic bias for negative prognostic information predicts hypothetical canine B-cell lymphoma treatment decision making. *Annals of Behavioral Medicine* 52, S54.

Spernak, S.M., Moore, P.J. and Hamm, L.F. (2007) Depression, constructive thinking and patient satisfaction in cardiac treatment adherence. *Psychology, Health & Medicine* 12(2), 172–189. DOI: 10.1080/10556790500465631.

Spitznagel, M.B. and Carlson, M.D. (2019) Caregiver burden and veterinary client well-being. *Veterinary Clinics of North America: Small Animal Practice* 49(3), 431–444. DOI: 10.1016/j.cvsm.2019.01.008.

Spitznagel, M.B., Ben-Porath, Y.S., Rishniw, M., Kogan, L.R. and Carlson, M.D. (2019a) Development and validation of a burden transfer inventory for predicting veterinarian stress related to client behavior. *Journal of the American Veterinary Medical Association* 254(1), 133–144. DOI: 10.2460/javma.254.1.133.

Spitznagel, M.B., Cox, M.D., Jacobson, D.M., Albers, A.L. and Carlson, M.D. (2019b) Assessment of caregiver burden and associations with psychosocial function, veterinary service use, and factors related to treatment plan adherence among owners of dogs and cats. *Journal of the American Veterinary Medical Association* 254(1), 124–132. DOI: 10.2460/javma.254.1.124.

Spitznagel, M.B., Marchitelli, B., Gardner, M. and Carlson, M.D. (2020) Euthanasia from the veterinary client's perspective: Psychosocial contributors to euthanasia decision making. *Veterinary Clinics of North America: Small Animal Practice* 50(3), 591–605. DOI: 10.1016/j.cvsm.2019.12.008.

Sweeny, K. and Shepperd, J.A. (2007) Do people brace sensibly? Risk judgments and event likelihood. *Personality and Social Psychology Bulletin* 33(8), 1064–1075. DOI: 10.1177/0146167207301024.

Torke, A.M., Petronio, S., Sachs, G.A., Helft, P.R. and Purnell, C. (2012) A conceptual model of the role of communication in surrogate decision making for hospitalized adults. *Patient Education and Counseling* 87(1), 54–61. DOI: 10.1016/j.pec.2011.07.027.

Tversky, A. (1977) Features of similarity. *Psychological Review* 84(4), 327–352.

Tyler, J.M. and Rosier, J.G. (2009) Examining self-presentation as a motivational explanation for comparative optimism. *Journal of Personality and Social Psychology* 97(4), 716–727. DOI: 10.1037/a0016231.

Uccheddu, S., Cataldo, L., Albertini, M., Coren, S., Graça Pereira, G. *et al.* (2019) Pet humanisation and related grief: Development and validation of a structured questionnaire instrument to evaluate grief in people who lost a companion dog. *Animals* 9(11), 933. DOI: 10.3390/ani9110933.

Uechi, M. (2012) Mitral valve repair in dogs. *Journal of Veterinary Cardiology* 14(1), 185–192. DOI: 10.1016/j.jvc.2012.01.004.

Verceles, A.C., Corwin, D.S., Afshar, M., Friedman, E.B., McCurdy, M.T. *et al.* (2014) Half of the family members of critically ill patients experience excessive daytime sleepiness. *Intensive Care Medicine* 40(8), 1124–1131. DOI: 10.1007/s00134-014-3347-z.

Waters, E.A., Klein, W.M.P., Moser, R.P., Yu, M., Waldron, W.R. *et al.* (2011) Correlates of unrealistic risk beliefs in a nationally representative sample. *Journal of Behavioral Medicine* 34(3), 225–235. DOI: 10.1007/s10865-010-9303-7.

Weinstein, N.D. (1980) Unrealistic optimism about future life events. *Journal of Personality and Social Psychology* 39(5), 806–820. DOI: 10.1037/0022-3514.39.5.806.

Zasloff, R.L. (1996) Measuring attachment to companion animals: A dog is not a cat is not a bird. *Applied Animal Behaviour Science* 47(1–2), 43–48. DOI: 10.1016/0168-1591(95)01009-2.

Wendler, D. and Rid, A. (2011) Systematic review: The effect on surrogates of making treatment decisions for others. *Annals of Internal Medicine* 154(5), 336–346. DOI: 10.7326/0003-4819-154-5-201103010-00008.

Zasloff, R.L. and Kidd, A.H. (1994) Loneliness and pet ownership among single women. *Psychological Reports* 75(2), 747–752. DOI: 10.2466/pr0.1994.75.2.747.

Zier, L.S., Sottile, P.D., Hong, S.Y., Weissfield, L.A. and White, D.B. (2012) Surrogate decision makers' interpretation of prognostic information: A mixed-methods study. *Annals of Internal Medicine* 156(5), 360–366. DOI: 10.7326/0003-4819-156-5-201203060-00008.

Zilcha-Mano, S., Mikulincer, M. and Shaver, P.R. (2011) An attachment perspective on human–pet relationships: Conceptualization and assessment of pet attachment orientations. *Journal of Research in Personality* 45(5), 345–357. DOI: 10.1016/j.jrp.2011.04.00.

9 Overcoming the Social Stigma of Losing a Pet: Considerations for Counseling Professionals

Michelle Kay Crossley[1]* and Colleen Rolland[2]

[1]Counseling, Educational Leadership, and School Psychology, Rhode Island College, RI, USA; [2]Association for Pet Loss and Bereavement, Albany, NY

Abstract

During the COVID-19 pandemic, individuals found themselves spending more time with their pets and relied on them to maintain normalcy and provide security during isolation. Pets play a significant role in the lives of their caregivers, taking on different attachment roles depending on the needs of the individual. Grieving the death of a pet continues to be disenfranchised in society. Perceptions of judgment can lead individuals to grieve the loss without social support. The present review builds on research in the field of pet loss and human bereavement and factors in the impact of the COVID-19 pandemic on human–animal attachment. A goal of the present review is to provide counselors with perspectives to consider in their practice when working with clients who have attachments to their companion animals and to acknowledge the therapeutic benefits of working through the grief process to resolution as a way to continue the bond with a deceased pet.

Keywords: pet loss, pet loss and human bereavement, pet grief, pet loss counseling, pet loss grief support, disenfranchised grief, attachment roles, COVID-19

Overcoming the Social Stigma of Losing a Pet: Considerations for Counseling Professionals

The stigma associated with openly grieving a loss can complicate the healing process. With life comes death and therefore, it is reasonable to expect that clients will come in to discuss important losses in therapy sessions, especially during the COVID-19 pandemic. While empathy may come more naturally when discussing human loss, there are other types of loss that are not acknowledged or given a similar amount of attention by society. Grief due to these socially unendorsed losses is referred to as disenfranchised grief and can include death by suicide, a lost pregnancy/miscarriage, and death from AIDS (Lenhardt, 1997) in addition to the death of a pet (Attig, 2004; Cordaro, 2012; Sife, 2014). Doka (2008) defined disenfranchised grief as a grief reaction after a loss that is important to the individual though unacknowledged as important enough to grieve or ask for social support. When relationships are not valued by society, individuals are more likely to experience disenfranchised grief after a loss that cannot be resolved and may become complicated grief. It is important for counselors to recognize their

*Corresponding author: mcrossley@ric.edu

own biases regarding the types of losses that are worth an empathetic response as individuals are better able to heal from a loss through social support and recognition (Cordaro, 2012). This article will focus specifically on the complex nature of losing a pet based on the roles ascribed to the animal companion and the importance of resolving grief through individuals openly seeking support as they would a human death.

According to the American Veterinary Medical Association (2018), in the United States, 57% of households owned a pet with 66% owning more than one companion animal. Of the individuals surveyed, approximately 80% consider their pets to be family members, 17% consider them to be a companion and only 3% consider them property. The data indicate that more individuals were choosing companion animals even before the pandemic; a poll by the American Society for Prevention of Cruelty to Animals (American Society for the Prevention of Cruelty to Animals, 2021) noted that 19% of individuals acquired a cat or dog during the pandemic. With the increase of individuals and families obtaining a companion animal, it is expected that as we move away from remote work and companion animals age, we will need to discuss pet loss more than ever before.

The pet loss grief response can be exacerbated and intensified by a multitude of factors (Gosse and Barnes, 1994), especially as many pet owners ascribe human characteristics to their pets (Field *et al.*, 2009). The attachment bond and meanings of the human–animal relationship create complexities in the loss of the companion animal, and the grieving that follows this loss, as it can be as traumatic as the grief one experiences from the loss of a family member (Brown *et al.*, 1996; Field *et al.*, 2009) or even more in some cases than a human (Sife, 2014; Eckerd *et al.*, 2016). One factor that complicates one's psychological well-being after this loss is the belief of others that pets are not worthy of being grieved over because a companion animal may be viewed as replaceable, whereas a human is not (Crossley, 2013; Sife, 2014). The stigma associated with pet loss, compounded by the feeling of losing a part of the family, can lead individuals to avoid openly grieving the loss of their companion animals and can intensify symptoms of depression (Sife, 2014). The major goals of this review are to provide counselors with an aspect to consider in their therapeutic work with clients dealing with grief and loss, present different factors that may impact how one grieves the loss of a pet, and discuss considerations for counseling that can be utilized to foster a supportive and non-judgmental space where clients' expressions of grief are validated.

Understanding pet loss

Defining the human–animal bond and how different factors may impact such a bond can inform a counselor's therapeutic response to clients who experience this type of loss. The human–animal bond can be simply stated as the interaction that a human has with a non-human animal and the nature of the relationship between the human and animal (Beck and Katcher, 2003). Given this bond, pets can provide emotional attachment bonds that help promote security and well-being (Sharkin and Knox, 2003; Sife, 2014). As with many other relationships, it is believed that one's level of attachment can impact the grief that one experiences following the loss of an important figure (Gosse and Barnes, 1994; Brown *et al.*, 1996; Margolies, 1999; Podrazik *et al.*, 2000; Field *et al.*, 2009; Sife, 2014). Pets may also serve a function to individuals whose interpersonal relationships are lower in quality and therefore, the bond formed between the individual and the pet can be a strong one, where the pets occupy traditional human roles because they evoke similar patterns of emotions for the human (Field *et al.*, 2009; Sife, 2014).

Since humans can form an attachment bond with an animal that is similar to one with a human, the grieving process can also be seen as similar. Losing a pet can be an isolating experience for many. Not only is the individual stressed and possibly depressed, but many individuals do not feel comfortable openly grieving the loss of their pet due to societal pressure, even more so for males (Field *et al.*, 2009; Crossley, 2013; Sife, 2014). The literature points to varying levels of grief experienced by individuals. Researchers have attempted to answer the question as to why this phenomenon occurs in relation to the strength of attachment of pet owners (Gosse and

Barnes, 1994; Brown *et al.*, 1996; Margolies, 1999; Podrazik *et al.*, 2000; Field *et al.*, 2009).

It is believed that the more an individual feels attached to their companion animal, the more severe the grieving process will be (Sife, 2014). Counselors are tasked with understanding the unique relationship between clients and their companion animals (Barton-Ross and Baron-Sorenson, 2007; Hess-Holden *et al.*, 2017). For counselors who have not had this type of bond with a pet, there may be biases about recovering from this type of disenfranchised grief; these biases must be explored and bracketed before working with a client grieving from pet loss. Without providing time and space to heal and resolve the pain associated with the death of a pet, a counselor can cause more pain to the client by not understanding or honoring the depth of the bond shared between the client and the pet (Sife, 2014). The distress that one can experience secondary to the loss of a companion animal can be intense, and it is critical to serving these clients in the same manner that we would have had they been grieving the loss of a human.

Background of Pet Loss and Human Bereavement

The statistics on pet ownership (American Veterinary Medical Association, 2018) provide evidence that the number of households that are acquiring companion animals continues to increase and has significantly increased with required isolation due to COVID-19 (American Society for the Prevention of Cruelty to Animals, 2021). As the shift to remote work and quarantine occurred, the relationship and time spent with companion animals increased (Bussolari *et al.*, 2021). While many pet owners already considered their companion animal a part of the family, and experienced serious grief when they died (Gosse and Barnes, 1994; Brown *et al.*, 1996; Wrobel and Dye, 2003; Dunn *et al.*, 2005; Pointon, 2006; Hunt *et al.*, 2008; Field *et al.*, 2009; Walsh, 2009a) given the length of the "new normal" since the pandemic began, we can expect to see more reports of intense grief as individuals' pets die. Social norms of grieving impact how an individual will mourn the death of their companion animal if they feel comfortable openly mourning them at all (Field *et al.*, 2009). Resolving loss in isolation or without support can intensify strong depressive feelings for the bereaved (Cordaro, 2012). Having a safe space to discuss the meanings associated with the companion-animal relationship is beneficial for moving through the loss in a supportive environment, leading to the resolution of the pain of the loss.

Findings from companion animal attachment research over the past 30 years suggest that individuals do form attachment bonds with their pets (Barton-Ross and Baron-Sorenson, 2007). Bowlby's (1969) work acknowledged that when attachments are no longer available, a certain level of distress may be expected. Given that companion animals have a shorter life expectancy than humans, it is not uncommon for the death of a companion animal to not only be the first encounter one has with death but is also something that can happen multiple times in one's lifetime (Sife, 2014). The grieving process is an important experience that one must face when the death of an important relationship occurs and a factor that has been found to impact this process is one's level of attachment (Bowlby, 1969; Bowlby, 1982). Researchers have investigated if attachment theory can also be used as a predictor for the grieving process of losing a companion animal (Gosse and Barnes, 1994; Brown *et al.*, 1996; Margolies, 1999; Podrazik *et al.*, 2000; Field *et al.*, 2009) and the findings have suggested that the stronger the attachment to companion animals, the more severe the grieving process will be parallelling findings of grief associated with losing a human (Eckerd *et al.*, 2016). Understanding a client's strength of attachment to a companion animal can equip counselors with a hypothesis of how devastating a change in the relationship will be in the future.

Attachment and loss

Much of what is understood about the reaction to the loss of an important companion animal bond is informed by literature about attachment and grief. Attachment theory describes an emotional bond to another person and explains the connectedness between human beings (Bowlby, 1969; Bowlby, 1973; Bowlby, 1980). These bonds are typically formed in the earlier years between children and their caregivers and can have a great impact on fostering secure relationships throughout the lifespan. Attachment, as it was originally studied, described how an individual will navigate their environment and relationships with other individuals (anxiously, securely, or avoidantly) based on their perceptions of safety and security in that environment. Researchers have linked attachment theory to the relationship one has with their companion animal (Gosse and Barnes, 1994; Brown *et al.*, 1996; Margolies, 1999; Podrazik *et al.*, 2000; Field *et al.*, 2009) as well as to the nature of the relationship and reasons for pet ownership (Sharkin and Knox, 2003; Pointon, 2006). Investigators have attempted to determine if the type of attachment style (Field *et al.*, 2009) or the strength of attachment bond (Gosse and Barnes, 1994; Brown *et al.*, 1996; Serpell, 1996; Wrobel and Dye, 2003; Field *et al.*, 2009; Walsh, 2009a) of individuals in relation to the death of their companion animals can effectively determine the level of stress and grief experienced. The findings suggest that the stronger the attachment bond and role of the companion animal, the more devastating the loss of the pet will be for the owner.

Bowlby's work on attachment posited that as certain attachments end there would be an imbalance in perceptions of safety within environments (Bowlby, 1980); humans work to maintain these relationships to live in balance and with safety in mind (Zentella, 2009). The understanding that life is finite and reasonable consequences can be expected after an important relationship is lost, be it by death or other types of loss (Sife, 2014; Applebaum *et al.*, 2020) is helpful in our understanding of how clients will react to the end of the relationship. The early study of death and dying has provided pet loss professionals with a basis for understanding how one will respond to the death of a companion animal. Grief is a response that one experiences after a major loss, or perhaps death. The Kübler-Ross model was created as a way to understand and cope with dying (Burglass, 2010) and describes five stages that one will encounter when experiencing a loss: *denial, anger, bargaining, depression, and acceptance.* These stages do not always happen in that order and not every individual who experiences a loss will encounter each stage. The time one spends in a particular stage is not consistent either; individual differences cause the process to differ across grieving persons. This model can be used in relation to an emotional response to trauma and is not necessarily and exclusively related to death. Some say that the loss or death of a companion animal can evoke the five stages of grief that also surface secondarily to the loss of an individual (Brown *et al.*, 1996; Field *et al.*, 2009).

There are many specific pet loss models of grief that have been developed since Kübler-Ross' work, just as other models of grief and mourning have been applied to pet loss. Cordaro (2012) work provides an overview of not only Kübler-Ross' model but also loss adaptation models (the dual-process model and adaptive grieving styles) in an effort to conceptualize pet loss and grief through a thorough application of the models to this specific type of disenfranchised grief. Having a basis for understanding ways in which individuals may process their grief provides opportunities for others to develop theories specific to pet loss. While many of the models overlap with previously mentioned models of grief and loss, they present factors unique to the experiences of an individual who is tasked with keeping their companion animal safe.

Models specific to pet loss arrive at similar ideas about the processes one may go through soon after a loss. One model that presents the grief process as a cycle was developed by Blue Cross for Pets in the U.K. (D. James, personal communication, March 8, 2021). The Blue Cross for Pets Grief Cycle starts with *anticipatory grief* where expressions of shock and denial are common; this type of grief is difficult as individuals are preparing for something that will be painful rather than dealing with the pain of something that has already happened. Self-blame is common in *responsibility grief*; here individuals hover in the mental space of what more they could have done to extend the time with their pet. *Anger and bargaining* are usually directed at the veterinary professionals providing care during this difficult time. Attention to physical symptoms comes at the onset of *depression, reflection, and loneliness*. This is also a time when an individual is adapting to a new lifestyle, one that is a little lonelier with more time to honor the memories of the deceased. Once through these stages, individuals will begin to socialize more by making *new beginnings* and move toward deeper healing through fostering *acceptance and hope*.

Other pet loss models represent stage models similar to Kübler-Ross' work. Barton-Ross and Baron-Sorenson (2007) describe their model to include the stages of *denial, bargaining, anger, guilt, sorrow,* and *resolution*. The Stages of Bereavement (Sife, 2014) describe similar stages and processes that serve as a roadmap for what an individual may experience after the loss of a pet. Sife's stages of pet loss include *shock, disbelief and denial, anger, alienation and distancing, guilt, depression, and resolution*. While Sife is credited for developing this model in the early 1990s it has had revisions along the way. One particular note about these models is that the language moves away from closure and more toward a resolution of the grief associated with the death of a companion animal. Through resolution, individuals are able to reorganize a relationship with the deceased (Field, 2008) and find comfort through displaying continuing bond expressions (Packman *et al.*, 2011).

Understanding Pet Loss Grief

Conceptualizing how an individual will grieve a loss depending on the strength of their attachment is helpful in counseling. Pets can play a significant role in the lives of their caregivers; especially more so since the start of the pandemic. The onset of the pandemic and the need for quarantine and isolation from other humans changed the amount of time that people were spending with their companion animals, therefore intensifying the relationship and bond (Applebaum *et al.*, 2020; Bussolari *et al.*, 2021). Past research has shown that some people believe that their companion animals serve as a support system in their lives (Flom, 2005; Schneider, 2005; Murphy, 2006; Pointon, 2006; Hara, 2007; Watt and Pachana, 2007;), and others consider their pets to be a member of the family (Murphy, 2006; Hara, 2007; Knight and Edwards, 2008; Walsh, 2009b). The role that the companion animal serves for an individual can impact the intensity in which one grieves when the relationship ends or changes in some way.

Companion animal roles

The COVID-19 pandemic has contributed to a change not only in the number of people adopting new pets (American Society for the Prevention of Cruelty to Animals, 2021) but also in the amount of time that individuals spent with their pets (Bussolari *et al.*, 2021). As some individuals shifted to remote work and school and others lost their jobs, pets served a different role; they were now co-workers and full-time companions. Pets are known to be therapeutic to their caregivers, offering psychological, physical, and social well-being (Murphy, 2006; Pointon, 2006). During this unprecedented time, individuals were spending more time with their pets while also navigating threats to their own safety as well as physical and mental health (Bussolari *et al.*, 2021; Mueller *et al.*, 2021). The responsibility of pet ownership helped to mitigate loneliness for some by allowing for a sense of normalcy by taking the pet for a walk (Lee *et al.*, 2022) and the increase in time spent at home strengthened the bond with their pets (Bussolari *et al.*, 2021). While most of the research post-pandemic points to the positive impact of living with pets has had on individuals, it has also contributed to individuals refusing medical care due to the concern of what will happen to the pet if the owner dies (Applebaum *et al.*, 2020).

A dual caregiver relationship between companion animals and human is not new; wall paintings of dogs helping humans navigate their environment date back to the Common Era of the 1st Century (Brown, 2019). Since the Americans with Disabilities Act of 1990, service animals have been recognized to provide physical assistance and safety and share the role of caregivers to their owners. Animals are trained to assist individuals with daily functioning, especially those who are blind, wheelchair-bound, may be apt to have seizures, have food allergies, or have other medical and/or mental health conditions. The time and resources to train a service animal factors into the importance of the human–animal bond. Individuals are tasked with recognizing traits for suitable service animals as an important first step in the process of training such animals, as well as the teamwork between the animals and trainers (Lucidi *et al.*, 2005). The relationship one has with a service animal is one built on trust—the human relies on their service animal to safely navigate the world around them. Individuals who rely on guide or service dogs have varying types of loss that they can experience secondary to their companion animals, most likely anticipatory loss. Schneider (2005) highlights the three goodbyes that owners of service animals must face: the decision-making goodbye, the working relationship goodbye, and the goodbye of death. As service animals age, they become less able to provide the needed services that were once rendered to their owners. Since human life expectancy traditionally exceeds that of a service animal, death is expected due to illness or old age (Schneider, 2005; Van de Pol, n.d.). Service animal owners are likely to experience loss multiple times over the course of their life. As can be imagined, the bond that one has with a service animal is powerful and, therefore, losing that helper can be devastating for any reason.

Adolescents (Flom, 2005) and elderly persons (McGolgan and Schofield, 2007; Watt and Pachana, 2007; ; Knight and Edwards, 2008; Winefield *et al.*, 2008; Rock and Babinec, 2010) find a social support system with companion animals. For these specific populations, the bond with pets can provide a range of benefits. Important life lessons and relationship skills can be learned, across the lifespan, when owning a companion animal. Children can benefit from the experience of pet ownership—as it can teach them responsibility and allow them to have a friend, confidant, and security base (Wanser *et al.*, 2019). Pets are non-judgmental and accepting and children are able to share their emotions with them. This can help children increase their emotional control and expression (Sato *et al.*, 2019), increase social competence, communication, and play (Purewal *et al.*, 2017), and develop a positive sense of self (Bodsworth and Coleman, 2001) as well as self-esteem and purpose (Vidović *et al.*, 1999) when caring for the pet. Companion animals for older individuals allow for a balance between an independent lifestyle and emotional dependence on their pets (Hara, 2007). Older individuals live alone more often and owning a companion animal can be seen to provide social support and companionship in the absence of others (McGolgan and Schofield, 2007; Watt and Pachana, 2007). In addition to social support and companionship, there are many benefits that can be seen as secondary to pet ownership, such as increasing exercise and illness prevention (Knight and Edwards, 2008) and having positive effects on human health (Rock and Babinec, 2010).

Pets are oftentimes seen as family members by their owners and are treated and sometimes pampered as such. Some owners even take the time to shop at trendy bakeries and buy high-end clothing, toys, and beds for their "fur babies" (Greenebaum, 2004). The bonds that owners form with their animals create this family-like relationship in many cases. Companion animals can be seen as surrogate children or grandchildren and make the lives of their owners richer and more fulfilling (Knight and Edwards, 2008). When working with families, it is important that the role of the pet within the family be identified (Barton-Ross and Baron-Sorenson, 2007). Not only do pet owners benefit and react to the behavior of their companion animals, but companion animals can oftentimes react to the stress and anxiety of the family (Walsh, 2009b).

Types of loss

Pets within one's life can lead to many, many years of joy and well-being. Many times, the death of a pet is the first experience a child may have with death and dying. For older individuals who may have experienced the death of many loved ones and friends, the death of a pet can be something that is seen as a component of the cycle of life. While death is the ultimate loss and end of a relationship, other scenarios lead to a separation between the individual and pet leading to grief and bereavement (Gitterman and Knight, 2019). These other types of loss can include forced removal or relinquishment of the pet for housing and/or safety reasons, ownership changes with divorce or romantic relationships that end, and missing and lost pets (Sife, 2014).

As work and school settings go back to in-person, individuals may be grappling with their own anxieties about leaving their pets at home (Sicurella, 2021). The human–animal bond has received more attention since the onset of the pandemic; with results pointing to both the positive and negative aspects of the time spent with pets. As these relationships have shifted and changed over the past two years, it is assumed that there will be anxiety and guilt on the part of humans who need to return to in-person work and school settings. Some companies have attempted to get ahead of these anxieties for their workers by allowing pets to come to the office as more businesses re-open (Case, 2021). In a poll, 24% of respondents indicated that they are concerned about how their pet will respond to their return to work out of the home and 27% reported that it was likely they would suffer emotionally with their return to work (Halpin, 2021). These reports underscore the fact that even without death, the attachments developed through quarantine have strengthened the bond and individuals are concerned about how their pets and themselves will respond to the loss of their pandemic routine.

The grief associated with pet loss has been highlighted during tragic weather events; namely in the wake of natural disasters. The need to abandon a pet due to a natural disaster has been further studied since Hurricane Katrina leading to positive changes in policies requiring relief shelters and hotels to make special accommodations for individuals fleeing with companion animals (Barton-Ross and Baron-Sorenson, 2007). Research has pointed to the psychological effects experienced by post-natural disasters can be great due to the loss of companion animals (Hunt *et al.*, 2008; Lowe *et al.*, 2009). Hunt *et al.* (2008) found that the impact of pet loss can be long-term as seen in post-traumatic stress disorder (PTSD) and depression, or short-term as seen with acute stress and peritraumatic dissociation. In these cases, the development of a PTSD diagnosis can be accounted for by the trauma that is experienced secondary to having to abandon their animals. If emergency agencies were prepared to help find suitable shelters for pets in order to reunite owners with their companion animals, there could be an added level of relief and support for victims of natural disasters. Lowe *et al.* (2009) also found that a stressful situation, such as a natural disaster, can be exacerbated when individuals must abandon their support system as they will be less able to emotionally get through this life-altering event. Recognizing the importance of keeping companion animals safe and/or with their owners during these events, the Human Animal Bond Research Institute (HABRI) created the Pet Giving Network through collaboration with Greater Good Charities to connect the pet care community with frontline rescuers helping pets to lessen the distress for pets and people (Human Animal Bond Research Institute, 2021).

Working through pet loss and human bereavement

How society views pet ownership and the grief that pet owners can experience after a loss impacts the bereavement process (Cordaro, 2012). Addressing the sociological understanding of companion animals in the lives of their owners is an important component that counselors must assess when creating treatment plans for individuals who are grieving such a loss (Morley and Fook, 2005). Counselors are trained to employ skills that help clients resolve challenges in their lives. In order to better identify clients who have strong attachments with their pets, these types of relationships should be assessed at initial intakes with clients (Donohue, 2005; Barton-Ross and Baron-Sorenson, 2007). Additionally, counselors are able to deliver a range of inventories to assess the connectedness between a pet and the client (Zilcha-Mano *et al.*, 2011; Ucceddu *et al.*, 2019) to get more information about how attached they are to their pets and the roles pets are ascribed.

When an individual loses a pet, it can be a traumatic experience, especially given the strength of attachment, the role the pet played in the life of the individual, as well as the circumstances and type of loss. While some stage models look to address the grieving process with an end-point of closure, this does not provide individuals with the opportunity to continue the bond with the lost family member; resolution in this case better addresses the need to maintain a connection with the departed pet (Field *et al.*, 2009; Sife, 2014). For some, resolution can lead owners to seek out religious ceremonies to honor, bless, and celebrate the life of the pet, further proving how animals are seen as members of the family unit (Holak, 2008). Children will, most likely, experience the loss of a pet early on and it can be their first experience with death, whereas elderly individuals may have experienced many previous losses in their lifetime (Kastenbaum, 2009); for the reasons provided previously, individuals in these cases may experience heightened grief after the loss of a pet.

Different strategies have been studied to assist grieving pet owners with the process of loss. Dunn *et al.* (2005) developed a bereavement support group for pet owners who were experiencing grief in a veterinary hospital setting. While the use of teaching hospitals can be frequent, these facilities are not always equipped to help pet owners through the difficult process of having to euthanize or treat a terminal illness. The creation of support groups for individuals can be a great benefit in the early stages of healing from the loss (Hess-Holden *et al.*, 2017). Dunn *et al.* (2005) found that the support group allowed the clients to get through a very difficult time by sharing their stories and becoming a support system for other members of the group. Without similar groups, either within or outside the veterinary hospitals, it is difficult for pet owners to fully heal from the grief they experience secondary to losing their pets. Society does not always recognize how important and detrimental the loss can be to an owner, and therefore support groups are an added benefit to the pet owner population (Sife, 2014; Hess-Holden *et al.*, 2017).

Morley and Fook's (2005) research was pivotal in recognizing the importance of providing services to grieving pet owners; although this phenomenon has received support in the literature, grieving the loss of a pet is still trivialized in today's society (Cordaro, 2012). It is important that society stop defining the human-pet relationship in comparison to human relationships because it can cause additional stress to grieving individuals and misunderstanding the experiences of those who lose companion animals. Radical changes need to take place in order to help resolve this issue because more and more pet owners will experience the loss of their pets in the future. As with many stressors and given the increase of individuals adopting "pandemic pets", it is likely that counselors will have clients come in to discuss their reactions to loss, and providing space and resources is needed.

Pet loss interventions

Giving a voice to individuals grieving a disenfranchised loss is one way in which counselors can help clients through pet loss. It is also important to integrate pet loss work into counseling interventions and coping strategies that are already being used in the therapeutic space. While cognitive behavioral therapy can be effective in grief work, clients may not be in a space when they are early in their grief to challenge the thoughts and beliefs they have about the loss. It has been noted that group counseling can be an effective strategy to navigate the anxiety, guilt, and depression that one experiences after the loss of a pet (Turner, 2003; Dunn *et al.*, 2005). Group counseling practices that are facilitated by empathetic leaders are helpful to those navigating difficult life events as being around others in similar situations normalizes the emotional response one has and makes the experience less isolating (Jordan and Neimeyer, 2003), however, with the disenfranchised nature of pet loss grief individuals may be less likely to participate due to fear of judgment. For this reason, the use of web-based chatrooms where individuals are able to read and write messages simultaneously while reducing the stress associated with speaking about a topic (Bohlke, 2003); in this case, pet loss chatrooms can be a healing space for those working through their grief.

Other interventions that can be incorporated when working through the loss of a pet come from expressive therapy practice. Play therapy can be helpful for individuals who lack the cognitive or emotional ability to fully process their experiences with grief and loss (Webb, 2011). Counselors can engage both children and adults who are navigating pet loss by providing them with supplies and space to paint, draw, or use figures to draw out their anxieties and fears about the loss. Other expressive approaches can be helpful in the process of healing that Attig (1996, as cited in Bowman, 2021) describes as relearning the world after an important loss. Therapeutic storytelling, narrative therapy, and bibliotherapy is a technique that is used to build the foundation from which a counselor can work (Bowman, 2021). There are a number of books that counselors can provide for their clients to read in addition to their grief work; this can be especially helpful for children who are grasping the ideas of death and dying. Other techniques, such as letter writing or role-playing can be beneficial as well. For example, a counselor may invite their client to write a letter to their companion animal as well as a letter from the companion animal to the client to resolve any guilt that is being experienced or conduct a role play to diffuse any anger they may be feeling.

Considerations for Counselors

Given statistics on pet ownership (American Veterinary Medical Association, 2018; American Society for the Prevention of Cruelty to Animals, 2021), the potential for counselors to work with clients who are experiencing intense distress over the loss of a companion animal is very likely, and the counseling profession is challenged to be prepared to help these clients through the grieving process just as they would if the lost loved ones were humans. Additionally, counselors are tasked with utilizing counseling strategies that align with the phenomenon surrounding the type of loss experienced and outside factors impacting their psychological well-being (Barton-Ross and Baron-Sorenson, 2007). It is in the accepting and understanding counseling space that bereaved pet owners are able to foster resolution; promoting adaptive coping and becoming invested once again in life (Clements *et al.*, 2003). Resolution can be a vehicle for continuing the bond and relationship with a companion animal and honoring the time that was spent together as a way to continue a connection with the deceased pet (Podrazik *et al.*, 2000).

The human–animal bond has been receiving increasing attention for approximately 30 years now, and even though it has emerged as an important component in counseling practice how to navigate distress when that bond ends has not received an adequate amount of attention. Many in the helping profession recognize the impact that losing companion animals can have on individuals; however, there is not enough support and education about how to best address this in counseling. There are many gaps in the current literature on helping individuals with pet loss and human bereavement. Given the time since the COVID-19 pandemic began and now, it is unclear how people will eventually navigate the loss of a companion animal who provided safety and security through uncertain times (Zilcha-Mano *et al.*, 2012). It is also unclear how the death of a pet might impact counselors who deliver services through telemental health; it is likely that companion animals have been introduced to the counselors throughout the pandemic. Future research about this aspect of pet loss can be helpful for the development of self-care strategies for counselors in addition to clients.

Helping professionals are trained to work with clients through various stressors, however, learning about pet loss work is disenfranchised here as well. Fortunately, there are organizations that provide certifications to individuals looking to provide these services as well as community resources for clients to receive additional social support through their loss. Individuals will not discuss their pain due to the fear of sharing something that is often invalidated by society. It is important for helping professionals to get more information about the power of the bond that individuals have with their animals and to set aside any biases that they may have about the relationships. Counselors can be influential in the healing of their clients through learning more about attachment and loss and about the struggles that an invalidating society presents to grieving pet owners (Morley and Fook, 2005). This is where helping clients resolve their loss can be influential in healing from the loss.

There are more individuals today who include their pets as part of the family. Due to the pandemic and virtual counseling, it is likely that they have even been a part of therapy. The human–animal bond and pet loss and human bereavement literature highlight the importance of pets in the lives of people, therefore, grief after a loss is an important topic that should be addressed in counseling literature, continuing education, and practice in the future. Not all individuals will grieve the same, and it is important to be responsive to the individual needs of the client. Understanding the grief process of pet owners can better prepare professionals to foster non-judgmental spaces where clients can feel open to display their grief. Providing empathy and validating the feelings that any type of loss of a pet can create for the clients may lead to more open sharing among the community further enhancing the healing process and a possible societal shift in the recognition of grieving pet loss as a normative experience.

Conflicts of Interest

The authors have no conflicts of interest to declare.

Funding

There are no funders to report for this article.

Ethics Statement

The authors confirm that the research meets any required ethical guidelines, including adherence to the legal requirements of the study country.

Authors' Contributions

All authors contributed equally to the development of this article.

References

American Society for the Prevention of Cruelty to Animals (2021) ASPCA Pandemic Pet Ownership Survey Memo. ASPCA. Available at: https://aspca.app.box.com/s/v4t7yrwalwk39mf71a857ivqo xnv2x3d

American Veterinary Medical Association (2018) *AVMA Pet Ownership and Demographics Sourcebook*, 2017th–2018th edn. American Veterinary Medical Association, Schaumburg, IL.

Applebaum, J.W., Tomlinson, C.A., Matijczak, A., McDonald, S. and Zsembik, B.A. (2020) The concerns, difficulties, and stressors of caring for pets during COVID-19: Results from a large survey of U.S. pet owners. *Animals* 10(10), 1882–1896.

Attig, T. (2004) Disenfranchised grief revisited: discounting hope and love. *OMEGA: Journal of Death and Dying* 49(3), 197–215.

Barton-Ross, C. and Baron-Sorenson, J. (2007) *Pet Loss and Human Emotion*, 2nd edn. Routledge, New York, NY.

Beck, A.M. and Katcher, A.H. (2003) Future directions in human-animal bond research. *American Behavioral Scientist* 47, 79–93. DOI: 10.1177/0002764203255214.

Bodsworth, W. and Coleman, G.J. (2001) Child-companion animal attachment bonds in single and two-parent families. *Anthrozoös* 14(4), 216–223. DOI: 10.2752/089279301786999391.

Bohlke, O. (2003) A comparison of student participation levels by group size and language stages during chatroom and face-to-face discussions in German. *CALICO Journal* 21(1), 67–87. Available at: https://www.jstor.org/stable/24149481

Bowlby, J. (1969) *Attachment and Loss*, Vol. 1. Basic Books, New York, NY.

Bowlby, J. (1973) *Attachment and Loss*, Vol. 2. Anxiety and Anger, Separation.

Bowlby, J. (1980) *Attachment and Loss*, Vol. 3. Basic Books, New York, NY.

Bowlby, J. (1982) Attachment and loss: Retrospect and prospect. *American Journal of Orthopsychiatry* 52(4), 664–678. DOI: 10.1111/j.1939-0025.1982.tb01456.x.

Bowman, T. (2021) Lessons from the field. family grief care and bibliotherapy: A call for models and studies. *Family Relations* 70(2), 402–407. DOI: 10.1111/fare.12539.

Brown, B.H., Richards, H.C. and Wilson, C.A. (1996) Pet bonding and pet bereavement among adolescents. *Journal of Counseling and Development* 74, 505–509.

Brown, S.A. (2019) *Individuals with Disabilities and Their Assistance Animals: A Brief History and Definitions*. ADA Knowledge Translation Center Legal Brief no.2.3. Available at: https://adata.org/legal_brief/individuals-disabilities-and-their-assistance-animals-brief-history-and-definitions
Burglass, E. (2010) Grief and bereavement theories. *Nursing Standards* 24, 44–47.
Bussolari, C., Currin-McCulloch, J., Packman, W., Kogan, L. and Erdman, P. (2021) I couldn't have asked for a better quarantine partner!": Experiences with companion dogs during Covid-19. *Animals* 11, 330–344.
Case, T. (2021) *'Pet anxiety is real': More Employers Willing to Allow Pandemic-Pets When Staff Return to the Office*. Digiday Media. Available at: https://digiday.com/media/pet-anxiety-is-real-more-employers-willing-to-allow-pandemic-pets-when-staff-return-to-the-office
Clements, P.T., Benasulti, K.M. and Carmone, A. (2003) Support for bereaved owners of pets. *Perspectives in Psychiatric Care* 39(2), 49–54.
Cordaro, M. (2012) Pet loss and disenfranchised grief: Implications for mental health professionals. *Journal of Mental Health Counseling* 34(4), 285–294.
Crossley, M.K. (2013) Pet loss and human bereavement: A phenomenological study of attachment and the grieving process. [Doctoral Dissertation, North Carolina State University].
Doka, K.J. (2008) Disenfranchised grief in historical and cultural perspective. In: Stroebe, M.S., Hansson, R.O., Schut, H. and Stroebe, W. (eds) *Handbook of Bereavement Research and Practice: Advances in Theory and Intervention*. American Psychological Association, pp. 223–240. DOI: 10.1037/14498-011.
Donohue, K.M. (2005) Pet loss: implications for social work practice. *Social Work* 50, 187–190.
Dunn, K.L., Mehler, S.J. and Greenberg, H.S. (2005) Social work with a pet loss support group in a university veterinary hospital. *Social Work in Health Care* 41, 59–70. DOI: 10.1300/J010v41n02_04.
Eckerd, L.M., Barnett, J.E. and Jett-David, L. (2016) Grief following pet and human loss: closeness is key. *Death Studies* 40(5), 275–282. DOI: 10.1080/07481187.2016.1139014.
Field, N.J., Orsini, L., Gavish, R. and Packman, W. (2009) Role of attachment in response to pet loss. *Death Studies* 33, 334–355. DOI: 10.1080/07481180802705783.
Field, N.P. (2008) Whether to relinquish or maintain a bond with the deceased. In: Stroebe, M.S., Hansson, R.O., Schut, H. and Stroebe, W. (eds) *Handbook of Bereavement Research And Practice: Advances in Theory and Intervention*. American Psychological Association, Washington, DC, pp. 113–132. DOI: 10.1037/14498-006.
Flom, B.L. (2005) Counseling with pocket pets: Using small animals in elementary counseling programs. *Professional School Counseling* 8, 469–471.
Gitterman, A. and Knight, C. (2019) Non-death loss: Grieving for the loss of a familiar place and for precious time and associated opportunities. *Clinical Social Work Journal* 47, 147–155. DOI: 10.1007/s10615-018-0682-5.
Gosse, G.H. and Barnes, M.J. (1994) Human grief resulting from the death of a pet. *Anthrozoos: A Multidisciplinary Journal of the Interactions of Pets and Animals* 7, 103–112.
Greenebaum, J. (2004) t's a dog's life: Elevating status from pet to "fur baby" at yappy hour. *Society and Animals* 12, 117–135.
Halpin, R. (2021) MSPCA Angell Poll: Owners Worried about How Pets Will Adjust to Our "New Normal". *MSCPA Angels News*, Available at: https://www.mspca.org/news/mspca-angell-poll-owners-worried-about-how-pets-will-adjust-to-our-new-normal
Hara, S. (2007) Managing the dyad between independence and dependence: Case studies of the American elderly and their lives with pets. *International Journal of Japanese Society* 16, 100–114. DOI: 10.1111/j.1475-6781.2007.00102.x.
Hess-Holden, C.L., Monaghan, C.L. and Justice, C.A. (2017) Pet bereavement support groups: A guide for mental health professionals. *Journal of Creativity in Mental Health* 12(4), 440–450. DOI: 10.1080/15401383.2017.1328291.
Holak, S. (2008) Ritual blessings with companion animals. *Journal of Business Research* 61, 534–541. DOI: 10.1016/j.jbusres.2007.07.026.
Human Animal Bond Research Institute (2021) HABRI Partners with Greater Good Charities to Match Frontline Disaster Needs with Providers of Pet Food, Medicine and Supplies. [Press Release]. Available at: https://habri.org/pressroom/20210816
Hunt, M., Al-Awadi, H. and Johnson, M. (2008) Psychological sequelae of pet loss following Hurricane Katrina. *Anthrozoos: A Multidisciplinary Journal of the Interactions of Pets and Animals* 21, 109–121. DOI: 10.2752/75303708X305765.

Jordan, J.R. and Neimeyer, R.A. (2003) Does grief counseling work? *Death Studies* 27(9), 765–786. DOI: 10.1080/713842360.

Kastenbaum, R. (2009) *Death, Society, and Human Experience*. Pearson Education, Inc, Boston, MA.

Knight, S. and Edwards, V. (2008) In the company of wolves: The physical, social, and psychological benefits of dog ownership. *Journal of Aging Health* 20, 437–455. DOI: 10.1177/0898264308315875.

Lee, H., Song, J. and Lee, J. (2022) Influences of dog attachment and dog walking on reducing loneliness during the COVID-19 pandemic in Korea. *Animals* 12, 483–493. DOI: 10.3390/ani12040483.

Lenhardt, A.C. (1997) Grieving disenfranchised losses: Background and strategies for counselors. *The Journal of Humanistic Education and Development* 35(4), 208–216.

Lowe, S.R., Rhodes, J.E., Zwiebach, L. and Chan, C.S. (2009) The impact of pet loss on the perceived social support and psychological distress of hurricane survivors. *Journal of Traumatic Stress* 22, 244–247. DOI: 10.1002/jts.20403.

Lucidi, P., Bernabo, N., Panunzi, M., Villa, P.D. and Mattioli, M. (2005) Ethotest: A new model to identify (shelter) dogs' skills as service animals or adoptable pets. *Applied Animal Behaviour Science* 95, 103–122. DOI: 10.1016/j.applanim.2005.04.006.

Margolies, L. (1999) The long good-bye: Women, companion animals, and maternal loss. *Clinical Social Work Journal* 27, 289–304.

McGolgan, G. and Schofield, I. (2007) The importance of companion animal relationships in the lives of older people. *Nursing Older People* 19, 21–23.

Morley, C. and Fook, J. (2005) The importance of pet loss and some implications for services. *Mortality* 10, 127–143. DOI: 10.1080/13576270412331329849.

Mueller, M.K., Richer, A.M., Callina, K.S. and Charmaraman, L. (2021) Companion animal relationships and adolescent loneliness during COVID-19. *Animals* 11, 885–898. DOI: 10.3390/ani11030885.

Murphy, S.A. (2006) Consumer health information for pet owners. *Journal of the Medical Library Association* 92, 152–158.

Packman, W., Field, N.P., Carmack, B.J. and Ronen, R. (2011) Continuing bonds and psychosocial adjustment in pet loss. *Journal of Loss and Trauma* 16(4), 341–357. DOI: 10.1080/15325024.2011.572046.

Podrazik, D., Shackford, S., Becker, L. and Heckert, T. (2000) The death of a pet: Implications for loss and bereavement across the lifespan. *Journal of Personal and Interpersonal Loss* 3, 364–395.

Pointon, C. (2006) Animal bereavement. *Therapy Today* 17, 36–38.

Purewal, R., Christley, R., Kordas, K., Joinson, C., Meints, K. *et al.* (2017) Companion animals and child/adolescent development: A systematic review of the evidence. *International Journal of Environmental Research and Public Health* 14(3), 234–259.

Rock, M. and Babinec, P. (2010) Prototypes connect human diabetes with feline and canine diabetes in the context of animal-human bonds: An anthropological analysis. *Anthrozoos: A Multidisciplinary Journal of the Interactions of Pets and Animals* 23, 5–20.

Sato, R., Fujiwara, T., Kino, S., Nawa, N. and Kawachi, I. (2019) Pet ownership and children's emotional expression: Propensity score-matched analysis of longitudinal data from Japan. *International Journal of Environmental Research and Public Health* 16, 758–770. DOI: 10.3390/ijerph16050758.

Schneider, K.S. (2005) The winding valley of grief: When a dog guide retires or dies. *Journal of Visual Impairment and Blindness* 99, 368–370.

Serpell, J.A. (1996) Evidence for an association between pet behavior and owner attachment levels. *Applied Journal of Behaviour Science* 47, 49–60. DOI: 10.1016/0168-1591(95)01010-6.

Sharkin, B.S. and Knox, D. (2003) Pet loss: Issues and implications for the psychologist. *Professional Psychology: Research and Practice* 34, 414–421. DOI: 10.1037/0735-7028.34.4.414.

Sicurella, S. (2021) *You Adopted a Pandemic Pet. Now You're Going Back to the Office. What Next?* National Public Radio. Available at: https://www.npr.org/2021/07/22/1016522446/you-adopted-a-pandemic-pet-now-youre-going-back-to-the-office-what-next

Sife, W. (2014) *The Loss of A Pet: A Guide to Coping with the Grieving Process When A Pet Dies*, 4th edn. Wiley Publishing, Inc, Hoboken, NJ.

Turner, W.G. (2003) Bereavement counseling: Using a social work model for pet loss. *Journal of Family Social Work* 7(1), 69–81.

Ucceddu, S., De Caraldo, L., Albertini, M., Coren, S., Pereira, G.D. *et al.* (2019) Pet humanisation and related grief: Development and validation of a structured questionnaire instrument to evaluate grief in people who have lost a companion dog. *Animals* 9, 933–947. DOI: 10.3390/ani9110933.

Van de Pol, W. (n.d.) Mourning the Loss of Your Service Dog. Center for Pet Loss Grief. Available at: https://centerforpetlossgrief.com/mourning-the-loss-of-your-service-dog

Vidović, V.V., Štetić, V.V. and Bratko, D. (1999) Pet ownership, type of pet and socio-emotional development of school children. *Anthrozoös* 12(4), 211–217. DOI: 10.2752/089279399787000129.

Walsh, F. (2009a) Human-animal bonds I: The relational significance of companion animals. *Family Process* 48, 462–480. DOI: 10.1111/j.1545-5300.2009.01296.x.

Walsh, F. (2009b) Human-animal bonds II: The role of pets in family systems and family therapy. *Family Process* 48, 481–499. DOI: 10.1111/j.1545-5300.2009.01297.x.

Wanser, S.H., Vitale, K.R., Thielke, L.E., Brubaker, L. and Udell, M.A. (2019) Spotlight on the psychological basis of pet attachment and its implications. *Psychology Research and Behavior Management* 12, 469–479.

Watt, D. and Pachana, N.A. (2007) The role of pet ownership and attachment in older adults. *Australian Journal of Rehabilitation Counseling* 13, 32–43.

Webb, N.B. (2011) Play therapy for bereaved children: Adapting strategies to community, school, and home settings. *School Psychology International* 32(2), 132–143. DOI: 10.1177/0143034311400832.

Winefield, H.R., Black, A. and Chur-Hansen, A. (2008) Health effects of ownership and attachment to companion animals in older populations. *International Journal of Behavioral Medicine* 15, 303–310. DOI: 10.1080/10705500802365532.

Wrobel, T.A. and Dye, A.L. (2003) Grieving pet death: Normative, gender, and attachment issues. *Omega: Journal of Death and Dying* 47, 385–393. DOI: 10.2190/QYV5-LLJ1-T043-U0F9.

Zentella, Y. (2009) Developing a multi-dimensional model of hispano attachment to and loss of land. *Culture Psychology* 15(2), 181–200. DOI: 10.1177/1354067X08099621.

Zilcha-Mano, S., Mikulincer, M. and Shaver, P.R. (2011) An attachment perspective on human-pet relationships: Conceptualization and assessment of pet attachment orientations. *Journal of Research in Personality* 45, 345–357. DOI: 10.1016/j.jrp.2011.04.001.

Zilcha-Mano, S., Mikulincer, M. and Shaver, P.R. (2012) Pets as safe havens and secure bases: The moderating role of pet attachment orientations. *Journal of Research in Personality* 46, 571–580. DOI: 10.1016/j.jrp.2012.06.005.

10 Older Adults and Companion Animal Death: A Survey of Bereavement and Disenfranchised Grief

Cary A. Brown[1]*, Donna M. Wilson[2], Eloise Carr[3], Douglas P. Gross[4], Maxi Miciak[5] and Jean E. Wallace[6]

[1]Department of Occupational Therapy, Faculty of Rehabilitation Medicine, University of Alberta, Edmonton, Alberta, Canada; [2]Faculty of Nursing, University of Alberta, Edmonton, Alberta, Canada; [3]Faculty of Nursing, University of Calgary, Calgary, Alberta, Canada; [4]Department of Physical Therapy, Faculty of Rehabilitation Medicine, University of Alberta, Edmonton, Alberta, Canada; [5]Faculty of Rehabilitation Medicine, University of Alberta, Edmonton, Alberta, Canada; [6]Faculty of Arts, University of Calgary, Calgary, Alberta, Canada

Abstract

Background: The number of older adults living with companion animals (pets) is increasing worldwide. While evidence revealing positive relationships between companion animals and healthy aging is well established, there is a dearth of research regarding companion animal death and subsequent human grieving. Some emerging research suggests that grief over companion animal death is often discounted or even unrecognized (disenfranchised) by others. The extent and consequences of disenfranchised grief (DG) are poorly understood. This study deepens our understanding of older adults' experiences of DG in relation to companion animal death.

Methods: Participants from Alberta, Canada, were recruited through social media platforms to participate in an online questionnaire that collected demographic information and standardized measures of companion animal attachment, bereavement, and DG.

Results: The majority of the 98 participants were between 60 and 70 years of age, female, and living alone. Following their companion animal's death, 38.1% identified a decrease in physical activity, and 47% reported that their emotional health had declined. One-third identified that they needed to be careful about who they disclosed their grief, as they were not certain that they would be supported. This group had a significantly greater likelihood of perceived decrease in physical health, and they were more likely to score higher on the Pet Bereavement Questionnaire.

Conclusions: This study adds weight to the emergent body of evidence highlighting companion animal bereavement as a legitimate and impactful health and well-being issue. The study found that DG is experienced by a sizable group of older adults following their companion animal's death and that many participants perceived that socially legitimized recognition of loss and accompanying bereavement resources were lacking. These shortfalls contribute to health risks that negatively affect older adults' ability to successfully age in the community.

*Corresponding author: cary1@ualberta.ca

Keywords: companion animal, pet, death, grief, older adult, disenfranchised grief, aging in place, well-being

Introduction

Research clearly shows that living with a pet (increasingly called a companion animal (CA) is a growing Canadian and international phenomenon (Canadian Animal Health Institute, 2020; LEK Consulting, 2021). Some recent studies attribute part, but not all, of this growth in households that include CAs to be a result of the COVID-19 pandemic and most predict that the CA trend will continue to rise (LEK Consulting, 2021). In Canada, where this study was carried out, immediate and extended families are now smaller as compared to those in past decades (Milan, 2000), and it appears that CAs may be fulfilling a number of emotional support needs for older adults living alone (Stanley *et al.*, 2014). Surveys report that CAs are often considered an important family member (Canadian Animal Health Institute, 2020), and there is robust evidence that living with a CA can play a strong role in promoting physical activity and ensuring emotional well-being (Scoresby *et al.*, 2021). This CA/human relationship can be particularly meaningful for older adults, where opportunities for physical activity, sense of purpose, emotional bonds, and social engagement are often more limited due to barriers associated with aging, such as living alone, reduced income, increased mobility challenges, geographically dispersed family members, and narrowing social circles (Bibbo *et al.*, 2019; Enders-Slegers and Hediger, 2019; Tang *et al.*, 2019). As such, it is logical to assume that the death of a CA that provided activity, emotional connection, and a sense of companionship and purpose can be experienced as a deep and significant loss. Although research in the area of CA death and bereavement is sparse, it supports the concern that CA death can be a major life event with consequent deterioration of the bereaved person's physical and emotional health (Davis, 2011; Cordaro, 2012; Kemp *et al.*, 2016; Reisbig *et al.*, 2017; Cowling *et al.*, 2020; Kogan and Erdman, 2020). It has been suggested that older adults experience stronger attachment and evidence shows that the degree of attachment to a CA contributes to the magnitude of grief (Adams *et al.*, 2000; Barnard-Nguyen *et al.*, 2016).

However, CA deaths are not often recognized for their immediate or ongoing effects. A study of older adult women residing alone in the community who experienced the death of a companion dog during the pre-COVID months of 2019 revealed that unrecognized or disenfranchised grief (DG) may be prevalent (Wilson *et al.*, 2021). Disenfranchised grief is defined by the American Psychological Association (APA) as 'grief that society (or some element of it) limits, does not expect, or may not allow a person to express. Examples include the grief of parents for stillborn babies, of teachers for the death of students, and of nurses for the death of patients. People who have lost an animal companion are often expected to keep their sorrow to themselves. Disenfranchised grief may isolate the bereaved individual from others and thus impede recovery.' (APA, 2022, para. 1). Disenfranchised grief is now considered to be a contributing factor to complicated grief (CG) (Bruinsma *et al.*, 2015; Thimm *et al.*, 2020), a state in which the painful emotions of grief do not reduce with time and the individual has difficulty resuming prebereavement activity and roles. There is some evidence that CG is not unique to the death of human (Adams *et al.*, 2000; Adrian and Stitt, 2017). Spain *et al.* (2019) concluded that there is a complex relationship between DG and post-traumatic growth following CA death. They encouraged greater attention to this poorly understood area, particularly in determining how it contributes to older adult well-being and ability to live independently. While interest in this area of study is growing, our literature search was unable to locate any CA grief studies that used a standardized DG measure, which is another gap in existing evidence.

Our study explored DG in relation to CA death through the involvement of a sample of community-dwelling older adults. Specifically, the study sought to determine the prevalence of DG following CA death and whether other demographic aspects of the individual's life or bond with the CA were related to the experience of DG following their companion animal's death.

Methods

Participants and recruitment

Our study included community-dwelling adults aged 60 years or older who had experienced the death of a dog or cat between January and December 2021. All methods were performed in accordance with the relevant guidelines and regulations. Following ethics approval (University of Alberta Health Research Ethics Board (Pro00101778), an invitation to complete an anonymous online survey was circulated across Alberta, a western Canadian province with a population distribution of approximately 80% urban dwellers and 20% rural, in January and February 2022. The invitation was distributed *via* senior organizations' communication tools (e.g. newsletters and email blasts) and posted extensively on a wide range of Facebook pages of relevant Albertan organizations and groups. As rural areas are typically more difficult to access and recruit participants from, an extensive geographic search for Facebook groups that would have relevant members was conducted. Consequently, the invitation was posted on the Facebook pages of libraries, coffee shops, service clubs (e.g. Lions Club, Elks, and Kinettes), agricultural societies, 'buy and sell' and 'community news' groups, as well as pet services, dog and cat rescues, and pet interest groups in communities across Alberta. It was not posted on Facebook groups for lost animals to avoid emotional distress.

There is some evidence that men are less likely to participate in survey research (Smith, 2008) and so to maximize gender representation in the survey, the study made a particular effort to identify and post to Facebook groups most typically identified with men (e.g. Royal Canadian Legion branches, Men's Shed, Kinsmen, snowmobile clubs). Facebook messages in response to the participant invitation were monitored and responded to by the Principal Investigator. Queries were typically from people asking if they could participate, although they did not meet the age inclusion criteria. The survey was closed on March 15, 2022, after a repeat round of invitations was sent out *via* the same Facebook groups. A total of 98 responses that met the inclusion criteria were received.

Survey tools

The invitations to participate in the Grief after Pet Loss study included a URL to an anonymous online survey hosted on the University of Alberta administered Google Forms ® platform. The survey took approximately 20 min to complete and included a consent form, prescreening inclusion questions, questions for basic descriptive demographic data (age, gender, geographic location, when the CA died, and whether they were a cat or dog), and three standardized measures (described below), and provided a separate email address for those wishing to request a copy of the final report. Asking participants to email a request for the report kept their survey responses separate from their contact details and maintained their anonymity.

The first standardized measure collected was the pet attachment and life-impact scale (PALS) (Cromer and Barlow, 2013), a psychometrically tested tool assessing owner attachment and perceived negative and positive impact of the CA relationship on the CA guardian's life. The PALS has 35 questions asking each participant's level of agreement with statements on a five-point scale ranging from '1 = not at all' to '5 = very much' about their pet in regards to four factors: 'Love,' 'Regulation,' 'Personal Growth,' and 'Negative Impact.' Higher scores indicate a greater endorsement of the impact. The PALS has no normative data.

The second measure was the pet bereavement questionnaire (PBQ) (Hunt and Padilla, 2006), which includes 16 questions and uses a four-point Likert response scale (0 = Disagree strongly, 1 = Disagree, 2 = Agree, 3 = Agree strongly). Higher scores signify a higher degree of bereavement distress. The PBQ has no normative data. The PBQ has 16 questions comprising three distinct domains: Grief (items: 2, 3, 5, 7, 10, 12, and 15), Anger (items: 1, 4, 11, 13, and 14), and Guilt (items 6, 8, 9, and 16). The PBQ is a brief, widely used, well-validated instrument, and the tool developers describe it as having good internal reliability (Cronbach's alpha = .87), factor structure, and construct validity (Hunt and Padilla, 2006).

The third data collection tool was the witnessing of disenfranchised grief measure (WDG) (St Clair, 2013). The WDG measures the degree to which the bereaved individual perceives their loss to be witnessed. A witness is defined at the start of the questions as 'someone who lets you know that your loss was real and that you had a right to grieve.' The WDG is a 22-item questionnaire, each ranked on a five-point Likert scale (5 = strongly agree to 1 = strongly disagree). The WDG measure has inter-item correlations reported to range from $p < .01$ to $p < .05$, and a Cronbach's alpha of .91 (St Clair, 2013).

Data were also collected through multiple-item, tick-box questions regarding what participants found supportive or unsupportive in relation to their grief. The listed items and activities were identified through a background literature review. To ensure key data that were potentially not covered in the questions with multiple-choice options were not missed three open-ended questions were included to gather more specific details: Q17. *Were there other people or activities not listed above that were helpful?* Q19. *Can you give us examples of what people did to make you feel your grief WAS NOT recognized and supported?* and Q20. *Can you give us examples of what people did to make you feel your grief WAS recognized and supported?* An open-ended question was also included at the end of the survey for participants who wanted to add additional information about CA grief that they felt had not been covered in the survey.

Analysis

All data from the Google Forms ® platform were imported into Excel for data cleaning and saved in the .csv file format required by the statistical analysis software program, JASP (JASP Team, 2022). Quantitative data analysis, examining the relationship between demographic characteristics and measures of CA attachment, grief, and perceived unwitnessed grief, was carried out using chi-square tests for dichotomous data (e.g. cat or dog guardian) and relevant independent samples t-tests or one-way between groups ANOVA for other data. The p-values were set as $p < .05$ and 95% for confidence intervals.

Text responses to open-ended questions were categorized and grouped in the order of the most common to least commonly occurring comments. These open-ended questions were not designed to elicit the depth of narrative data required for thematic analysis. Rather, the data were treated as descriptive. The research team lead read all of the data and then similar comments were grouped together. Two team members then reviewed the groupings, and any disagreements were resolved through discussion.

Results

Participant demographics and relationship with CA

Demographics are detailed in Table 10.1; 98 participants remained after one incomplete survey's responses were removed from the data set. Despite extensive efforts to recruit across genders, 92 (93.9%) participants identified as female and only 6 (6.1%) as male or other. Most participants were 70 years of age or less (60–64 = 42.9%; 65–70 = 40.8%), four participants (4.1%) were 76–80 years of age, and one (1.0%) was over 80 years. Most (74.5%, n = 73) participants lived alone when their CA died, and 80.6% (n = 79) reported the death of a dog compared to only 19.4% (19) reporting a cat. Companion animal age at death ranged from 0 to 5 years (3.1%, n = 3), 6–10 years (18.4%, n = 18), 11–15 years (58.2%, n = 57), to 16 years + (20.4%, n = 20). The number of years participants had lived with their companion animal predeath ranged from 0 to 5 years (10.2%, n = 10), 6–10 years (31.6%, n = 31), 11–15 years (43.3%, n = 43), to 16 years + (14.3%, n = 14).

Background of CA'S death

In response to Question 10, '*Was your CA's death expected?*' 29 (29.6%) identified it was sudden (e.g., '*While she had been in heart failure for the last 2 years, the day her heart gave out it was completely unexpected and a shock*'), 45 (45.9%) stated it was expected (e.g., '*I had her at the vet for treatment and blood work. Before the results came back, 3 days later, I knew she was not recovering and that the time to consider euthanasia had arrived*'), and eight (8.2%) did not respond to this question. A further 16 (16.3%) wrote a comment indicating that death expectation was a complicated matter and was not answerable with a simple yes or no. They typically related that they realized their CA was aging and that death was closer, but there were no particular warning signs that it was imminent (e.g., '*She was very old, she was still strong and in good spirits. Then suddenly she began having seizures at 4pm and lost motor control of her hind end around midnight and I had to have her euthanized the next morning. She was old, but her passing was sudden*').

A small majority of participants (50/94, 53.2%) who responded to the question '*How did your CA die?*' indicated that their CA had been euthanized. Two participants mentioned that the vet had come to their home for this procedure. Additional causes of death that were identified included heart attack, poison, and fatal attack by another animal.

Memorializing activities

Ninety participants (91.8%) responded to question 12: '*What, if anything, did you do to mark their passing or to keep as a memorial to them?*' While six participants stated that they did not feel the need for anything beyond their memories, 88 (93.6%) of the participants listed multiple activities and ways they memorialized their CA. Most commonly, participants (n = 38, 42.2%) identified tangible items, such as favorite photographs placed around the home, or items such as plaques, paw prints, keychains, and ornaments that they had created or purchased specifically as ways to remember their deceased CA. Some noted how family members or friends had painted a CA portrait or crafted a needlework blanket or cushion. The second most common postdeath activity (n = 29, 32.2%) involved their CA's cremation ashes. Typically, these were scattered in favorite places (e.g., '*I spread them at her favorite hiking trail*'), kept in a commemorative urn in a spot associated with positive memories of the CA (i.e., '*placed in his favorite spot by the fireplace*'), or had small amounts encapsulated in memorial jewelry or embedded in statues. Three participants noted that they had left instructions that the CA's ashes should be buried along with their own when they died.

The next most common activity (n = 15, 16.7%) was to keep a collection of the CA's belongings (collars, favorite toys, lock of fur) as memorials. Following this, the activities of having a funeral/ memorial service, placing a social media announcement of the CA's death, and receiving a commemorative item from the veterinarian (e.g. paw print in plaster) were identified by equal numbers (n = 12) of participants. Burial was mentioned by eight of the participants, and talking to family and friends about the CA was identified by four participants as an activity to mark their CA's death. One participant stated that she felt pressure to make a costly decision about how her CA's death and remains were handled at a time when she was not prepared (e.g., '*In my grief, I chose the one option...needless to say this was the most expensive option. It was very difficult for me to pay for the $411.00 fee. I wish I'd been more clear-minded to be able to choose one of the other options*').

Self-perceived health and activity level following the CA death

As detailed in Table 10.1, more than half of the participants stated that they felt there was no change in their level of physical activity (56.7%), physical health (72.2%), or emotional health (52.1%) following their CA's death. However, this means a significant number of participants did perceive a decrease in physical activity (38.1%), physical health (23.7%), and, markedly, emotional health (46.9%). Only three participants reported improvement in any of these variables; therefore, for statistical analysis, the three response categories ('improved,' 'stayed the same,' and 'decreased') were collapsed into two ('better/same' and 'decreased').

Table 10.1. Demographics and well-being self-report (n = 98).

Location				
Large city with population of 200,000+	33.7% (33)	Town with population between 1000 and 50,000		25.5% (25)
City with population between 100,001 and 200,000	4.1% (4)	Town with population of less than 1000		7.1% (7)
City with population between 50,001 and 100,000	11.2% (11)	Rural		18.4% (18)
Activity since CA death (n = 97)	more active 5.2% (5)	less active 38.1% (37)	the same 56.7% (55)	
Physical health since CA death (n = 97)	more healthy 4.1% (4)	less healthy 23.7% (23)	the same 72.2% (70)	
Emotional health since CA death (n =96)	more healthy 1.0% (1)	less healthy 46.9% (45)	the same 52.1% (50)	
Perceived grief recognized and supported		68.4% (65/95)		
Perceived unsupported and need for caution around disclosure		31.6% (30)		

Table 10.2. Perceived helpfulness and availability of CA grief resources (n = 98).

	a	b	c	d	Columns a+c	Columns b+d
Resource (n)	Available/ helpful	Available/not helpful	Not available/ would be helpful	Not available/ would not be helpful	% who found this helpful or perceived it would be helpful (%)	% who found this was not helpful or perceived it would not be helpful (%)
Family and friends (96)	76.0% (73)	9.4% (9)	9.4% (9)	5.2% (5)	85.4	14.6
Plaques and pictures (93)	63.4% (59)	17.2% (16)	4.3% (4)	15.1% (14)	67.7	32.3
Veterinarian (92)	54.3% (50)	9.8% (9)	15.2% (14)	20.7% (19)	69.5	30.5
Commemorative donation (89)	43.8% (39)	24.7% (22)	10.1% (9)	21.3% (19)	53.9	46.1
Social media post (91)	26.4% (24)	28.6% (26)	5.5% (5)	39.5% (36)	31.9	68.1
Website info and videos (91)	17.6% (16)	23.1% (21)	25.3% (23)	34.1% (31)	42.9	57.1
Memorial/funeral service (89)	16.7% (15)	21.4% (19)	21.4% (19)	40.5% (36)	38.1	61.9
Information booklets (91)	12.1% (11)	14.3% (13)	29.7% (27)	43.9% (40)	41.8	58.2
Pet loss counselor (91)	8.8% (8)	3.4% (3)	43.9% (40)	43.9% (40)	52.7	47.3
Pastoral care/general counselor (90)	6.7% (6)	10.0% (9)	27.7% (25)	55.6% (50)	34.4	65.6
Pet loss support groups (91)	4.4% (4)	5.4% (5)	45.1% (41)	45.1% (41)	49.5	50.5

Sources of help

For Question 16: *'what people or activities, if any, were most helpful to you after your CA died?'* participants were asked to rank items on a predetermined list as *available and helpful, available and not helpful, not available but potentially helpful,* and *not available but likely not helpful* (Table 10.2). The four highest occurring resources that participants identified as having been or likely to be helpful were: family and friends (85.4%), veterinarians (69.5%), plaques and pictures (67.7%), and commemorative donations (53.9%). The four lowest occurring resources identified as not having been or not likely to be helpful were information booklets (41.8%), memorial/funeral service (38.1%), pastoral care/general counselor (34.4%), and social media posts (31.9%). The two resources most often identified as 'not available but potentially helpful' were pet loss support groups (45.1%) and pet loss counselor (43.9%). Several participants wrote in the 'other' box that being with other people's dogs or cats or having another CA already living in the home was helpful to them. The most commonly added-in comment (six participants) was *'adopting another dog/cat.'*

Supported and unsupported grief

Question 18 asked, *'Did you feel that your grief was recognized and supported or that you had to be careful because some people would not understand?'* While 65 of the 95 participants (68.4%) who responded stated their grief was recognized and supported, a notable number (n = 30, 31.6%) stated that they were careful about disclosure and they were not certain of being recognized and supported.

Supported grief

Eighty-four (85.7%) participants gave examples of what people did, or could have done, to make them feel that their grief was recognized and that they felt supported. The most frequently occurring examples involved being listened to and feeling free to talk about the CA (e.g., *'sympathetic listened; listened to me talk; talked about it'*). A number of participants used language conveying that they felt they were 'allowed to' or had permission to talk about their CA (e.g., *'they let me talk about her and listened; just letting me say what I wanted to about him and understanding; just letting me talk about him; allowed me to share good memories of her'*). Several participants noted that people communicated an understanding that the grief they felt was valid and deep (e.g., *'she understood the depth of my grief- it was comforting to hear that she said that we never forget or stop missing our pets and that it's okay to do so indefinitely; they would totally be enveloped in my pain as they truly understood; recognized my sadness at the beginning; cried with me; validated my feelings'*). A few participants stated people around them shared stories of their own grief when their own CA had died as a way to demonstrate empathy and understanding (e.g., *'listening and giving their stories about their dog losses over the years and how they coped. How they went through the grieving process; each of them has lost one of their dogs in recent years and I know how they grieved their losses, so their support was heartfelt'*). Most, however, spoke of the support they felt when other people shared stories of the participant's CA (e.g., *'they shared pictures and memories; they told me they missed her very much as well, funny stories about her antics'*).

Tangible examples of support that were reported included receiving phone calls, flowers, condolence cards, memorial ornaments and jewelry, and donations to charity (e.g., *'sent flowers with cards and very thoughtful words; cards; phone calls; Christmas ornaments commemorating him; stuffed animal as a gift; made donations in his name, many messages and phone calls to me'*) and invitations to participate in activities (e.g.*'took me places; tried to keep me busy; inviting me on walks'*). Several participants mentioned that others showed support by visiting them with their own CA along, assuming that the CA would provide a form of comfort (e.g., *'my daughter offered to leave her dog with me for a few days, brought their dog to help visit, my granddaughter brought her cat over to visit me'*). Two participants mentioned the support and compassion of their veterinarian in 'bending' COVID public health restrictions to allow them to be present in the clinic when their CA was euthanized, and one participant stated being referred to a counselor by their veterinarian after the death was a very supportive act.

Unsupported grief

Over 60% (n = 61) participants felt unsupported when grieving. Participants' most frequent comments involved feeling unsupported when other people suggested or implied they were over-reacting (e.g., *'I was told 'It was just a dog' and that others have had far worse losses, so that I should be focusing more on others; People would say things such as 'It's just a cat' and expect me to either not feel the loss of my beloved fur friend's passing or that I should be over it in a few days; my loss should be less because my dog was not a person; they told me to move on, get over it')*. The next most frequent comments related to feeling shut down, as they were not encouraged to talk about the loss (e.g., *'Didn't want to talk about it and didn't want me to talk about it; Not really listening to my story; seemed indifferent; Doing other things while I talked'*) and they received advice to get a replacement CA, which made them feel their relationship with the decreased CA was not seen as significant (e.g., *'there are lots of cats, just get another one'*). Fifteen participants gave examples of being told about the 'positive' impact of their CA's death regarding, for example their having more free time (e.g., *'now you can spend more time with your family'*), less housework (e.g., *'commented how nice it was to not have cat hair in the house'*), and more freedom to move to other accommodations (e.g., *'now you can move into a better place')*. Four participants mentioned how, after their CA's death, people disclosed that they had not actually liked the CA (e.g., *'told me they never liked Charlie anyways'*) or that they did not personally like pets. One participant commented that she was at times not supportive of herself and she self-censored when talking about her loss (*'it was hard to talk about my grief over the loss of my dog when people were losing their family members'*).

Other comments

Over 65% of the participants added additional comments in response to Question 21: *Is there anything else you would like to share?* A large number of participants mentioned how hard the loss was and how they had not actually anticipated feeling so bereaved (e.g., *'It is the worst thing I have experienced in a long time. I did not realize how it affected me; I never understood before how truly painful the loss of a cherished pet is-but I do now; I lost my best friend and companion. I have never cried so much in a long time; the grief runs so very deep. And it takes a really long time to come back from that...')*. They also mentioned that they encountered grief triggers (e.g., *'Christmas Eve and Christmas will forever be overshadowed by our loss; he was such a part of my life-all kinds of things remind me of him and make me sad'*).

One participant reflected on how certain objects and places, that had originally been triggers for grief, had over time softened to trigger happy memories and positive feelings. Six other participants also mentioned that grief decreased with time and that death was an accepted part of life (e.g., *'I was very sad but she was 16 so I accepted it...just get on with life'*) but this was not a feeling shared by the majority of participants (e.g., *'I have lost many, many pets and it doesn't get any easier')*. Nine participants mentioned that society in general does not prepare us for CA loss (e.g., *'people seem reluctant to talk about what to expect before, and also what happens after')*. Some felt this lack of awareness contributed to feelings of guilt for having potentially made a bad decision for their CA (e.g., *'...felt so guilty that panic and acting without a lot of thought resulted instead'*). Over half (n = 37) of the participants who responded to this question talked about the loss of meaningful roles they experienced when their CA died (e.g., *'...I don't know who I am without her; she gave me something to focus on, to care and be responsible for, to protect and cook for and talk to....'*) and several mentioned the role their CA had played in supporting them through the grief associated with other deaths (e.g., *'T had been my son's treasured dog. My son... died suddenly. Losing T made me feel I was losing the last living connection to my son'*).

About a quarter (n = 14) of the participants mentioned challenges they would have now if they were to establish a new CA bond (e.g., *'one of my greatest fears is reaching a point where I have to move to some sort of facility and not being able to take my dog; with my age I do not want to leave an animal with no home'*). Seven participants also mentioned that COVID-19 public health restrictions had made their CA's death more difficult; two stated that (although the study asked specifically only about cats and dogs) the loss of a bird, rabbit, reptile, or other type of pet could lead to very significant grief as well; and five stated that there are logistical issues (such as limited vet availability and feeling hurried to decide about euthanasia) that could contribute to deeper grief.

Of final note is that over 10% (n = 11) of the survey participants thanked us for the opportunity to complete the survey and, in so doing, share their loss. They commented that this work was needed and that it is currently neglected. Some stated that the survey legitimized their grief (e.g., '*Thank you for validating my deep grief... Awareness, acceptance, and education is needed so people can grieve without having to be silent or ashamed*'), and a few took the opportunity to share CA grief resources with the researchers to pass along to others.

Standardized measures

The scores of the three measures (PALS, PBQ, and WDG) are detailed in Table 10.3. As previously stated, there are no normative data for these three measures. The PALS (Cronbach's alpha = .92), the PBQ (Cronbach's alpha = .86), and the WDG (Cronbach's alpha .90) all had acceptable internal consistency in this study.

The PALS's mean participant score (150.68 of a total possible 175) indicated an overall high level of attachment. While there was a range of scores in the PALS subcategories of Love, Regulation, and Personal Growth, the small standard deviation (1.81) in the Negative Impact subcategory reflected that the large majority of participants felt that their relationship with the CA had little negative impact on their life. Scores in the PBQ showed mid-range bereavement (mean = 22.69 of possible 48), with most of the variations occurring in the Grief subcategory. There were much lower scores and range in the subcategories of Anger and Guilt (mean = 3.28 and 3.47 of a possible 15 and 12, respectively). The mean WDG score was 77.54 out of a possible 110, and the standard deviation (14.46) reflects there was considerable variation in the degree to which people felt their grief was witnessed and supported.

Given that only six (6.12%) participants reported a gender other than female, the data were treated as a whole with no gender categorization or differentiation. Three statistically significant relationships emerged: (1) A chi-square test for independence (with Yates' Continuity Correction) indicated a significant association between older participants and the likelihood of living alone versus not living alone ($X^2 = 8.701$, df = 1, p = .013). There were no other significant relationships related to the

Table 10.3. Standardized measures of attachment, bereavement, and disenfranchised grief (n = 98).

	Mean	Median	Mode	Standard Deviation	Possible Range
Pet attachment and life-impact scale	150.68	155	162	19.37	35–175
Love (17 items)	76.05	80	81	11.78	17–85
Regulation (9 items)	36.04	38	45	8.02	9–45
Personal growth (5 items)	19.11	19	22	4.46	5–25
Negative impact (4 items)	18.67	19	20	1.81	4–20
Pet bereavement questionnaire	22.69	23	23	7.82	0–48
Grief (7 items)	15.90	17	20	4.26	0–21
Anger (5 items)	3.28	3	1	2.53	0–15
Guilt	3.47	3	0	3.18	0–12
Witnessing of disenfranchised grief	77.54	79	79	14.46	22–110

age of participants or whether they lived alone. (2) An independent samples t-test determined that the 79 participants whose CA was a dog (M = 153.89, SD = 16.21) compared to the 19 participants whose CA was a cat (M = 137.47, SD = 25.44) demonstrated significantly higher scores on the PALS (t (95) = −3.50, $p < .001$). There was no difference between the cat guardian and dog guardian groups in relation to any other variables.

Interestingly, the age of the CA and how long the participant had lived with the CA had no significant relationship with other variables, including the PALS and PBQ. (3) An independent samples t-test determined that the 30 participants who reported feeling unsupported and needing to be careful to whom they disclosed their grief to (M = 26.53, SD = 7.01), compared to the 66 participants who reported feeling supported and able to disclose (M = 20.95, SD = 7.57), demonstrated significantly higher scores on the PBQ (t (94) = 3.42, $p < .001$). (4) A chi-square test for independence (with Yates' Continuity Correction) indicated a further significant association between feeling unsupported and a perceived decrease in physical health since CA death ($X^2 = 7.43$, df = 2, p = .024). No other statistically significant relationships emerged related to perceptions of being supported/unsupported or between perceived changes in activity, physical health, mental health, and the PALS, PBQ, and WDG.

Summary of findings

The majority of participants were between 60 and 70 years of age, female, lived alone, and had been guardians of their (deceased) CA for 11 years or more. Most CAs died by euthanasia, and the participants identified a wide range of grieving and memorializing activities. While in the minority, a notable percentage identified a subsequent decrease in physical activity and health after their CA's death. Markedly, about half of the participants (46.9%) reported that their emotional health had declined. Participants identified a number of post-death resources and supports, most frequently from family and friends. Being 'listened to' was identified most often as helpful support for their grief. Being told by others that they were over-reacting and should 'get over it' was listed most often as a lack of support. One-third of the participants identified that they needed to be careful about who they disclosed their grief to and were not certain that they would be supported. These qualitative findings align with the quantitative survey data, which demonstrated overall high scores on pet attachment (particularly for participants whose CAs were dogs) as measured by the PALS and bereavement measured by the PBQ. The mean score for the WDG and the wide range in scores indicated that while a number of participants felt their grief was acknowledged, there were also many who did not feel their grief was recognized and respected. Finally, there was a significantly greater likelihood of a perceived decline in physical health following CA death for those who reported that they needed to be cautious about whom to disclose the death to and also among those who felt they were not always supported. This group was also more likely to have higher scores on the PBQ.

Discussion

The goal of this study was to explore DG in relation to older adults' experiences of death due to CA. Specifically, the study sought to determine the extent of DG following CA death, and whether other demographic aspects of the individual's life or bond with the CA were related to increased experience of DG following the CA's death. The notable findings are discussed below.

Living alone

The significant number of older participants in this study living alone reflects the current socio-demographic and housing trends in Canada, where this study was carried out (Tang *et al.*, 2019). It is interesting to note that there were no statistically significant differences related to the PALS, PBQ, and WDF measures and whether the participant lived alone or with another person. The question of whether living with others acts as a protective feature of grief is complex and understudied. Some evidence suggests that the intensity of grief experienced following CA death varies widely between cohabitating couples, and this can contribute to feelings of DG (Gage and Holcomb, 1991).

There are insufficient relevant data from our study to draw similar conclusions. However, it is clear from these findings that our original assumption, arising from the literature, that those living alone are more at risk of DG following CA death than those living with others, is not supported and further examination is needed.

Attachment

The high degree of attachment, indicated by the PALS scores and grief as measured by the PBQ, is consistent with other CA grief studies (Davis, 2011; Cordaro, 2012; Eckerd *et al.*, 2016; Kemp *et al.*, 2016; Reisbig *et al.*, 2017; Spain *et al.*, 2019; Cowling *et al.*, 2020; Kogan and Erdman, 2020; Wilson *et al.*, 2021). The authors speculate that the statistically significant difference between dog guardians' and cat guardians' PALS scores may be an artifact of the much larger representation of dog guardians in the study. In addition, given that the 9-item PALS subcategory 'regulation' includes items such as pet walking and other forms of regulation that are not required to the same extent by cat guardians, one would reasonably expect to see higher scores for dog guardians. There may be other contributing factors that could not be determined from the data and readers are cautioned against assuming that this statistically significant finding has any relevance in the degree of attachment of guardians to their cats or dogs.

Gendered grief

The participants in this study, similar to others, were largely consisted of females. As Packman *et al.* (2016) pointed out, this under-representation of male participants has contributed to the assumption in the literature that gender differences in CA bonds and grief are small. They stress that the phenomenon is likely to be more complex, perhaps related to gender-typical forms of communication and behavior. Findings from studies of gendered non-CA (human-to-human) grief have been reported to be inconsistent and at times conflicting, and recent researchers have called for more rigorous and longitudinal examinations (Park and Royal, 2020).

Currently, the authors of this study can only speculate that the gendered aspects of CA grief exist (e.g., socio-culturally influenced gender-mediated behaviors such as willingness to articulate feelings) and that they may contribute to the risk for DG. Further research is needed, particularly studies informed by contemporary understandings of gender identity (Lundorff *et al.*, 2020), and of the role of other social determinants of health (e.g., income, housing, social network) (Fernández-Alcántara *et al.*, 2021) into older adults' risk of DG. Although extensive efforts to achieve a higher representation of non-female participants were made, they were unsuccessful and recognized to be a shortcoming of the study.

Measuring disenfranchised grief

A notable percentage of participants perceived a decline in their activity level (38.1%), physical health (23.7%), and emotional health (46.9%) following their CA's death. While no statistically significant relationship emerged between these variables and WDG scores, it is known from other human-to-human grief studies that decreased physical activity and mental well-being (e.g., Lannen *et al.*, 2008; Trevino *et al.*, 2018), as well as increased utilization of healthcare resources (Lannen *et al.*, 2008), are consequences of unresolved grief. It has been proposed that the experience of DG is a risk factor for delayed or precluded grief resolution and complicated grief (Corr, 1999; Doka, 1999) and, as such, this requires closer examination. It is possible that the experience of DG is related to activity, physical health, and mental well-being, but our measure, the WDG (St Clair, 2013), was not sensitive to this for CA grief. To the best of our knowledge, there are no standardized measures specific to the DG experienced in the death of CA.

Given the extensive comments that the participants provided as examples of being unsupported and made to feel their grief was not real or exaggerated, it is possible that there is a disconnect between what was measured in the survey and the participants' lived experiences. Further study to develop a measure of DG specific to human–CA loss is called for. This is particularly warranted for its potential clinical relevance in screening bereaved CA guardians for risks to grief resolution and consequent health and well-being. The authors speculate that the need for effective screening tools to guide intervention is of particular concern, given the growing number of older adults who will experience CA bereavement in the coming years, concurrent with their advancement to older adulthood and their acquisition of additional age-related health and activity challenges to independent community living.

Euthanasia and disenfranchised grief

Most participants reported that they needed to make a decision about euthanasia to end the life of their CA. While there was no statistically significant relationship between the PBQ subscale for 'Guilt' or the WDG measure and electing euthanasia for their CA, some of the qualitative data reflected the complexity and emotional challenge of this decision. Vonk *et al.* (2022) found an apparent relationship between empathy and emotion regulation as predictors of guilt following decisions to euthanize a CA and cautioned that much more work needs to be done to better understand this important area. A recent American study of 340 CA guardians who had euthanized their CA found that 74.7% stated that they had mourned privately (Park and Royal, 2020). Park and Royal (2020) speculated that the decision to grieve privately might, for many, be a consequence of DG following CA loss and stressed that this is an alarming finding that has negative health and social consequences. Our April 2022 Google search revealed numerous online blog posts and articles about the experience of guilt following the decision to euthanize a CA; however, a formal database search was unsuccessful in identifying any research-informed intervention studies.

While this study did not ask specifically if participants grieved privately, typical manners of shared grieving such as memorial services and social media posts were identified by over 30% of the participants as not having been, or not believed to be helpful. These findings indicate that for a large number of participants, grieving was performed in private. Given the consequences to health and well-being of unresolved guilt compounded by the likelihood of self-imposed isolation consequent to DG, a deeper understanding of mental health support related to euthanasia is a key unmet need.

Memorialization

Participants in this study identified a large number of memorializing activities, such as plaques, pictures, and special places to store or scatter their CA's ashes after cremation. Researchers have proposed that memorializing activities may be important tools for maintaining a continuing bond with the deceased CA, and they also provide a way to revisit memories as the bereaved process their loss and new reality (Dickinson and Hoffman, 2017; Rémillard *et al.*, 2017; Fine, 2019; McKinney, 2019; Spain *et al.*, 2019; Park and Royal, 2020). Spain *et al.* (2019) proposed that memorializing activities and objects adds legitimacy to the grief experience and that these practices can help reduce the risk of DG. Park and Royal (2020) nuanced this further by pointing out that a lack of participation in memorialization may not be out of preference but rather self-disenfranchisement based on the strong social messages from some that these activities are over-reacting to the death of a CA and a consequent fear of judgment by others. As such, people may be denied the emotional support of continuing bonds, self-compassion (Bussolari *et al.*, 2021), and opportunities for post-traumatic growth that are facilitated through positive social interactions (Spain *et al.*, 2019).

In summary, there is robust evidence from this and other studies that memorialization is important, as it contributes to well-being. A brief review of social media on this topic and an examination of survey participants' comments reflect that memorialization opportunities and awareness about how to access them (particularly commercial products and services) are increasing. Social marketing research suggests that making a service or product more visible in a positive light contributes to overall societal acceptance (Wang *et al.*, 2021) and this is reflected in the ever-growing number of positive stories about the role of CAs as integral family members. This increased visibility should logically contribute to greater social acceptance and understanding of CA grief, thus reducing the risk of DG. However, this also potentially increases the risk of exploitive practices for those who see CA grief as an opportunity for financial gain. Notably, one survey participant noted: '*In my grief, I chose the one option XYZ. Needless to say this was the most expensive option. It was very difficult for me to pay for the $411.00 fee. I wish I'd been more clear-minded to be able to choose one of the other options.*' We believe this underlines the need for those close to, or who are providing services to, older adults grieving CA loss to encourage and support open communication around memorialization, avoid hasty decisions, and legitimize the loss as opposed to expressing judgment that can leave the bereaved isolated and emotionally vulnerable in decision making.

A 2017 meta-analysis revealed that, conservatively, one of every 18 cognitively intact, community-dwelling older adults had been the victim of a financial scam (Burnes *et al.*, 2017), and scams targeting bereaved older adults appear to be a growing concern (Finberg, 2003). Based on this evidence, we propose that DG may increase the risk of financial exploitation of vulnerable older adults, a further significant reason for developing and testing strategies to reduce the risk of DG following CA death.

Counseling, support groups, and pastoral care

Similar to other studies (Cowling *et al.*, 2020; Park and Royal, 2020), it was found that few participants identified pastoral care or general counseling services as something they had experienced to be useful or felt would be useful if available. Research has stressed that those providing pastoral care and counseling services in general poorly understand the significance of CA loss (Brown, 2006; Cordaro, 2012; Laing and Maylea, 2018; Leonhardt-Parr and Rumble, 2022). Interestingly, in a qualitative study of 68 Australians, 56% stated that they believed in an afterlife for their CA, and 46.8% reported praying for their CA (Davis, 2011). Given these relatively high numbers who felt comforted by their belief in an afterlife for their CA, it would most likely be of benefit for those who play pastoral roles to become more informed about CA grief and human–animal bonds in general. Some steps in this direction are apparent in Brown's (2006) review of religious thinking about the place animals occupy in relation to humans where he pointing out that 'there is a need for religious leaders, pastoral career, and practical theologians to consider the research results regarding CA grief, the impact of inappropriate counsel and comments, and contributing factors to DG' [p. 419].

It is striking that, of the nine participants who had direct access to a support group, five felt the support group process had not been helpful. An additional 41 participants who did not have access stated that they thought it would not be helpful. This means that 50.5% of the 91 participants responding to this question did not find or believe that pet loss support groups would be helpful. This is puzzling given that these support groups are predicated on the acknowledgement that CA grief is real. Therefore, one would assume that this type of nonjudgmental support would be perceived as helpful. Indeed, a growing number of veterinary, social, and mental health education programs and practices are establishing various forms of support (Miller *et al.*, 2014; Rémillard *et al.*, 2017; Park and Royal, 2020; Crossley and Rolland, 2022). Typically, the literature assumes that pet grief support groups are tools to reduce or eliminate the risk of grieving CA guardians experiencing DG and progressing to complicated grief. However, this is not yet a well-researched area and our literature search did not retrieve any outcome studies.

A qualitative study of older women living alone in a community whose CA had died (Wilson *et al.*, 2021) identified that grief coping strategies were highly idiosyncratic, and what was seen as very helpful by one participant was equally likely to be judged as unhelpful by another. The findings from this survey align with Wilson *et al.*'s findings and, as detailed in Table 10.2, demonstrate the diversity of endorsements for what were considered helpful or unhelpful coping strategies. The theoretical assumptions underpinning support groups have recently come under increasing scrutiny, and it has been proposed that some people perceive support group membership as undesirable, believing that these supports reinforce their membership in stigmatized groups (Crabtree *et al.*, 2010; Markowitz, 2015). For example, a study involving 73 mental health support group members across the UK determined that support group membership can have negative outcomes, such as reinforcement of the extent of social stigma, increased self-stigmatization, and reduced self-esteem (Crabtree *et al.*, 2010). It is also possible, from the scarce literature available, that those with greater resources (e.g., social capital, economic security, access to alternative support such as positive and involved family and friends) are less inclined to find support groups useful (Markowitz, 2015). This is a complex area, and as a full examination is beyond the scope of this paper, readers are referred to more in-depth reviews of emerging evidence (e.g., Markowitz, 2015). These broader findings indicate that pet loss support groups, depending on the individual, may serve either to reduce DG or to increase self-disenfranchisement. Evidently, support groups should not be considered the gold standard intervention, and a range of options are indicated.

Finally, the implications of DG were underlined by the statistically significant difference between those who reported feeling unsupported and those who were cautious about who they disclosed to, compared to those who felt supported. Those who felt unsupported had higher scores on the PBQ ($p < .001$) and reported a decrease in physical health ($p = .024$) (Table 10.1).

Limitations

The survey has limitations in relation to the sample lacking gender and other intersectorial diversity, lack of comparative numbers of participants living alone or with others, under-representation of participants who were 71 years of age or older, and possible exclusion of those without access to social media. Surveys are also limited by participant self-selection, and it is possible that people who were not as significantly affected by the death of the CA did not participate. It is also possible that, given the impact of COVID-19 on CAs and their guardians (Applebaum *et al.*, 2020), the findings were influenced by atypical circumstances during 2021, such as restrictions on access to veterinary and counseling services. Additionally, the presence of another CA in the home may have had an influence that the study failed to identify. Finally, the lack of a CA-specific DG measure may have obscured the existing relationships between the study variables. The authors believe that the development of a CA-specific tool is the fundamental next step for researchers in this domain.

Conclusions

The findings of this study add to the emergent body of evidence underlying CA bereavement as an impactful mental and physical health issue. The significance of health impacts consequent to CA death and the need for evidence-informed and tested screening tools and interventions will continue to grow, given the increasing international trend of CAs being considered integral family members, coupled with global improvement in human longevity. The findings of this study indicate that DG is experienced by a sizable group of older adults following CA death, and that many participants perceive that socially legitimized recognition of loss and accompanying bereavement resources are lacking. These shortfalls contribute to significant health risks that can decrease older adults' ability to successfully age in the community. The study also revealed new questions and gaps in the evidence base, and several key areas for further study and intervention development. Specifically, unanswered questions remain regarding the relationship between gender and CA bereavement, assumptions about successful grieving and living with others or alone, the prevalence of guilt as a result of euthanasia decisions and effective screening and intervention strategies, the role of social marketing in increasing the societal legitimization of CA grief, and outcome studies of CA bereavement support groups and counseling interventions. The development and testing of a DG screening tool specific to CA guardians is a priority.

Thank you for validating my deep grief. This research is so important.
Awareness, acceptance, and education is needed so people can grieve without having to be silent or ashamed. (Anonymous participant).

Conflict of Interest

The authors have no conflict of interest to report.

Funding

This study was funded by funded by the joint Kule Institute for Advanced Study (KIAS), University of Alberta and the Calgary Institute for the Humanities (CIH), University of Calgary – Alberta Humanities Research Grant. The funding sources had no role in the study design, data collection, analysis, and interpretation of the data, or writing of the manuscript.

Acknowledgements

We would like to thank the participants of this study and the organizations and groups that distributed our participant recruitment advertisements.

Authors' Contributions

CB, DW, EC, DG, MM, and JW contributed to study design. CB performed the primary analyses and interpretation of the data, which were discussed and refined with DW, EC, JW, DG, and MM. CB drafted the initial manuscript, which has been refined and revised several times with the other authors. All authors contributed to the manuscript and have read and approved the final manuscript.

Data Availability Statement

The data set used in the current study is available from the corresponding author upon reasonable request.

Ethics Statement

Ethics approval for this study was obtained from the Human Research Ethics Board, University of Alberta (Pro00101778).

Abbreviations

CA	Companion animal
DG	Disenfranchised grief
PBQ	Pet bereavement questionnaire
PALS	Pet attachment and life-impact scale
WDG	Witnessing disenfranchised grief

References

Adams, C.L., Bonnett, B.N. and Meek, A.H. (2000) Predictors of owner response to companion animal death in 177 clients from 14 practices in Ontario. *Journal of the American Veterinary Medical Association* 217(9), 1303–1309. DOI: 10.2460/javma.2000.217.1303.

Adrian, J.A.L. and Stitt, A. (2017) Pet loss, complicated grief, and post-traumatic stress disorder in Hawaii. *Anthrozoös* 30(1), 123–133. DOI: 10.1080/08927936.2017.1270598.

American Psychological Association (2022) *Definition – Disenfranchised Grief*. APA Dictionary of Psychology. Available at: https://dictionary.apa.org/disenfranchised-grief

Applebaum, J.W., Tomlinson, C.A., Matijczak, A., McDonald, S.E. and Zsembik, B.A. (2020) The concerns, difficulties, and stressors of caring for pets during COVID-19: Results from a large survey of U.S. pet owners. *Animals* 10, 1882. DOI: 10.3390/ani10101882.

Barnard-Nguyen, S., Breit, M., Anderson, K.A. and Nielsen, J. (2016) Pet loss and grief: Identifying at-risk pet owners during the euthanasia process. *Anthrozoös* 29(3), 421–430. DOI: 10.1080/08927936.2016.1181362.

Bibbo, J., Curl, A.L. and Johnson, R.A. (2019) Pets in the lives of older adults: A life course perspective. *Anthrozoös* 32(4), 541–554.

Brown, K. (2006) Pastoral concern in relation to the psychological stress caused by the death of an animal companion. *Mental Health, Religion & Culture* 9(5), 411–422. DOI: 10.1080/13694670500212208.

Bruinsma, S.M., Tiemeier, H.W., Heemst, J.V., van der Heide, A. and Rietjens, J.A.C. (2015) Risk factors for complicated grief in older adults. *Journal of Palliative Medicine* 18(5), 438–446. DOI: 10.1089/jpm.2014.0366.

Burnes, D., Henderson, C.R., Sheppard, C., Zhao, R., Pillemer, K. *et al.* (2017) Prevalence of financial fraud and scams among older adults in the United States: A systematic review and meta-analysis. *American Journal of Public Health* 107(8), e13–e21. DOI: 10.2105/AJPH.2017.303821.

Bussolari, C., Habarth, J.M., Phillips, S., Katz, R. and Packman, W. (2021) Self-compassion, social constraints, and psychosocial outcomes in a pet bereavement sample. *OMEGA – Journal of Death and Dying* 82(3), 389–408. DOI: 10.1177/0030222818814050.

Canadian Animal Health Institute (CAHI) (2020) *2020 Pet Population Survey*. Available at: https://www.globenewswire.com/fr/news-release/2021/02/16/2176264/0/en/2020-Canadian-Pet-Population-Figures-Released.html

Cordaro, M. (2012) Pet loss and disenfranchised grief: Implications for mental health counseling practice. *Journal of Mental Health Counseling* 34(4), 283–294. DOI: 10.17744/mehc.34.4.41q0248450t98072.

Corr, C.A. (1999) Enhancing the concept of disenfranchised grief. *OMEGA – Journal of Death and Dying* 38(1), 1–20. DOI: 10.2190/LD26-42A6-1EAV-3MDN.

Cowling, D.M., Isenstein, S.G.E. and Schneider, M.S. (2020) When the bond breaks: Variables associated with grief following companion animal loss. *Anthrozoös* 33(6), 693–708. DOI: 10.1080/08927936.2020.1824651.

Crabtree, J.W., Haslam, S.A., Postmes, T. and Haslam, C. (2010) Mental health support groups, stigma, and self-esteem: Positive and negative implications of group identification. *Journal of Social Issues* 66(3), 553–569.

Cromer, L.D. and Barlow, M.R. (2013) Factors and convergent validity of the pet attachment and life impact scale (PALS). *Human Animal Interaction Bulletin* 1(2), 34–56.

Crossley, M.K. and Rolland, C. (2022) Overcoming the social stigma of losing a pet: Considerations for counseling professionals. In: *Human-Animal Interactions*. CAB International, Wallingford, UK. DOI: 10.1079/hai.2022.0022.

Davis, H.L. (2011) Death of a companion animal: Understanding human responses to bereavement. In: *The Psychology of the Human-Animal Bond*. Springer, New York, pp. 225–242.

Dickinson, G.E. and Hoffman, H.C. (2017) Saying goodbye to family: Caretakers' experiences with euthanasia and honoring the legacy of companion animals. *Society and Animals* 25, 490–507. DOI: 10.1163/15685306-12341456.

Doka, K.J. (1999) Disenfranchised grief. *Bereavement Care* 18(3), 37–39. DOI: 10.1080/02682629908657467.

Eckerd, L.M., Barnett, J.E. and Jett-Dias, L. (2016) Grief following pet and human loss: Closeness is key. *Death Studies* 40(5), 275–282. DOI: 10.1080/07481187.2016.1139014.

Enders-Slegers, M. and Hediger, K. (2019) Pet ownership and human–animal interaction in an aging population: rewards and challenges. *Anthrozoös* 3(2), 255–265. DOI: 10.1080/08927936.2019.1569907.

Fernández-Alcántara, M., Kokou-Kpolou, C.K., Cruz-Quintana, F. and Pérez-Marfil, M.N. (2021) New perspectives in bereavement and loss: Complicated and disenfranchised grief along the life cycle. *Frontiers in Psychology* 12, 1–3. DOI: 10.3389/fpsyg.2021.691464.

Finberg, J. (2003) Financial Abuse of the Elderly in California. 36 Loy. L.A. L. Rev. 667. Available at: https://digitalcommons.lmu.edu/llr/vol36/iss2/3

Fine, A. (2019) The eternal bond. In: Kogan, L. and Erdman, P. (eds) *Pet Loss, Grief, and Therapeutic Interventions: Practitioners Navigating the Human–Animal Bond*. Routledge, New York.

Gage, M.G. and Holcomb, R. (1991) Couples' perception of stressfulness of death of the family pet. *Family Relations* 40(1), 103–105. DOI: 10.2307/585666.

Hunt, M. and Padilla, Y. (2006) Development of the pet bereavement questionnaire. *Anthrozoös* 19(4), 308–324. DOI: 10.2752/089279306785415493.

JASP Team (2022) JASP (Version 0.16.1) [Computer software]. Available at: https://jasp-stats.org

Kemp, H.R., Jacobs, N. and Stewart, S. (2016) The lived experience of companion-animal loss: A systematic review of qualitative studies. *Anthrozoös* 29(4), 533–557. DOI: 10.1080/08927936.2016.1228772.

Kogan, L. and Erdman, P. (2020) *Pet Loss, Grief, and Therapeutic Interventions: Practitioners Navigating the Human–Animal Bond*. Routledge, New York.

Laing, M. and Maylea, C. (2018) They burn brightly, but only for a short time: The role of social workers in companion animal grief and loss. *Anthrozoös* 31, 221–232. DOI: 10.1080/08927936.2018.1434062.

Lannen, P.K., Wolfe, J., Prigerson, H.G., Onelov, E. and Kreicbergs, U.C. (2008) Unresolved grief in a national sample of bereaved parents: impaired mental and physical health 4 to 9 years later. *Journal of Clinical Oncology* 26(36), 5870–5876. DOI: 10.1200/JCO.2007.14.6738.

LEK Consulting (2021) Pet Ownership to Keep Growing after Pandemic Bump. Available at: https://www.consulting.us/news/6322/pet-ownership-to-keep-growing-after-pandemic-bump

Leonhardt-Parr, E. and Rumble, B. (2022) Coping with animal companion loss: A thematic analysis of pet bereavement counselling. *OMEGA – Journal of Death and Dying* 1–17. DOI: 10.1177/00302228211073217.

Lundorff, M., Bonanno, G.A., Johannsen, M. and O'Connor, M. (2020) Are there gender differences in prolonged grief trajectories? A registry-sampled cohort study. *Journal of Psychiatric Research* 129, 168–175. DOI: 10.1016/j.jpsychires.2020.06.030.

Markowitz, F.E. (2015) Involvement in mental health self-help groups and recovery. *Health Sociology Review* 24(2), 199–212. DOI: 10.1080/14461242.2015.1015149.

McKinney, K. (2019) Emotion work of coping with the death of a companion animal. *Society and Animals* 27(1), 109–125. DOI: 10.1163/15685306-12341586.

Milan, A. (2000) *One Hundred Years of Families, Canadian Social Trends, Statistics Canada Catalogue no.11-008*.

Miller, T.A.K., Prout, M.F., Rourke, M., Lefkowitz, C. and Boyer, B. (2014) A therapist's guide to treating grief after the loss of a pet: A three-tier model. *Human-Animal Interaction Bulletin* 2(1), 38–58.

Packman, W., Bussolari, C., Katz, R. and Carmack, B.J. (2016) Continuing bonds research with animal companions: Implications for men grieving the loss of a dog. In: Blazina, C. and Kogan, L.R. (eds) *Men and Their Dogs: A New Understanding of Man's Best Friend*. Springer International Publishing AG, New York, pp. 303–320. DOI: 10.1007/978-3-319-30097-9_15.

Park, R. and Royal, K. (2020) A national survey of companion animal owners' self-reported methods of coping following Euthanasia. *Veterinary Sciences* 7(3), 89. DOI: 10.3390/vetsci7030089.

Reisbig, A.M.J., Hafen, M., Siqueira Drake, A.A., Girard, D. and Breunig, Z.B. (2017) Companion animal death: A qualitative analysis of relationship quality, loss, and coping. *OMEGA – Journal of Death and Dying* 75(2), 124–150. DOI: 10.1177/0030222815612607.

Rémillard, L.W., Meehan, M.P., Kelton, D.F. and Coe, J.B. (2017) Exploring the grief experience among callers to a pet loss support hotline. *Anthrozoös* 30(1), 149–161. DOI: 10.1080/08927936.2017.1270600.

Scoresby, K.J., Strand, E.B., Ng, Z., Brown, K.C., Stilz, C.R. *et al*. (2021) Pet ownership and quality of life: A systematic review of the literature. *Veterinary Sciences* 8(12), 332. DOI: 10.3390/vetsci8120332.

Smith, W.G. (2008) *Does Gender Influence Online Survey Participation? A Record-Linkage Analysis of University Faculty Online Survey Response Behavior*. Available at: https://files.eric.ed.gov/fulltext/ED501717.pdf

Spain, B., O'Dwyer, L. and Moston, S. (2019) Pet loss: Understanding disenfranchised grief, memorial use, and posttraumatic growth. *Anthrozoös* 32(4), 555–568. DOI: 10.1080/08927936.2019.1621545.

St Clair, J.S. (2013) The witnessing of disenfranchised grief: Reliability and validity. *Journal of Nursing Measurement* 21(3), 401–414.

Stanley, I.H., Conwell, Y., Bowen, C. and Orden, K.A. (2014) Pet ownership may attenuate loneliness among older adult primary care patients who live alone. *Aging and Mental Health* 18(3), 394–399. DOI: 10.1080/13607863.2013.837147.

Tang, J., Galbraith, N. and Truong, J. (2019) Living alone in canada. In: *Insights on Canadian Society. Statistics Canada Catalogue No.75-006-X, ISSN*. Available at: https://www150.statcan.gc.ca/n1/en/pub/75-006-x/2019001/article/00003-eng.pdf?st=qpDXRavj

Thimm, J.C., Kristoffersen, A.E. and Ringberg, U. (2020) The prevalence of severe grief reactions after bereavement and their associations with mental health, physical health, and health service utilization: A population-based study. *European Journal of Psychotraumatology* 11(1), 1844440. DOI: 10.1080/20008198.2020.1844440.

Trevino, K.M., Litz, B., Papa, A., Maciejewski, P.K., Lichtenthal, W. *et al*. (2018) Bereavement challenges and their relationship to physical and psychological adjustment to loss. *Journal of Palliative Medicine* 21(4), 479–488. DOI: 10.1089/jpm.2017.0386.

Vonk, J., Maria Corina Bouma, E. and Dijkstra, A. (2022) A time to say goodbye: empathy and emotion regulation predict timing of end-of-life decisions by pet owners. In: *Human–Animal Interaction Bulletin*. CAB International, Wallingford, UK. DOI: 10.1079/hai.2022.0013.

Wang, Y., Dai, Y., Li, H. and Song, L. (2021) Social media and attitude change: Information booming promote or resist persuasion. *Frontiers in Psychology* 12, 596071. DOI: 10.3389/fpsyg.2021.596071.

Wilson, D.M., Underwood, L., Carr, E., Gross, D., Kane, M. *et al*. (2021) Older women's experiences of companion animal death: Impacts on well-being and aging-in-place. *BMC Geriatrics* 21, 470. DOI: 10.1186/s12877-021-02410-8.

11 When Support is "Pawsed": Increased Attachment Mediates the Association Between Loss of Support and Pet Bereavement During the Pandemic

Victoria L. O'Connor[1], Jennifer Vonk[1]* and Katherine Compitus[2]

[1]Department of Psychology, Oakland University, Rochester Hills, MI, USA; [2]Silver School of Social Work, New York University, New York, NY, USA

Abstract

The COVID-19 pandemic has introduced and exacerbated innumerable stressors for Americans. Pet ownership has been shown to help individuals cope with stress and loneliness. However, given the shorter life spans of most pets compared to humans, many pet owners inevitably dealt with pet loss and its associated grief during the pandemic. We surveyed 284 community and college participants that had suffered the loss of a pet during the pandemic. We asked these pet owners about their pandemic-related experiences over the preceding year with regard to the types of losses they experienced, whether they experienced isolation through quarantine and their perception of social support. We also measured their general attachment to pets along with the grief they felt as a result of pet loss. We hypothesized that greater loss, increased isolation, and reduced social support would lead to increased attachment to pets, which would intensify the experience of grief. Mediated regression analyses revealed a direct effect of loss on grief that was not mediated through attachment. Unexpectedly, greater perceived social support showed an indirect effect on grief through stronger attachment to pets. Results confirm prior findings that greater pet attachment leads to more intense pet grief, but the attachment was not intensified through loss of support social or increased isolation as predicted. It is important to recognize the substantial impact of pet loss, especially during stressful times, and this topic deserves further investigation, perhaps with a greater focus on the type of pet and pet-specific measures of attachment.

Keywords: stress, pet loss, grief, attachment, isolation, social support

Introduction

The 2020 SARS-CoV-2 (COVID-19) virus emerged in the United States in December 2019, changing the dynamics of the country. Perhaps due to an increase in work-from-home orders, 2020 saw a rise in the pet population—estimated to be nearly 71 million pet-owning American households, representing a 4% growth in one year (Packaged Facts, 2020). According to the 2021 American Pet Products Association National Pet Owners Survey, approximately 70% of U.S. households own a pet (American Pet Products Association (APPA), 2021). Pet ownership bestows numerous benefits on owners (e.g., O'Haire, 2010; McConnell *et al.*,

*Corresponding author: vonk@oakland.edu

2011; Marsa-Sambola *et al.*, 2017). However, an unfortunate consequence of pet ownership is the inevitability of pet mortality. Millions of pets each year die of natural causes or are euthanized. Thus, the number of pet owners who experience pet loss voluntarily or involuntarily is high. We were interested in whether pet owners' increased time at home and potential loss of social support due to the pandemic might increase their attachment to their pet, which might, in turn, intensify grief felt for the loss of a pet during the pandemic. Thus, we examined pet owners' grief at the loss of a pet during the preceding year during the height of the COVID-19 pandemic as a function of loss, isolation, and support, mediated through attachment to the pet.

The attachment between humans and pets is a mutually beneficial and dynamic relationship (American Veterinary Medical Association, 2022) as pets readily provide companionship and affection (Levinson, 1969). This bond can be explained by the Human-Animal Attachment Theory (Bowlby, 1982), which suggests that a high level of attachment to animals allows humans to better cope with their environmental stressors (e.g., loss of financial stability, social isolation, increase in health risks, etc.). Research indicates that the human-pet relationship meets the four prerequisites for attachment—proximity seeking, safe haven, secure base, and separation distress (Bowlby, 1982). Pet owners feel and enjoy the closeness to their pets (Hall *et al.*, 2004) as they provide comfort and security (Pirrone *et al.*, 2015). Furthermore, research indicates improvement in general health and a reduction in loneliness with a higher attachment to pets in older adults (e.g., Krause-Parello and Gulick, 2013). Pets have a buffering effect on loneliness in older adults (Mueller *et al.*, 2021); loneliness can predict pet ownership while pet ownership can also predict loneliness (Pikhartova *et al.*, 2014). While pets may ease loneliness (Krause-Parello, 2012) and improve the mental health of pet owners (Ratschen *et al.*, 2020), overly strong attachment to pets has also been associated with poor psychological adjustment and health (McDonald *et al.*, 2021).

In March 2020, the World Health Organization sought to combat the spread of the respiratory illness, COVID-19, by encouraging social isolation and distancing (Lewnard and Lo, 2020). Many states issued a temporary stay-at-home orders and quarantine was mandated for infected individuals. These unfortunate consequences of the pandemic increased social isolation and negative psychological effects, such as loneliness, anxiety, and depression (e.g., Hawes *et al.*, 2021). Whereas some research suggests that pets have helped some individuals cope with the pandemic (Bowen *et al.*, 2020), and pet owners experienced lower levels of loneliness (Applebaum *et al.*, 2021), other findings suggest that pet owners faced unique hardships at the beginning of the pandemic, resulting in worsening mental health (Hawkins and Brodie, 2020). The strength of pet attachment can be predictive of the level of owner's grief (e.g., Field *et al.*, 2009) and can determine the psychological impact on the owner (Cowles, 1985). Higher levels of attachment are associated with greater grief at the loss of a pet in both children (Schmidt *et al.*, 2020) and adults (Gosse and Barnes, 1994), complicated by feelings associated with grief, depression, and trauma (Archer and Winchester, 1994).

Whereas levels of grief after pet loss are comparable to the loss of a human spouse (Packman *et al.*, 2011) or family member (Luiz Adrian *et al.*, 2009), bereavement after pet loss is often invalidated (Topál *et al.*, 2009). This may have been especially true during the COVID-19 pandemic, which saw a catastrophic human loss. Factors further complicating grief over the loss of a pet include the responsibility of owners to euthanize animals (Adams *et al.*, 2000; Vonk *et al.*, 2022), circumstances of death (Baydak, 2000), physical or financial restrictions (Meier and Maurer, 2022), attachment style (Henry, 2008; Field *et al.*, 2009), and social support (McCutcheon and Fleming, 2002). King and Werner (2012) found that higher levels of social support predicted lower levels of grief, depression, and anxiety. Research on Australian adolescents indicated that youth with less support from parents have stronger bonds with their dogs (Bodsworth and Coleman, 2001). Although those who experience grief associated with pet loss are more likely to seek social support (Nilsson, 2005), the pandemic made it more challenging to receive social support. Thus, we expected that lower perceived social support would predict greater grief at pet loss, which might be mediated by a greater attachment toward the pet. Others (Stallones *et al.*, 1990) have observed this relationship pre-pandemic as well.

Although most previous research dealing with pet loss and bereavement focuses on cat and dog owners, we recruited pet owners broadly. We surveyed community and college students that had lost a pet during the preceding year, which covered the height of the COVID-19 pandemic when lockdowns and social distancing protocols were in full effect. We asked respondents to report on their experiences related to the pandemic with particular attention to the types of losses they experienced during the pandemic, whether they experienced isolation through quarantine and their perception of social support. We measured their attachment to their pet along with the grief they felt as a result of pet loss. We hypothesized that greater loss, increased isolation, and reduced social support would lead to increased attachment to pets, which would then be associated with greater reported grief. Thus, our hypotheses were consistent with a direct and indirect effects model whereby support, isolation, and losses were associated with grief through attachment to the bereaved pet.

Method

Participants and procedure

Participants ($n = 413$) who had lost a pet during the previous year (i.e., at the height of the COVID-19 pandemic restrictions) were recruited from the Psychology Subject Pool at a university in the mid-western United States ($n = 284$) and social media outlets (e.g., Facebook, Reddit, Twitter; $n = 129$) from February through June of 2021. University students were recruited from introductory-level psychology classes and were compensated with class credit. To recruit participants from social media, the authors shared a link to the research with a brief summary of the study via their personal social media accounts.

All participants were asked to report about grief associated with the loss of a pet during the pandemic and their attachment to that pet. They also completed measures concerning their demographics, personality, social support, and experiences during the pandemic with particular attention to their relationship with other people and their pets via a secure website, Qualtrics.com. Data were excluded for 169 participants who did not complete at least 75% of the survey ($n = 65$), did not lose a pet during the pandemic (n=88), or failed one of the three attention checks ($n = 16$). Our final sample (n = 244) consisted of 206 cis gender females/trans-females, 31 cis gender males/trans-males, and 7 non-binary individuals and was composed of 81.2% 18–30 year-olds, 16% 31–54 year-olds, 2.8% individuals 55 and older. Participants' racial/ethnic composition was 76.2% White, 7.8% Black, 4.9% Latinx, 6.6% Other/Unknown, 3.7% Asian, and .8% Native Hawaiian/ Pacific Islander. A majority of participants ($n = 213$), though not all ($n = 30$ no, n=1 did not answer) quarantined during the pandemic. Participants provided information on which kind of pet died: Dog 47.1% ($n = 115$), Cat 23% ($n = 56$), Reptile 2.5% ($n = 6$), Fish 15.2% ($n = 37$), Bird 2.9% ($n = 7$), Rodent 4.5% ($n = 11$), Pig .8% ($n = 2$), Exotic 1.2% ($n = 3$), and Other 2.9% ($n = 7$).

Measures

Predictors

Losses

Participants were asked if they experienced any of the following losses in the previous twelve months: (0) none, (1) loss of social support, (2) loss of job, (3) loss or decrease in income, (4) loss of social opportunities, (5) loss of relationship, (6) death of family member, (7) death of friends, or (8) health suffered due to the virus. The predictor variable "loss" was created by counting how many categories were experienced as a proxy to represent the breadth of the pandemic's impact on the individual.

Isolation

Individuals that quarantined were asked two follow-up questions. In the first, individuals answered how long they quarantined for: 1 (1 week), 2 (2 weeks), 3 (3 weeks), or 4 (longer than 3 weeks). They were assigned a score of 1–4 to reflect the increased time in quarantine.

Subsequently, they were asked if they quarantined alone (scored as 2), or quarantined with others (scored as 1). Individuals' scores on these two questions were multiplied to create the "isolation" predictor variable to ascertain the impact of time spent quarantining.

Social support

The Multidimensional Scale of Perceived Social Support (MSPSS; Zimet *et al.*, 1988) measured social support of family (e.g., "My family really tried to help me"; $\alpha = .93$), friends (e.g., "I can count on my friends when things go wrong"; $\alpha = .94$), and significant others (e.g., "There is a special person who is around when I am in need"; $\alpha = .95$) on a seven-point Likert scale ranging from 1 (very strongly disagree) to 7 (very strongly agree).

The Duke Social Support and Stress Scale (DUSOCS; Parkerson *et al.*, 1989) assessed family and non-family support and stress using 24 questions equally divided over two subscales. The DUSOCS support ($\alpha = .64$) and stress ($\alpha = .68$) subscales were rated on a four-point Likert scale from 0 (there is no person) to 3 (a lot) when asked about individuals such as "Your wife, husband, or significant other person" or "Your children and grandchildren."

We created a composite variable to represent "support" by taking the average of the standardized total scores from these two measures.

Mediator

Attachment to pet

The Censhare Pet Attachment Scale (CENS; Holcomb *et al.*, 1985) consists of 27 items that are responded to using a four-point Likert scale from 0 (almost never) to 4 (almost always). An example statement is "You confide in your pet." Inter-item reliability was $\alpha = .94$. Participants were not asked to respond with regard to a specific pet; however, they responded to all attachment measures after the set of pet demographic questions in which they were instructed to respond to "the following questions" with regard to a pet they had lost during the past year.

The Lexington Attachment to Pet Scale (LAPS; Johnson *et al.*, 1992) examines an individual's emotional attachment to their pet via three subscales- general attachment (e.g., "My dog/cat understands me"; $\alpha = .96$), people substituting (e.g., "I love my dog/cat because it never judges me"; $\alpha = .90$), and animal rights/animal welfare (e.g., "Pets deserve as much respect as humans do"; $\alpha = .86$). Respondents report their level of agreement with 23 statements using a scale of 0 (strongly disagree) to 3 (strongly agree). Inter-item reliability was $\alpha = .97$. Participants were instructed to respond to this scale with regard to their favorite pet.

The modified version of the Pet Attitude Scale (PAS; Templer *et al.*, 1981) assesses participants' attitudes, both positive and negative, toward pets. It included 18 items such as, "I really like seeing pets enjoy their food." Participants responded using a Likert scale from 1 (strongly disagree) to 7 (strongly agree). Inter-item reliability was $\alpha = .89$. Scores on this scale are typically correlated with measures of attachment to animals including the CENS, CABS, LAPS, Pet Attitude Inventory, and Pet Relationship Scale (Blazina *et al.*, 2011). The PAS has also been associated with greater dog and cat grief (Planchon and Templer, 1996).

The Companion Animal Bonding Scale (CABS; Poresky *et al.*, 1987) measures a human–animal bond with eight questions regarding pet owner behavior (e.g., "How often were you responsible for your companion animal's care?"). Responses to items range from 1 (never) to 5 (always). Inter-item reliability was $\alpha = .85$. Participants responded to this scale specifically while thinking about the pet they had lost during the pandemic.

We created a composite variable to represent Pet Attachment by taking the average of the standardized total scores from these four measures, which were highly correlated (all p's $< .001$, see Table 11.1).

Outcomes

Grief

Grief was assessed using the Pet Bereavement Questionnaire (PBQ; Hunt and Padilla, 2006), which consists of 16 questions to measure grief (e.g., "I cry when I think about my pet"; $\alpha = .89$),

Table 11.1. Correlations among the variables that compose the predictors, mediators, and outcomes.

	1	2	3	4	5	6	7	8
1. MSPSS	-							
2. DUSOCS	.19**	-						
3. CENS	.17*	.18**	-					
4. LAPS	.16*	.20**	.74**	-				
5. PAS	.19**	.15*	.69**	.83**				
6. CABS	.06	.17**	.67**	.59**	.54**	-		
7. PBQ	–.11	.07	.42**	.48**	.32**	.46**	-	
8. CBS	.09	.12	.60**	.60**	.50**	.59**	.59**	-
Mean	5.24	.02	3.16	5.71	5.68	3.60	2.52	3.24
Standard Deviation	1.21	.01	.57	1.09	.71	.86	.55	.88

*p < .05. **p < .01.

anger (e.g., "I feel very angry at the veterinarian for not being able to save my pet"; $\alpha = .72$), guilt (e.g., "I feel bad that I didn't do more to save my pet"; $\alpha = .83$), and trauma (e.g., "I have had nightmares about my pet's death"; $\alpha = .73$) on a four-point Likert scale from 0 (disagree strongly) to 3 (agree strongly). Inter-item reliability was $\alpha = .73$.

The Continuing Bonds Scale (CBS; Field *et al.*, 2003) was developed to measure bereavement in spouses using 11 questions ($\alpha = .90$) asking how much a statement relates to themselves (e.g., "I seek out things to remind me of my pet") as 1 (not at all true) to 5 (very true). For the purpose of this study, the term "spouse" in the instruction was changed to "pet" so that it read, "Rate the extent to which each of the items is true with respect to your pet that died during the pandemic."

Respondents completed both of these measures with regard to a pet that they had lost during the previous year. The CBS and PBQ were highly correlated ($r = .60$, $p < .001$), standardized and averaged together to form the composite "Grief" outcome variable.

Analyses

We conducted three parallel mediation analyses using Model 4 of the PROCESS macro for SPSS (Hayes, 2013) to test the direct and indirect effects of loss, isolation, and social support, through pet attachment, on pet grief (see Fig. 11.1). The model used a bootstrap resampling method repeated 10,000 times to generate a 95% percentile bootstrap confidence interval (CI) for the direct and indirect associations. Cases of incomplete data were excluded from these analyses, leaving a sample of 241 for the effects of loss and 243 for both the effects of isolation and support. We used a seed command and included all predictors as covariates in each model in which they were not predictors.

Results

Descriptives and correlations

Zero-order correlations between the variables and descriptive statistics appear in Table 11.2. The loss was correlated positively with isolation and negatively with support. Support was correlated with attachment, which was correlated with grief. Grief was also positively correlated with isolation and negatively with support.

Mediation analyses

Loss

We conducted a mediation analysis for loss mediated by pet attachment to predict pet grief. In all models, attachment predicted grief ($b = .68$, $t = 13.31$, $p = .00$, $CI_{95\%}$ [–.58, .78]). The association between loss and attachment

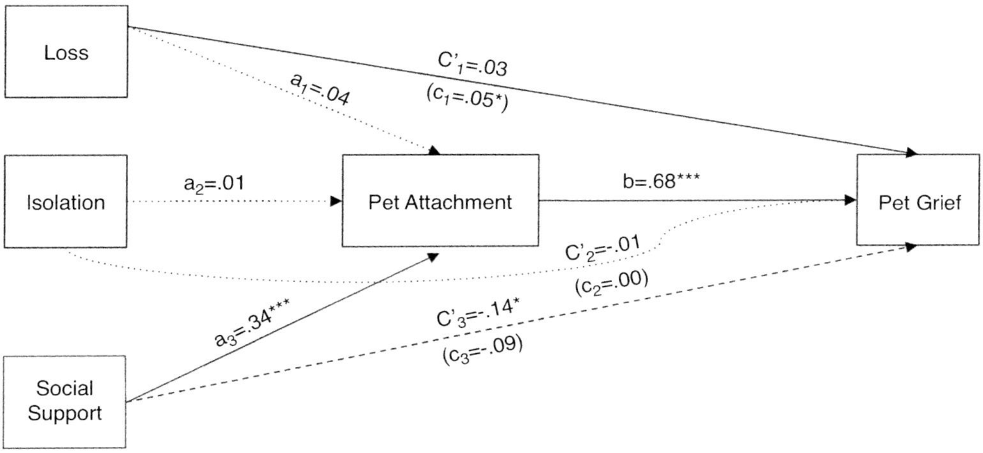

Fig. 11.1. Direct and indirect effects of loss, isolation, and social support on grief through attachment. *Note*. Dotted lines depict insignificant associations. Dashed lines depict significant negative associations. Solid lines depict significant positive associations. *Note*. *p = .05, **p < .01, ***p < .001.

Table 11.2. Correlations among the composite variables used in analyses.

	1	2	3	4	5
1. Loss	—				
2. Isolation	.16*	-			
3. Support	−.18**	.024	-		
4. Attachment	.08	.06	.13*	-	
5. Grief	.13*	.04	−0.01	.67**	—
Mean	2.51	2.91	2.64	4.54	2.88
Standard deviation	1.75	1.43	.63	.71	.64

*p < .05. **p < .01.

approached significance ($a_1 = .04$, $t = 1.78$, $p = .08$, $CI_{95\%}$ [−.00, .08]) and loss had a significant positive association with pet grief ($c_1 = .05$, $t = 2.30$, $p = .02$, $CI_{95\%}$ [.01, .10]). However, this effect disappeared when controlling for attachment, ($c'_1 = .03$, $t = 1.48$, $p = 0.14$, $CI_{95\%}$ [−.01, .06]). The indirect effect of loss on pet grief through attachment approached significance ($a_1b = .03$, $z = 1.76$, $p = .08$, $CI_{95\%}$ [−.00, .06]).

Isolation

Isolation was not a significant predictor of pet attachment ($a_2 = -.01$, $t = -.50$, $p = .62$, $CI_{95\%}$ [−.05, .03]) or pet grief, ($c_2 = .00$, $t = .04$, $p = .97$, $CI_{95\%}$ [−.05, .05]). There was no significant indirect effect of isolation through attachment ($a_2b = .01$, $z = 0.63$, $p = .53$, $CI_{95\%}$ [−.03, .05]).

Social support

Social support had a positive association with pet attachment ($a_3 = .34$, $t = 3.86$, $p = .00$, $CI_{95\%}$ [.17, .51]). There was no total effect of support on pet grief ($c_3 = .09$, $t = .95$, $p = .34$, $CI_{95\%}$ [−.09, .26]), but a negative association emerged when attachment was controlled for ($c'_3 = -.14$, $t = -2.03$, $p = .04$, $CI_{95\%}$ [−.28, −.00]).

There was an indirect effect of support on grief through attachment ($a_3b = .22$, $z = 3.70$, $p = .00$, $CI_{95\%}$ [.10, .37]).

Discussion

We were able to survey pet owners during a unique time in American history when many pet owners were experiencing additional loss and stress due to the COVID-19 pandemic. We asked owners to reflect on their experiences during a year when the restrictions in place to curb the spread of disease were at their height. This was a period in which most of our respondents quarantined for at least a short period of time and experienced other losses, such as loss of job and social support. Research has verified the intuition that these stressors posed significant mental health risks for a number of Americans, such as increased anxiety and depression (Hawes *et al.*, 2021; Huato and Chavez, 2021; Mojtahedi *et al.*, 2021).

It was also a time when many individuals spent more time at home, presumably interacting more frequently with pets (Bolstad *et al.*, 2022). The presence of pets has been shown to improve coping with stress (Allen *et al.*, 2002), maintain regularity with exercise and healthy eating behavior (Vesnaver and Keller, 2011), and enhance social connectedness (Curl *et al.*, 2017). Companion animals are consistent, reliable sources of social support for humans (Serpell, 2003). For adolescents during the pandemic, pets served as resources for social and emotional support and facilitated their online friendships (Charmaraman *et al.*, 2022). However, the COVID-19 pandemic also brought new hardships to pet owners with many surveyed participants indicating they had issues meeting pets' social and behavioral needs and concerns for the functioning of their own households (Applebaum *et al.*, 2020). Additionally, while there was an initial surge in pet adoption and ownership, it proved unsustainable with many animals abandoned in shelters post-quarantine (Ho *et al.*, 2021). Pets act as substitutes for human-human interactions (Veevers, 1985), which might facilitate greater attachment to pets when human interactions are lacking. Although we have noted several positive impacts of attachment to pets, a strong attachment is also predictive of intense grief when pets pass away (Cowles, 1985; Gosse and Barnes, 1994; Brown *et al.*, 1996; Field *et al.*, 2009; Schmidt *et al.*, 2020). Additionally, those pet owners that feel strongly attached to their pets may feel "responsibility grief," or feelings of profound guilt (Dawson, 2010). We found further evidence here that greater attachment to pets led to increased grief. We were concerned that aspects of the pandemic might intensify both attachment to pets and grief for pets that passed away during this time.

We gathered information about various aspects of participants' COVID-19 pandemic experience and pet relationships to assess the extent to which loss, especially loss of social support, would impact attachment to pets, and therefore, grief at the loss of a pet that passed away during this time. Inconsistent with our predictions, increased perceptions of social support predicted greater attachment to pets, and this attachment mediated the relationship between perceived social support and grief. It is possible that if we had asked specifically about changes in social support during the pandemic, rather than general perceptions of support, we might have seen a different pattern of results. Our results were somewhat consistent with prior findings that pet relationships can increase bonds with other people as well (Charmaraman *et al.*, 2022). This information aids our understanding of the complex interplay between attachments and support within human and nonhuman animal companionship.

Contrary to our predictions, increased loss and isolation did not predict greater pet attachment, so attachment did not significantly mediate the associations between these predictors and grief, although the indirect effects of loss on grief approached significance. The number of different types of loss also predicted greater grief for the loss of a pet. This finding makes sense as loss in general might intensify the feeling of grief with the idea that "there is only so much an individual can take." But, these types of loss may not lead directly to an increased reliance on or attachment to a pet. Interestingly, Bolstad *et al.* (2022) found that whereas the pandemic led to increased physical contact with dogs and cats, it did not lead to changes in time spent caring for the pet or attachment to the pet.

It is somewhat surprising that we did not observe the effects of isolation as measured. There is strong evidence that a human–animal bond reduces isolation and loneliness as it provides stress-buffering effects (Virués-Ortega and

Buela-Casal, 2006). Thus, due to the pandemic, we expected the effects of isolation to impact owners' relationships with their animal companions and the subsequent grief due to the loss of those companions. However, it is important to note that our measure of isolation simply asked if individuals had quarantined, for how long, and if they did so alone. The quarantine may not have been lengthy, and they may not have spent it with their pets. In addition, it may have occurred early in the pandemic, months before they completed our survey. In future work, we would ask individuals to attempt to quantify the amount of time spent alone with pets versus in the company of others.

Limitations and future directions

Our data are correlational and self-reported so, as with any similar data, we cannot infer causality. Although we focused on a period of time during which American pet owners were dealing with the COVID-19 pandemic, we do not have comparable data from a different period of time with which to compare pet owners' attachment and grief. Thus, we must exert caution when attributing the pattern of results to the pandemic. However, we were able to examine the extent to which individual pet owners experienced different aspects of the pandemic and how these experiences related to their attachment to their pets and subsequent grief at their loss. Future research will be required to determine whether the patterns reported here were specific to the pandemic context.

Our sample size was modest and not representative of the broader population. Although we recruited community participants, most of our participants were university students, and 70% of them owned a traditional pet. We surveyed owners of a variety of pets rather than restricting our focus to dog and cat owners, as most previous research on grief has done. Thus, although we aimed to extend the research to pets defined more broadly, our sample size limited the extent to which we could examine differences with regard to the type of pet. At the same time, the inclusion of pets other than cats or dogs may have impacted our results. Prior research has found that dog and cat owners are more attached to their pets than owners of other pet types (Vidović *et al.*, 1999). In the current study, during the pandemic, owners may not have spent more time physically with animals such as fish, birds, and reptiles that spend more time enclosed compared to cats and dogs that they may interact with more freely. Pets, such as dogs and cats, are commonly deemed grievable, while experiencing grief at the loss of other species such as reptiles, birds, and fish is specific to the owner (Hirschman, 1994; Redmalm, 2015). In a separate study, we examined the bereavement of exotic pet owners in a larger community sample and found whether the pet was caged and the role of the pet predicted attachment and grief (Jordan and Vonk, unpublished). Level of education has also been correlated with attachment to pets (both negatively, e.g., Martens *et al.*, 2016 positively, e.g., Wong *et al.*, 2019), so the fact that the majority of our sample had completed some college may have biased the results as well. College students may have been better equipped than the general population to maintain social support during the pandemic due to their proficiency with technology for online communication. Our sample was predominantly female, which is common for this type of research, but females tend to show greater attachment to their pets in general (e.g., Brown *et al.*, 1996), so this was also a biasing factor.

Importantly, we did not ask participants to complete all of the attachment measures with the specific pet that they had most recently lost in mind. Although we did ask participants to complete all questions with regard to the pet they had lost, we had not reminded participants of this specific requirement at the beginning of each attachment measure, and for the Lexington Attachment to Pet Scale, we asked them to respond with regard to their favorite pet. We did not specify a target for the Pet Attitude Scale because this scale is framed toward pets in general. We included this measure because it was more appropriate for a broader variety of pet owners compared to many existing attachment measures. Initially, we wished to examine the associations of general attachment style toward pets and general attachment style toward humans with grief, although we did not analyze the latter data here in the interest of parsimony. In retrospect, we would have had respondents complete all of the measures with the one specific pet that they lost in mind. However, we are not concerned that failing to do so for two of the attachment measures invalidates our results given the strong positive correlations between all attachment measures (all correlations, $r > 0.55$, all $ps < 0.001$) and the strong positive association between attachment and grief for the specific pet that was lost. Given that others have found attachment style to contribute to pet grief, above and beyond the strength of attachment (Field *et al.*, 2009), we plan to examine specific attachment styles in future work as well.

Despite its limitations, we think the current data are valuable in capturing a unique time in history in which pets may have become the primary companions for many individuals that experienced extra stressors and less support than they typically experienced. Although we were not able to capture the intensity of perceived loss, we were able to capture a broad spectrum of experiences during the pandemic. Future studies should ask participants to rate the extent to which they felt negatively impacted by the pandemic.

Conclusions

The literature on pet attachment and social support is limited (see Stallones *et al.*, 1990), particularly with regard to pets other than cats and dogs. Therefore, the current findings make an important contribution and add to existing data that support the idea that humans rely on companion animals for support during times of stress, but that increased attachment to pets can intensify the experience of grief. Because bereaved pet owners often do not receive adequate support for their loss (Sharkin and Bahrick, 1990; Topál *et al.*, 2009; Tzivian *et al.*, 2014), even though the death of a pet can induce a similar grief response to a human loss (e.g., Quackenbush, 1985; Cowles, 1985; Luiz Adrian *et al.*, 2009; Rujoiu and Rujoiu, 2014; Habarth *et al.*, 2017), it is important to recognize factors contributing to grief so that adequate resources are provided to support individuals. Our data confirm the idea that this may be particularly important during times of stress. Our data suggest that perceived lack of social support and cumulative loss are stronger predictors of intense feelings of grief following pet loss compared to isolation itself.

Conflict of Interest

The authors have no conflicts of interest to declare.

Funding

There are no funders to report for this article.

Authors' Declaration

This study was reviewed and approved by the Oakland University Institutional Review Board Protocol # IRB-FY2021-245.

Authors' Contributions

VO and JV conceived of the study, collected and analysed the data and wrote the paper. KC contributed background literature and advice on measures and commented on a draft of the paper.

References

Adams, C.L., Bonnett, B.N. and Meek, A.H. (2000) Predictors of owner response to companion animal death in 177 clients from 14 practices in Ontario. *Journal of the American Veterinary Medical Association* 217(9), 1303–1309.

Allen, K., Blascovich, J. and Mendes, W.B. (2002) Cardiovascular reactivity and the presence of pets, friends, and spouses: The truth about cats and dogs. *Psychosomatic Medicine* 64(5), 727–739.

American Pet Products Association (APPA) (2021) 2021–2022 APPA National Pet Owners Survey. Available at: https://www.americanpetproducts.org/pubs_survey.asp

American Veterinary Medical Association (2022) AVMA Guidelines for Pet Loss Support Services. Available at: https://www.avma.org/KB/Policies/Pages/AVMA-Guidelines-for-Pet-Loss-Support-Services.aspx

Applebaum, J.W., Tomlinson, C.A., Matijczak, A., McDonald, S.E. and Zsembik, B.A. (2020) The concerns, difficulties, and stressors of caring for pets during COVID-19: Results from a large survey of US pet owners. *Animals* 10(10), 1882.

Applebaum, J.W., Ellison, C., Struckmeyer, L., Zsembik, B.A. and McDonald, S.E. (2021) The impact of pets on everyday life for older adults during the COVID-19 pandemic. *Frontiers in Public Health* 9, 292.

Archer, J. and Winchester, G. (1994) Bereavement following death of a pet. *British Journal of Psychology* 85(2), 259–271.

Baydak, M.A. (2000) Human grief on the death of a pet (Unpublished Master's Thesis), University of Manitoba, Winnipeg, Manitoba, Canada.

Blazina, C., Boyra, G. and Shen-Miller, D.S. (2011) *The Psychology of the Human-Animal Bond*. Springer Publications, New York, NY.

Bodsworth, W. and Coleman, G. (2001) Child-companion animal attachment bonds in single and two-parent families. *Anthrozoös* 14, 216–223.

Bolstad, C.J., Grayson, E.E., Gardner, A. and Nadorff, M.R. (2022) Pets and a pandemic: An exploratory mixed method analysis of how the COVID-19 pandemic affected dogs, cats, and owners. *Human Animal Interaction Bulletin* 11(2), 65–78.

Bowen, J., García, E., Darder, P., Argüelles, J. and Fatjó, J. (2020) The effects of the Spanish COVID-19 lockdown on people, their pets, and the human-animal bond. *Journal of Veterinary Behavior* 40, 75–91.

Bowlby, J. (1982) Attachment and loss: retrospect and prospect. *American Journal of Orthopsychiatry* 52(4), 664.

Brown, B.H., Richards, H.C. and Wilson, C.A. (1996) Pet bonding and pet bereavement among adolescents. *Journal of Counseling & Development* 74(5), 505–509.

Charmaraman, L., Cobas, S., Weed, J., Gu, Q., Kiel, E. *et al.* (2022) From regulating emotions to less lonely screen time: Parents' qualitative perspectives of the benefits and challenges of adolescent pet companionship. *Behavioral Sciences* 12(5), 143.

Cowles, K.V. (1985) The death of a pet: Human responses to the breaking of the bond. *Pets and the Family* 8, 135–161.

Curl, A.L., Bibbo, J. and Johnson, R.A. (2017) Dog walking, the human–animal bond and older adults' physical health. *The Gerontologist* 57(5), 930–939.

Dawson, S.E. (2010) Compassionate communication: Working with grief. In: Gray, C. and Moffett, J. (eds) *Handbook of Veterinary Communication Skills*. Wiley-Blackwell, pp. 62–99.

Field, N.P., Gal-Oz, E. and Bonanno, G.A. (2003) Continuing bonds and adjustment at 5 years after the death of a spouse. *Journal of Consulting and Clinical Psychology* 71(1), 110.

Field, N.P., Orsini, L., Gavish, R. and Packman, W. (2009) Role of attachment in response to pet loss. *Death Studies* 33(4), 334–355.

Gosse, G.H. and Barnes, M.J. (1994) Human grief resulting from the death of a pet. *Anthrozoös* 7(2), 103–112.

Habarth, J., Bussolari, C., Gomez, R., Carmack, B.J., Ronen, R. *et al.* (2017) Continuing bonds and psychosocial functioning in a recently bereaved pet loss sample. *Anthrozoös* 30(4), 651–670.

Hall, M.J., Ng, A., Ursano, R.J., Holloway, H., Fullerton, C. *et al.* (2004) Psychological impact of the animal-human bond in disaster preparedness and response. *Journal of Psychiatric Practice* 10(6), 368–374.

Hawes, M.T., Szenczy, A.K., Klein, D.N., Hajcak, G. and Nelson, B.D. (2021) Increases in depression and anxiety symptoms in adolescents and young adults during the COVID-19 pandemic. *Psychological Medicine* 1–9.

Hawkins, R.D. and Brodie, Z.P. (2020) The role of human-pet attachment on people's mental health over time during COVID-19 lockdown. In: *NRS Mental Health 2020 Annual Scientific Meeting*, United Kingdom.

Hayes, A.F. (2013) *Introduction to Mediation, Moderation, and Conditional Process Analysis: A Regression-Based Approach*. Guilford Press, New York, NY.

Henry, C.M. (2008) Risk indicators for grief symptoms after the death of a pet: does quality of attachment make a difference, Purdue University West, Lafayette, IN.

Hirschman, E.C. (1994) Consumers and their animal companions. *Journal of Consumer Research* 20(4), 616–632.

Ho, J., Hussain, S. and Sparagano, O. (2021) Did the COVID-19 pandemic spark a public interest in pet adoption. *Frontiers in Veterinary Science* 8, 647308.

Holcomb, R., Williams, R.C. and Richards, P.S. (1985) The elements of attachment: Relationship maintenance and intimacy. *Journal of the Delta Society* 2, 28–34.

Huato, J. and Chavez, A. (2021) Household income, pandemic-related income loss, and the probability of anxiety and depression. *Eastern Economic Journal* 47(4), 546–570.

Hunt, M. and Padilla, Y. (2006) Development of the pet bereavement questionnaire. *Anthrozoös* 19(4), 308–324.

Johnson, T.P., Garrity, T.F. and Stallones, L. (1992) Psychometric evaluation of the lexington attachment to pets scale (LAPS). *Anthrozoös* 5(3), 160–175.

King, L.C. and Werner, P.D. (2012) Attachment, social support, and responses following the death of a companion animal. *OMEGA-Journal of Death and Dying* 64(2), 119–141.

Krause-Parello, C.A. (2012) Pet ownership and older women: The relationships among loneliness, pet attachment support, human social support, and depressed mood. *Geriatric Nursing* 33(3), 194–203.

Krause-Parello, C.A. and Gulick, E.E. (2013) Situational factors related to loneliness and loss over time among older pet owners. *Western Journal of Nursing Research* 35(7), 905–919.

Levinson, B.M. (1969) *Pet-Oriented Psychotherapy*. Charles C. Thomas Publisher, Springfield, IL.

Lewnard, J.A. and Lo, N.C. (2020) Scientific and ethical basis for social-distancing interventions against COVID-19. *The Lancet Infectious Diseases* 20(6), 631–633.

Luiz Adrian, J.A., Deliramich, A.N. and Frueh, B.C. (2009) Complicated grief and posttraumatic stress disorder in humans' response to the death of pets/animals. *Bulletin of the Menninger Clinic* 73, 176–187.

Marsa-Sambola, F., Williams, J., Muldoon, J., Lawrence, A., Connor, M. *et al.* (2017) Quality of life and adolescents' communication with their significant others (mother, father, and best friend): The mediating effect of attachment to pets. *Attachment and Human Development* 19(3), 278–297.

Martens, P., Enders-Slegers, M.J. and Walker, J.K. (2016) The emotional lives of companion animals: Attachment and subjective claims by owners of cats and dogs. *Anthrozoös* 29(1), 73–88.

McConnell, A.R., Brown, C.M., Shoda, T.M., Stayton, L.E. and Martin, C.E. (2011) Friends with benefits: On the positive consequences of pet ownership. *Journal of Personality and Social Psychology* 101(6), 1239.

McCutcheon, K.A. and Fleming, S.J. (2002) Grief resulting from euthanasia and natural death of companion animals. *OMEGA-Journal of Death and Dying* 44(2), 169–188.

McDonald, S.E., O'connor, K.E., Matijczak, A., Tomlinson, C.A., Applebaum, J.W. *et al.* (2021) Attachment to pets moderates transitions in latent patterns of mental health following the onset of the COVID-19 pandemic: Results of a survey of US adults. *Animals* 11(3), 895.

Meier, C. and Maurer, J. (2022) Buddy or burden? Patterns, perceptions, and experiences of pet ownership among older adults in Switzerland. *European Journal of Ageing* 1–12.

Mojtahedi, D., Dagnall, N., Denovan, A., Clough, P., Hull, S. *et al.* (2021) The relationship between mental toughness, job loss, and mental health issues during the COVID-19 pandemic. *Frontiers in Psychiatry* 11, 1668.

Mueller, M.K., Richer, A.M., Callina, K.S. and Charmaraman, L. (2021) Companion animal relationships and adolescent loneliness during COVID-19. *Animals* 11(3), 885.

Nilsson, K.M. (2005) Pet bereavement and avenues of support (Unpublished Doctoral Dissertation), The Wright Institute, Chicago, IL.

O’Haire, M. (2010) Companion animals and human health: Benefits, challenges, and the road ahead. *Journal of Veterinary Behavior* 5(5), 226–234.

Packaged Facts (2020) 68 Million U.S. Households Have Pets, Expect 4% Growth in 2020, Reports Packaged Facts. CISION: PR Newswire. Available at: https://www.prnewswire.com/news-releases/68-million-us-households-have-pets-expect-4-growth-in-2020-reports-packaged-facts-301119637.html

Packman, W., Field, N.P., Carmack, B.J. and Ronen, R. (2011) Continuing bonds and psychosocial adjustment in pet loss. *Journal of Loss and Trauma* 16(4), 341–357.

Parkerson Jr, G.R., Michener, J.L., Wu, L.R., Finch, J.N. and Muhlbaier, L.H. (1989) Associations among family support, family stress, and personal functional health status. *Journal of Clinical Epidemiology* 42(3), 217–229.

Pikhartova, J., Bowling, A. and Victor, C. (2014) Does owning a pet protect older people against loneliness? *BMC Geriatrics* 14(1), 1–10.

Pirrone, F., Albertini, M., Mazzola, S.M., Pierantoni, L. and Bavagnoli, F. (2015) Correlation between the size of companion dogs and the profile of the owner: A cross-sectional study in Italy Marian. *Dog Behavior* 1(2), 32–43.

Planchon, L.A. and Templer, D.I. (1996) The correlates of grief after death of pet. *Anthrozoös* 9(2–3), 107–113.

Poresky, R.H., Hendrix, C., Mosier, J.E. and Samuelson, M.L. (1987) The companion animal bonding scale: Internal reliability and construct validity. *Psychological Reports* 60(3), 743–746.

Quackenbush, J. (1985) The death of a pet—how it can affect owners. *Veterinary Clinics of North America: Small Animal Practice* 15(2), 395–402.

Ratschen, E., Shoesmith, E., Shahab, L., Silva, K., Kale, D. *et al.* (2020) Human-animal relationships and interactions during the COVID-19 lockdown phase in the UK: Investigating links with mental health and loneliness. *PLoS One* 15(9), e0239397.

Redmalm, D. (2015) Pet grief: When is non-human life grievable? *The Sociological Review* 63(1), 19–35.

Rujoiu, O. and Rujoiu, V. (2014) Pet loss and human emotion: Romanian students’ reflections on pet loss. *Journal of Loss and Trauma: International Perspectives on Stress and Coping* 19, 474–483.

Schmidt, M., Naylor, P.E., Cohen, D., Gomez, R., Moses Jr, J.A. *et al.* (2020) Pet loss and continuing bonds in children and adolescents. *Death Studies* 44(5), 278–284.

Serpell, J. (2003) Anthropomorphism and anthropomorphic selection—beyond the "cute response". *Society & Animals* 11(1), 83–100.

Sharkin, B.S. and Bahrick, A.S. (1990) Pet loss: Implications for counselors. *Journal of Counseling and Development* 68(3), 306–308.

Stallones, L., Marx, M.B., Garrity, T.F. and Johnson, T.R. (1990) Pet ownership and attachment in relation to the health of U.S. adults, 21 to 64 years of age. *Anthrozoös* 4(2), 100–112.

Templer, D.I., Salter, C.A., Dickey, S., Baldwin, R. and Veleber, D.M. (1981) The construction of a pet attitude scale. *The Psychological Record* 31(3), 343–348.

Topál, J., Miklósi, Á., Gácsi, M., Dóka, A., Pongrácz, P. *et al.* (2009) The dog as a model for understanding human social behavior. *Advances in the Study of Behavior* 39, 71–116.

Tzivian, L., Friger, M. and Kushnir, T. (2014) Grief and bereavement of Israeli dog owners: Exploring short-term phases pre- and post-euthanization. *Death Studies* 38, 109–117.

Veevers, J.E. (1985) The social meaning of pets: Alternative roles for companion animals. *Marriage and Family Review* 8(3–4), 11–30.

Vesnaver, E. and Keller, H.H. (2011) Social influences and eating behavior in later life: A review. *Journal of Nutrition in Gerontology and Geriatrics* 30(1), 2–23.

Vidović, V.V., Štetić, V.V. and Bratko, D. (1999) Pet ownership, type of pet and socio-emotional development of school children. *Anthrozoös* 12(4), 211–217.

Virués-Ortega, J. and Buela-Casal, G. (2006) Psychophysiological effects of human-animal interaction: Theoretical issues and long-term interaction effects. *The Journal of Nervous and Mental Disease* 194(1), 52–57.

Vonk, J., Bouma, E.M. and Dijkistra, A. (2022) A time to say goodbye: Predictors of end-of-life decisions by pet owners. *Human Animal Interaction Bulletin* 13(1), 146–165. DOI: 10.1079/hai.2022.0013.

Wong, P.W., Yu, R.W. and Ngai, J.T. (2019) Companion animal ownership and human well-being in a metropolis—The case of Hong Kong. *International Journal of Environmental Research and Public Health* 16(10), 1729.

Zimet, G.D., Dahlem, N.W., Zimet, S.G. and Farley, G.K. (1988) The multidimensional scale of perceived social support. *Journal of Personality Assessment* 52(1), 30–41.

12 "We Lost a Member of the Family": Predictors of the Grief Experience Surrounding the Loss of a Pet

Anna Maria C. Behler[1]*, Jeffrey D. Green[2] and Jennifer Joy-Gaba[2]
[1]North Carolina State University, NC, USA; [2]Virginia Commonwealth University, VA, USA

Abstract
Pets play an important role in their owners' lives and are often viewed as family members. However, research on human–animal relationships suggests that pet owners often receive relatively less emotional support when experiencing grief after the death of a beloved pet, a phenomenon known as disenfranchised grief. In this internet-based survey study, we explored how people experienced grief surrounding the loss of their pets, and how this experience mirrors emotions that result from the death of a human loved one. We examined how factors such as anthropomorphism, attachment to a pet, and social support influence the grief experience. We also explored how feelings of guilt and shame play a role when grieving the loss of a pet. We found that grief over the loss of a pet is similar to grieving a human loved one in large part due to the anthropomorphic qualities attribute that owners attribute to their pets. Avenues for future exploration of the psychological impact of pet ownership are discussed.

Keywords: disenfranchised grief, attachment, anthropomorphism

Introduction

In the most recent survey conducted by the American Pet Products Association (APPA, 2018), sixty-eight percent (or 85 million) of U.S. households report owning a pet. This statistic is twelve percent higher than the initial survey conducted thirty years earlier. The most common household pets include dogs and cats, with 60.2 million households reporting dog ownership and 47.1 million households reporting cat ownership. With such a large number of pet owners in the population, it is worth examining the psychological and emotional impact that pet ownership may have on individuals.

Pet ownership is a unique experience, in that pet owners not only care for the animal's basic needs, but also often come to view pets as companions, confidants, and part of the family (McConnell *et al.*, 2017). Indeed, research suggests that pets play an extremely meaningful role in their owners' lives and that individuals form deep emotional bonds with them (e.g. Green *et al.*, 2009, 2018). As such, the loss of a pet can also invoke intense grief.

*Corresponding author: acbehler@ncsu.edu

Anthropomorphism: The Psychological and Biological Phenomena Underlying Human-Animal Emotional Bonding

Feelings of attachment to animal companions is associated with increased anthropomorphism, which is the assignment of a human identity or characteristics to a non-human animal or object (Albert and Bulcroft, 1988). For example, an owner may look over to their pet and believe that the animal looks content or guilty, may ascribe personality traits to their pet and use relationship names (e.g. daughter, brother), and may even incorporate their pet into family celebrations, such as birthday parties for the pet.

Beyond simply attributing a unique identity to their pets, research has found that if faced with a hypothetical ethical dilemma, people who view a pet as family would even choose to allocate resources (such as a rare but life-saving medicine) to the pet over a human who is not kin (Cohen, 2002). Similarly, a study in Australia found that considering a pet to be a part of the family predicted an increased likelihood of including the pet in considerations for emergency planning in the event of a natural disaster (Trigg *et al.*, 2015). Because individuals may assign their animal companions human-like characteristics and thus elevate them to the status of family members in many respects, we propose that anthropomorphism is one mechanism that explains why people grieve so strongly over the loss of their pet.

In addition to psychological experiences, researchers have also pointed to evolutionary mechanisms and biological changes that may also be the underlying causes of this attachment. Specifically, research has shown that dogs and cats were some of the first animals to be domesticated, and thus have co-evolved alongside humans over several thousand years, increasing our interdependence with them (Green *et al.*, 2009). Other recent work has showed that there are similar neurobiologic bonding mechanisms between human-human and owner-dog pairs, including evidence of increased levels of oxytocin, beta-endorphin, prolactin, beta-phenylethylamine, and dopamine in pet owners and their dogs during and after positive interactions (Handlin *et al.*, 2011). Affiliative hormones like prolactin and oxytocin have been shown to promote mother-child bonding (Numan and Young, 2016), and oxytocin has also been found to promote more positive paternal behaviors in men, including greater positive affect and increased physical contact with their infants (Weisman *et al.*, 2014). Thus, the hormone increases revealed in human–animal interactions indicates that people and their pets are forming attachment bonds as parents and children do, bolstering our contention that people often bond with their pets because they assign human characteristics to them and treat them like humans in some respects. This anthropomorphizing, in turn, will increase the depth and extent of grief experienced on the loss of the pet.

Further, fMRI evidence suggests similarities in patterns of brain activation in the affiliation and reward centers of the brain among women who were asked to view photos of their own children and own dogs (Stoeckel *et al.*, 2014). Notably, these similar patterns of activation did not appear when the women were asked to view photos of children or dogs not belonging to them, suggesting that people are uniquely attached to their own animal companions. In addition to brain activation, self-reports provide converging evidence showing that mothers rated pictures of their own children and dogs with similar levels of arousal and pleasantness. Taken together, these findings indicate that people may view their relationship with their pets similarly to the way they view a relationship with a child, especially since the pet is entirely dependent upon them to receive care.

Pet Ownership and Grief

Given the extensive research support for the depth and importance of bonds between humans and their animals, it follows that losing a pet may trigger similar feelings of grief to losing another human loved one. However, these emotions following the death of a pet are often not given the same validation or empathy by close others (e.g. those who do not have pets) relative to the support one might receive if the deceased were a human loved one. This lack of support is known as *disenfranchised grief*, and leaves people feeling isolated and unsupported (Packman *et al.*, 2011; Cordaro, 2012). This sense of isolation can inhibit one's willingness to disclose feelings to close others (Rémillard *et al.*, 2017). In fact, research suggests that people will even weigh the costs and benefits of posting about the loss of a pet on social media, as they fear they may be ignored, or worse, derided (Vitak *et al.*, 2017). Most importantly, this lack of support exacerbates the already challenging grief process, leaving people feeling that their emotions are illegitimate, resulting in increased distress and reduced quality of life (Spain *et al.*, 2019).

Though there has been some research examining the grief surrounding the loss of a pet, a majority of this work approaches grief over a pet from a counseling or social work perspective. Thus, most research focuses on the emotional impact and the types of services that should be provided to an individual during these times (Hess-Holden *et al.*, 2017). There is far less work that attempts to theoretically and empirically describe the psychological experience and its aftermath. Greater understanding of the psychological experience, in turn, will better inform interventions to ameliorate the grief.

In a survey of participants who had recently lost an animal companion, 30% of individuals reported severe grief in the aftermath of their loss (Adams *et al.*, 1999). The authors proposed that the experience of grief varied by how attached people were to their pets, and whether or not the pet had been euthanized. Interestingly, the authors discussed that societal attitudes towards pet death was a contributing factor for experiencing severe grief. This suggests that people may be forced to express grief over a pet differently than grief over a human (e.g. immediately went back to their everyday routines) because social norms may dictate that an extended mourning period for pets is not appropriate. They also reported that over half of participants reported feeling as though society did not view the loss of a pet as an appropriate reason to grieve. However, they assessed these feelings in the days and weeks immediately following the loss.

In the current study, we did not limit our survey only to participants who had experienced the recent death of a pet, with the rationale that grief in the immediate aftermath of a loss may be more pronounced than it would be after some time has passed. By including a wider range of participants, we were able to avoid the element of time as a potential confounding factor. This also allowed pet owners to provide a longer-term picture of the amount of social support they had received following the death of their pet; they might have received support in the immediate aftermath of the loss, but may have felt that this tapered off rather quickly if the people around them did not fully recognize or acknowledge the magnitude of grief associated with the death of a pet.

Grief is a complicated emotion, with multiple factors determining how strongly it may influence an individual. For example, the circumstances surrounding the death, the individual's closeness to the deceased, and how much social support received (Lobb *et al.*, 2010; Bellet *et al.*, 2018) can affect the depth and duration of an individual's grief. Thus, we expect that these factors will also play a role when losing an animal companion, especially for pet owners who report a strong bond to their pets. The sudden or accidental death of a loved one can result in greater depression during the grief process versus a prolonged illness or death due to natural causes, suggesting that these types of deaths are a distinct type of trauma (Kaplow *et al.*, 2014). However, there has been mixed research regarding the most critical situational factors that might surround the death of a beloved pet (Davis, 2011). For example, whereas some research suggests that the decision to euthanize a pet might result in a less negative emotional experience relative to circumstances in which pets die suddenly or accidentally, other findings support the notion that being faced with this decision is actually more stressful for owners. This increased stress is attributed to the anticipatory grief that pet owners face when trying to determine if euthanasia is an appropriate decision for their pet, and this negative experience can be exacerbated without the proper social and emotional support (Lagoni, 2011).

Adams *et al.* surveyed participants about how the decision to euthanize their pet influenced their grief and found that doubts over this choice predicted a stronger grief experience. The authors concluded that because of the different societal perspectives surrounding mourning the loss of a pet versus a person, and the fact that euthanasia plays a much more prominent role in the loss of a pet, grief over the loss of an animal may differ from grief experienced over the loss of a human and should not be studied using the same models. However, they did not directly examine feelings of guilt or shame, which we believe factor directly into the lingering feelings of doubt surrounding decisions to euthanize a pet, as they play a role in the mental well-being of those individuals caregiving for their human loved ones (Losada *et al.*, 2010; Roach *et al.*, 2013). More specifically, guilt is typically viewed as involving emotional discomfort over a specific offense committed, whereas shame is typically viewed as seeing oneself as bad or flawed (Marschall *et al.*, 1994; Tangney *et al.*, 1996; Griffin *et al.*, 2016). In the case of our pets, owners struggle with making decisions about end of life care just as they would for a human loved one (Testoni *et al.*, 2017). Thus, guilt may stem from feeling as though we did not do enough to care for them, and shame may be triggered by the thought that we directly contributed to their deaths by deciding to euthanize. Because human–animal relationships are more asymmetrical (e.g. inability to communicate verbally, greater responsibility for pets due to their reduced agency), experiences of shame and/or guilt may be qualitatively different and quite influential in the unfolding experience of guilt. Taken together, these emotional experiences may exacerbate the grief experience surrounding an already difficult loss, especially when we feel responsibility in a caregiver-type role. Moreover, we argue that the need for social support surrounding the death of a pet and doubt over how to manage caring for a pet in their final stages of life means that these processes are actually more similar than previously suggested, especially when pets are treated and viewed as family members.

Research suggests that the more bonded a person is to their pet, the more profoundly they experience grief (e.g. Ryan and Ziebland, 2015). In one such study, researchers surveyed a small sample of adolescents (n=55) who had recently lost a pet and found that grief was amplified among those who viewed the pet as a companion (Brown *et al.*, 1996). Other research has found that receiving understanding from others plays an important role in buffering feelings of grief when a pet dies (Gosse and Barnes, 1994), just as social support plays an integral role in helping us cope with the loss of a human loved one (Villacieros *et al.*, 2014).

More recent research also lends further support to our argument. In secondary analyses of video interviews of participants with chronic illnesses, Ryan and Ziebland (2015) found that individuals discussed pets as being similarly important as human family members, but did not receive the same type of responses from the researchers performing the interviews. The authors concluded that the influence of pets often was downplayed or ignored in research examining people's health. They further argued that because animals offer a number of benefits to an individual's health and well-being, including being a source of unwavering emotional support, they should be considered when assessing individuals' health. Other researchers have deemed grief surrounding the loss of a pet as a "destabilizing emotion" (Redmalm, 2015), because grieving owners fluctuate between whether or not they feel their emotions are acceptable. Participants interviewed for this research indicated that this vacillation stems from the influence of societal attitudes that contend that the lives of pets are not as valuable as the lives of people.

Further research shows that pets can serve as attachment figures and sources of social support in the same way that human companions do (Meehan *et al.*, 2017; Green *et al.*, 2018), even in the most traumatic circumstances (Flynn, 2000). In fact, the attachment bond among pets and their owners has been found to be comparable in strength to that between romantic partners, and also more likely to be categorized as secure (Beck and Madresh, 2008; Green *et al.*, 2018). Research also has found that we are more motivated to anthropomorphize our pets when we feel less socially connected to other people (Paul *et al.*, 2014), suggesting that the loss of a pet can simultaneously involve the loss of a significant source of comfort and security for many individuals. Taken together, these findings underscore the importance of our current research, and why it is crucial to gain a better understanding of how to offer support to those experiencing the loss of a pet.

Overview of the Current Research

We examined the role of anthropomorphism as a mediational variable in the relationship between how attached pet owners are to their pets and the grief they feel over their loss. In addition, we explored whether owners perceive adequate social support surrounding the loss of a pet relative to a human loved one. Not all people will experience the loss of a pet in their lifetimes. Thus, some people might underestimate or even dismiss the emotional significance of this type of loss. Consequently, many who have lost an animal companion may not receive the same quantity or quality of social support from others, though the grief may be as profound as the grief in the aftermath of losing a human companion. Third, we wanted to examine how shame and guilt played a role in the grief experience, as people are caregivers for their pets, and these emotions typically are associated with caregiving in the end of life.

Hypotheses

We predicted:

Hypothesis 1) That participants would report feeling less support from others after experiencing the death of a pet compared to after experiencing the death of a human loved one, consistent with the literature on disenfranchised grief (Packman *et al.*, 2011; Cordaro, 2012).

Hypothesis 2) The circumstances surrounding the death of the pet would influence grief, shame, and guilt, such that these emotions will be stronger for those whose pets died due to an accident or due to being euthanized versus those that died of natural causes.

Hypothesis 3a) Anthropomorphism, guilt, shame, and attachment to one's pet would all positively predict the experience of grief. Thus, the more one attributes personality characteristics and human-like qualities to their pet, and the greater one feels guilty or ashamed regarding their pet's death, the more profound the sense of loss would be.

Hypothesis 3b) Receiving increased social support after a pet dies from a variety of sources (significant other, family, friends) would be associated with reduced grief, consistent with findings surrounding the loss of a human loved one (Lobb *et al.*, 2010; Bellet *et al.*, 2018).

Hypothesis 4) Anthropomorphism would mediate the relationship between attachment and grief, given the existing literature on the similarities between human–animal bonds and attachment bonds between people. That is, we hypothesized that the attribution of personality characteristics and human-like qualities to the deceased pet would explain the relationship between attachment to a pet and the grief surrounding their loss.

Method

Participants

Participants (n=328)[1] were recruited from Facebook pet groups (n=170) and from the undergraduate research pool at a large, urban research university (n=158). Participants must have experienced the loss of a pet dog (n=253) or cat (n=56) in order to qualify for the study. Our rationale for including only dog or cat owners is that individuals typically form stronger bonds with these types of pets and more interdependent behaviors and routines evolve with cats and dogs, whereas relationships with other types of animals such as fish are relatively parasocial (i.e. one-sided; Green *et al.*, 2009; Brown *et al.*, 2015). There were no additional exclusion criteria.

Participants reported a wide variety in the length of time since the pet had passed away, ranging from less than 1 year (19.8%) to more than 5 years ago (37.5%). Additionally, approximately 43% of our participants reported that they had owned this pet for 10 or more years, underscoring the significant roles these companions play in the lives of their owners.

We included seven attention check items at various points throughout the questionnaires, (e.g. "*To show that you are paying attention, select strongly agree and move to the next question.*"), and any participant who answered more than 2 incorrectly was excluded. Of the 328 individuals who completed the online survey, 19 failed attention check measures, leaving a final sample of 309 participants (235 women).

All participants were 18 years of age or older (M_{age} = 29.08). Of the sample reporting, 68.3% reported being White, 9.4% reported being Hispanic/Latino, 6.5% reported Black/African-American, 2.9% reported being Asian, 5.9% reported being more than one race, and 7.0% reported Other.

Procedure

All participants completed an online survey that contained items pertaining to their experience dealing with the loss of a pet. Participants were asked to name a pet whose loss had a significant impact on them and to think of that pet when answering items in the survey. They then completed the following self-report measures in this order:

Measures

PET DEMOGRAPHICS. At the beginning of the study, participants responded to a number of questions regarding the pet that had passed away. More specifically, they were asked to provide the pet's name and to select the type of pet (i.e. dog or cat) so that the pet's name could be auto-populated in the to-be-completed questionnaires (i.e. the subsequent questions they answered contained the name of their deceased pet). In the event that participants had experienced the loss of more than one pet, they were asked to select the one that had the most significant emotional impact. They were also be asked to provide the length of time that they had had the animal, how long ago the pet died, and the circumstances surrounding the pet's death (i.e. accidental, natural causes, euthanasia, etc.).

ANTHROPOMORPHISM SCALE. The widely-used, 10-item Anthropomorphism Scale ($\alpha = 0.79$; Albert and Bulcroft, 1988) measured the extent to which pet owners anthropomorphize their dogs, ranging from *0 (doesn't describe me at all)* to *10 (describes me exactly)*. Sample items include "I celebrate my dog's birthday" and "I assign my dog a role, such as son or daughter." Higher levels of personification are likely to result in greater feelings of loss and grief surrounding the death of the pet. This scale is frequently cited in the human–animal interaction literature as a strong measure of the anthropomorphism construct (Trigg *et al.*, 2019); we slightly modified the scale to feature the pet's name rather than merely a specific type of pet in order to ensure that it would be applicable to all of our participants.

PET BEREAVEMENT QUESTIONNAIRE. This 16-item measure ($\alpha = 0.85$; PBQ; Hunt and Padilla, 2006) assesses feelings of grief following the loss of a pet, and all items were written such that they asked participants to reflect on their experience at the time their pet passed away. Items are rated on a 4-point scale from *1 (Disagree Strongly)* to *4 (Agree Strongly)*. An example item would be *"My life felt empty without my pet."*

MULTI-DIMENSIONAL SOCIAL SUPPORT SCALE. This 12-item measure ($\alpha = 0.94$; MDSSS; Zimet *et al.*, 1988) was intended to assess one's perceived level of social support from friends ($\alpha = 0.91$), family ($\alpha = 0.91$), or a significant other ($\alpha = 0.90$) surrounding the loss of their pet at the time of the loss. The scale contained items such as *"My family provides me the emotional support that I need"*, and all responses ranged from *1 (Very Strongly Disagree)* to *10 (Very Strongly Agree)*.

In addition to the MDSSS, we also included two single-item measures (presented in counterbalanced order): one to assess the overall level of social support that participants felt surrounding the loss of their pet and one to assess how well supported they felt surrounding the loss of a human loved one (e.g. *"Overall, how supported did you feel when your pet/human loved one passed away?"*). These items were rated on a *1 (Completely Unsupported)* to *7 (Completely Supported)*.

THE STATE SHAME AND GUILT SCALE. This 10-item measure (SSGS; Marschall *et al.*, 1994) assessed one's state feelings of shame ($\alpha = 0.79$) and guilt $\alpha = 0.87$) at the time of their pet's death. This scale ranged from *1 (Not feeling this way at all)* to 5 *(Feeling this way strongly)*.

Finally, we measured feelings of emotional closeness and attachment to a pet in two ways:

INCLUSION OF OTHER IN THE SELF SCALE. This scale is a single item measure that involves selecting a pictorial representation of how connected one feels to another, such that more overlap signifies greater psychological connectedness (IOSS; Aron *et al.*, 1992). In this study, the "other" was the pet listed by the participant at the beginning of the study. Greater psychological connectedness will likely be positively related to greater reported grief surrounding the loss of the pet. The IOSS is a widely-used and validated measure of closeness and has been applied to individuals, groups, the environment, and pets (e.g. Davis *et al.*, 2009).

PET ATTACHMENT AND LIFE IMPACT SCALE. This 35-item measure was used to assess overall attachment to one's pet, because it purports to assess several facets of the emotional bond and interdependence that owners may feel toward their pets ($\alpha = 0.93$; PALS; Cromer and Barlow, 2013). More specifically, the scale measures how close people felt to their pets and how much they viewed them as members of the family ($\alpha = 0.87$; love subscale), how much the pet helped them manage their emotions ($\alpha = 0.91$; regulation subscale), how much the pet influenced their personal growth ($\alpha = 0.85$; growth subscale), and how negatively the pet affected their life ($\alpha = 0.66$; negative impact subscale).

Results

Principal dependent measures

HYPOTHESIS 1. We used a paired samples *t*-test to determine whether there were differences between the amount of support felt over the loss of a pet vs a human loved one. Given the nature of the questions, only participants who had experienced both types of loss were able to answer items in this section of the survey. However, approximately 91% of individuals fell into this category (n=281), and nearly every eligible participant responded to all items in this section (n=266). Participants reported feeling more supported after having experienced the loss of a human (M=6.02, SD=1.25) compared to the support received after losing a companion animal (M=5.41, SD=1.56), $t(265)$ = 7.01, p<0.001, 95% CI [.47, .83], d=0.43. Notably, using the IOS self-other overlap measure, participants reported similar feelings of connectedness to their pet (M= 5.62, SD=1.29) as to their human loved one (M= 5.47, SD= 1.53), $t(280)$ = 1.30, p=0.19, 95% CI [−.08, .37], d=.11.

HYPOTHESIS 2. We used standard multiple regression analyses to examine the relationship between circumstances surrounding the pet's death and feelings of grief, shame, and guilt participants experienced. We expected stronger feelings of grief, shame and guilt to be associated with pets that died due to euthanasia (n=85) or accidental death (n=46) than those who died of natural causes (n=152). The circumstances surrounding the pet's death were dummy coded and entered into the model as predictors, and grief, shame, and guilt were assessed as outcomes. This hypothesis was partially supported: there was a significant difference between the groups on the outcome of grief, R^2=.05, $F(2, 280)$ = 8.04, p<.001, with participants feeling significantly more grief if a pet's death were the result of the decision to euthanize (M=2.63, SD=.48), β=.14, $t(280)$ = 2.05, p=.042, and the highest levels of grief if the death was unexpected (M=2.85, SD=0.50), β=.27, $t(280)$ = 4.01, p<.001, relative to if it were due to natural causes (M=2.48, SD=.50). Pet owners also reported differences in their feelings of shame depending upon the circumstances surrounding their pet's death, R^2=.02, $F(2, 273)$ = 3.09, p=0.047. They felt most ashamed when a pet's death was accidental (M=2.85, SD=0.95), relative to when their pet had to be euthanized (M=2.47, SD=1.01), β=0.14, $t(273)$ = 2.27, p=.024 or died due to natural causes (M=2.42, SD=.95), β=.14, $t(273)$ = 2.32, p=0.021. Interestingly, guilt did not vary as a function of the circumstances surrounding the death of a pet, R^2=.02, $F(2, 271)$ = 2.56, p=.079. This suggests that while people may not consider blameworthy specific decisions and behaviors related to the death of their pets (thus the lack of a significant relationship with guilt), they may feel bad about not being able to do more to have prevented an accidental or unexpected death from occurring. Future research should investigate this possibility and examine the potentially unique aspects of shame versus guilt in these experiences.

As a more stringent test of the hypothesis, we also used a hierarchical linear regression to assess the differences in grief and shame after controlling for the length of ownership and the length of time since the pet's death. Both of these covariates were assessed as continuous variables and entered into the first step of the model. The relationship with grief remained significant even when controlling for these variables, $\Delta R^2 = .04$, $F\Delta(2, 278) = 5.94$, $p < .001$. Grief was stronger when a pet died unexpectedly or accidentally, even when accounting for how long the person had owned their pet and how much time had passed since the pet had died, $R^2 = .08$, $F(4, 278) = 6.16$, $p < .001$. However, the relationship between shame and circumstances surrounding a pet's death was no longer significant when the covariates were entered into the model, $R^2 = .03$, $F(4, 271) = 2.15$, $p = .08$.

HYPOTHESES 3A AND 3B. We used a hierarchical multiple regression analysis to assess the relationship between our predictors (anthropomorphism, social support, guilt, shame, and attachment) and grief, while controlling for length of pet ownership and how much time had elapsed since the pet's passing. In this model, attachment was assessed via the overall mean scores of the PALS scale (See Table 12.1 for full descriptive statistics).

Overall, the duration of pet ownership and the length of time since the pet's death significantly predicted how much grief pet owners reported feeling, $R^2 = 0.06$, $F(2, 288) = 9.30$, $p < 0.001$. Their grief was stronger when the death of the pet was more recent, $\beta = 0.20$, $t(288) = 3.55$, $p < 0.001$. Interestingly, however, length of ownership negatively predicted grief, $\beta = -0.16$, $t(283) = 2.80$, $p = 0.005$, suggesting that owners who had their pets for shorter periods of time may not have been as prepared for the emotional ramifications of the loss. To examine this finding further, we used a chi-square analysis to determine whether there was a difference between the manner in which a pet died and the amount of time they had with their owners. Data on length of ownership was collected on an ordinal scale ranging from 1 (Less than 1 year) to 7 (More than 10 years). Thus, a chi-square analysis was appropriate to further examine the differences between groups. We found that there was a significant difference in ownership length when participants were grouped based on the manner in which their pet had died, $X2\ (12) = 91.37$, $p < 0.001$. Further, among those who reported that the death had been unexpected, approximately 80.4% had owned their pet for less than 6 years. However, most pet owners whose pets were euthanized or died of natural causes reported owning their pets for 10 years or more, at rates of 60.0% and 49.3%, respectively.

Table 12.1. Correlations and descriptive statistics.

	1	2	3	4	5	6	7
1. Anthropomorphism	–						
2. Pet Bereavement	.42[b]	–					
3. Multi-Dimensional Social Support	.31[b]	–.04	–				
4. Guilt	.14[a]	.41[b]	–.03	–			
5. Shame	.29[b]	.51[b]	–.04	.65[b]	–		
6. Self-Other Overlap	.61[b]	.33[b]	.21[b]	.06	.24[b]	–	
7. Pet Attachment Life Impact Scale	.70[b]	.44[b]	.24[b]	.25[b]	.38[b]	.58[b]	–
M	7.86	2.62	5.56	2.5	2.56	5.6	4.08
SD	1.46	0.51	1.29	1.11	1.01	1.28	0.57

[a]Correlation is significant at the 0.05 level (1-tailed),
[b]Correlation is significant at the 0.01 level (1-tailed); $n = 309$.

When anthropomorphism, social support, guilt, shame, and attachment were added to the model, they significantly improved the prediction of grief, $\Delta R^2=.35$, $F\Delta$ (5, 283) = 33.92, $p<.001$. All variables together significantly predicted grief $R^2=.41$, F(7, 283) = 28.40, $p<.001$, accounting for 41% of the variance in how severely one experienced grief surrounding the loss of one's pet. Both parts of Hypothesis 3 were fully supported, as each of our predictors was significantly related to grief in the expected directions. More specifically, higher levels of anthropomorphism ($\beta=.21$, t(283) = 3.24, $p=.001$), guilt ($\beta=.15$, t(283) = 2.38, $p=.018$), shame ($\beta=.27$, t(283) = 4.19, $p<.001$), and attachment ($\beta=.16$, t(283) = 2.42, $p=.016$) all predicted greater feelings of grief. In addition, receiving greater social support when a pet died negatively predicted experiencing grief, $\beta=-.12$, t(283) = −2.56, $p=.011$.

HYPOTHESIS 4: THE EXPLANATORY ROLE OF ANTHROPOMORPHISM. *Why* does greater attachment to a pet lead to feeling more grief? We wanted to further explore the role of anthropomorphism in the relationship between attachment to a pet and grief surrounding the pet's death. We conducted a bootstrapping analysis to examine the indirect effect of attachment to one's pet on grief via anthropomorphism using PROCESS (Hayes, 2012). We used a mediation model, whereby attachment was modeled to affect grief through anthropomorphism. The overall model was significant, $R^2=0.22$, $F(2, 297) = 41.83$, $p<.001$, accounting for 22% of the variance in grief (see Fig. 12.1). Feelings of attachment to one's pet shared a strong positive relationship with levels of anthropomorphism ($\beta=.71$) and with grief ($\beta=.40$, both *p's* < 0.001). Anthropomorphism was also positively related to how strongly pet owners experienced grief following the loss of their pets ($\beta=.21$, $p=.004$). This model, conducted with 5000 bootstraps, yielded a mean bootstrap estimate of the indirect effect of 0.13 (SE = .05). Because the 95% confidence interval did not include 0 (0.04–0.22), we concluded that the indirect effect of anthropomorphism on the association between attachment and grief was significant. That is, greater attachment predicted higher levels of anthropomorphism, which, in turn, led people to experience more severe grief when their pet died.

As an alternative explanation for the experience of grief, we examined whether assessing attachment as a mediator would provide a better fitting model than our original mediation. Thus, we assessed whether anthropomorphism affected grief through attachment. When considered this way, the indirect effect was smaller, at just .07 (*SE* = 0.02, 95%CI [0.02, .12]), suggesting that our original model provided a stronger explanation for the relationship among these variables and the experience of grief.

Exploratory Analyses

We conducted several exploratory analyses regarding gender differences on our measures related to closeness (self-other overlap, anthropomorphism, and attachment to a pet),

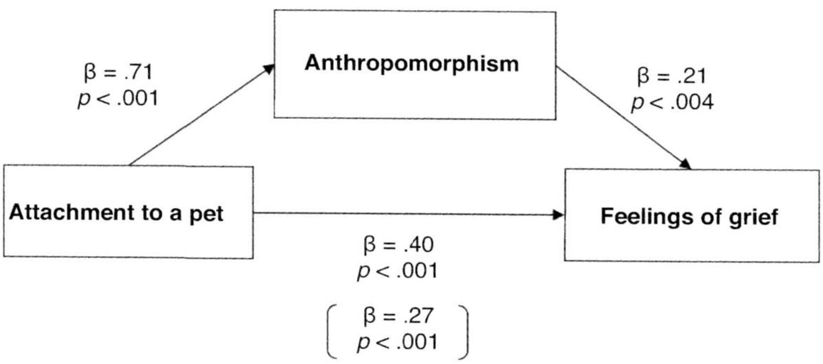

Fig. 12.1. Mediation analysis depicting the relationships between attachment to one's pet, and self-reported levels of grief via anthropomorphism.

Table 12.2. Sample descriptives using t-test for equality of means.

	Women		Men			
	M	*SD*	*M*	*SD*	*t*	*p*
Self-Other Overlap (Pet)	5.69	1.26	5.15	1.36	2.96	.003
Self-Other Overlap (Human)	5.44	1.55	5.6	1.47	0.66	.51
Anthropomorphism	7.96	1.39	7.31	1.55	3.18	.002
Pet Bereavement	2.66	0.51	2.42	0.47	3.35	.001
Social Support	5.65	1.28	5.17	1.26	2.57	.011
Pet Attachment Life Impact Scale	4.14	0.54	3.86	0.48	3.48	.001

bereavement, and social support, as woman are more relationally interdependent than men (Gabriel and Gardner, 1999; Cross *et al.*, 2003) and thus may exhibit differences in how they are bonded with their pets and their resulting grief when the pet dies. We found that women reported greater scores on all measures of closeness to a pet, felt more severe grief after the pet's death, and perceived greater social support after the pet's death (see Table 12.2). However, it was interesting to note that both women ($M = 5.44$, $SD = 1.55$) and men ($M = 5.60$, $SD = 1.47$) reported feeling equally close to their human loved ones, $t(268) = 0.66$, $p = 0.51$.

Discussion

Participants recalled and assessed, via online questionnaire, the grief they had experienced after losing an animal companion. Participants selected a specific pet at the start of the survey, so that every item was autopopulated to be specifically about the identified pet. This was a key strength of our study, as it was intended to facilitate recall, increase the vividness of the experience, ensure that participants identified a pet whose death had a significant impact on them, and confirm that they were thinking about the same pet for each response.

Most of our hypotheses were supported, providing empirical evidence that pet loss has a profound emotional and psychological impact on pet owners and helping to further our understanding of the role pets play in people's lives. To be specific, we provided quantitative evidence that grief over the loss of a pet is comparable to grief that is experienced surrounding the loss of a human, in large part due to the human-like qualities that owners attribute to their pets. As expected, anthropomorphism played a major role in the severity of a pet owner's grief following the loss of their pet. Specifically, anthropomorphism not only predicted stronger feelings of grief, but actually mediated the relationship between attachment and grief. This was a particularly significant finding, as it suggests that ascribing human-like qualities to our pets results in our considering them to be just as important as human companions, and that the death of a pet may be felt similarly as the loss of a human friend or family member to the bereaved.

Despite the importance of the human–animal bond, our sample of pet owners felt less supported by others when grieving over the death of a pet relative to a human, providing converging evidence with previous research on disenfranchised grief (Packman *et al.*, 2011; Cordaro, 2012). We also provided evidence that social support plays a significant role in reducing feelings of grief surrounding the loss of a pet, underscoring the importance of validating a person's emotions when their pet has died, just as when a human loved one has passed. This converges with research regarding the grief process following the death of a human loved one, which suggests that adequate social support is crucial in one's ability to move forward and strive for growth following the trauma of a loss (Bellet *et al.*, 2018).

Interestingly, individuals reported less guilt and more shame over the loss of a pet, suggesting that while they may not feel responsible for their animal's death, they may question whether they did enough to prevent it. Future research should attempt to replicate and investigate more closely the experience of these two self-conscious emotions in the context of grief. In addition, women reported higher feelings of bondedness than men, providing evidence that converges with previous research (Cohen, 2002). However, women also reported greater feelings of grief over the loss of their pets than men, and more severe grief overall. It may be interesting to further examine the differences in how men and women perceive their relationships with their pets, and to explore the different ways in which they look to their pets as a source of comfort, support, and connectedness. Taken together, our results speak to the fact that grief is a complicated emotion, especially when it is not fully recognized or validated by those around us.

Limitations and Future Directions

The proposed study is limited in that is it non-experimental, using self-report data. Given the variables being assessed (i.e. grief over loss of a pet), experimental research may be neither feasible nor ethical, though other methodologies (e.g. longitudinal) should be employed. Future work might continue to examine the parallels between the grief experienced by pet owners who are faced with the decision to euthanize, and individuals having to make end of life decisions for their human loved ones. It may be that the guilt and shame surrounding the loss of a pet may be exacerbated depending on a person's view of their pets' agency, and the fact that pets cannot communicate their wishes ahead of time nor provide reassurances (or be verbally reassured) at the end in the way that a human loved one might.

Another limitation of the study was that we chose to include only cat and dog owners. This is not because other types of pet owners do not experience attachment to their pets or grief over a pet's loss. Rather, we expected and found that dog and cat owners would anthropomorphize their pets to a relatively high degree, especially given that pet owners are able to engage with these animals more often and more directly. However, broadening the types of pets included in research could be a potential avenue for future work.

Future research also might explore how children experience the death of a pet, and how these events may be seen as significant teaching periods in a child's development. Specifically, how does a child experience grief, and what may be the role of anthropomorphism? In addition, research might examine whether the presence of children in a household predicts a decreased grief response for pet owning parents, as attentional resources may be reallocated towards childcare responsibilities, thus reducing the time spent ruminating over the death of a pet.

Affective forecasting, or how individuals predict their future emotional experiences, may also influence the experience of grief (e.g. Green *et al.*, 2013). While affective forecasting typically involves overestimating our anticipated feelings in a particular situation, it is possible that pet owners may be more susceptible to inaccurate forecasting in the opposite direction (i.e. underestimate the forecasted grief, particularly compared to anticipated grief over the loss of a human companion). They may be under the impression that "it's just a pet," a refrain commonly heard by pet owners experiencing loss (Cowles, 2016), and therefore be less aware of how connected they have become to their pet or how significant the changes will be after the pet's loss. Thus, this forecasting inaccuracy may result in a lack of emotional preparedness when the pet dies, and a decreased ability to properly cope with the feelings of loss, especially if the owner is faced with the decision of having to euthanize their pet without preparation, or if the pet dies unexpectedly. Indeed, our results show that pet ownership was inversely related to feelings of grief, suggesting that the less time an individual owned a pet, the more they reported feelings of grief. In such instances, social support would likely be even more invaluable for the bereaved pet owner.

Another avenue for continued exploration is how pets, like children, influence relationship satisfaction among romantic partners. Pets may increase or inhibit relationship satisfaction, either strengthening the bond between partners or inhibiting it if both members of the dyad are not equally invested in caring for the pet. The death of a pet in these situations may exacerbate existing tensions, especially if one partner does not provide adequate support for the other after the pet has died.

Conclusion

Our participants reported similar feelings of bondedness and bereavement to their animal companions as to their human loved ones. Importantly, our results are the first to provide quantitative data suggesting that anthropomorphism actually accounts for the relationship between attachment and grief: greater attachment to animal companions is associated with ascribing more human qualities to them, and this, in turn, is associated with more grief in the aftermath of their loss. Put another way, individuals may experience the same levels of grief regarding departed pets as they do human companions because they see those pets as having human qualities. Despite these feelings, however, individuals may not experience the same levels of social support, underscoring the importance of seeking out connection with others who value human–animal bonds in the same manner. Ultimately, we contend that high anthropomorphism coupled with a lack of appropriate social support interact, leading to a more difficult experience of grief over a pet.

Notes

[1] An a priori power analysis was conducted using G*Power software (Faul *et al.*, 2009). Assuming a small effect size for even our most complex regression model ($r^2 = .04$), we found that 265 participants would be sufficient to detect an effect (power > 0.90, alpha < 0.05). A separate post-hoc power analysis was conducted for Hypothesis 4 (Kenny, 2017), as we wanted to ensure that the mediation analysis was sufficiently powered based on our sample size and obtained effect sizes. We found that power ranged from .81–.99 for all paths in the model.

[2] We used the mean scores of the overall PALS scale in accordance with how the scale's creators have used the scale in previous research (Barlow *et al.*, 2012).

References

Adams, C.L., Bonnett, B.N. and Meek, A.H. (1999) Owners' response to companion animal death: Development of a theory and practical implications. *Canadian Veterinary Journal* 40, 33–39.

Albert, A. and Bulcroft, K. (1988) Pets, families, and the life course. *Journal of Marriage and the Family* 50, 543–552.

American Pet Products Association (2017-2018) *National Pet Owners Survey.*

Aron, A., Aron, E.N. and Smollan, D. (1992) Inclusion of other in the self scale and the structure of interpersonal closeness. *Journal of Personality and Social Psychology* 63, 596–612.

Barlow, M.R., Cromer, L.D., Caron, H.P. and Freyd, J.J. (2012) Comparison of normative and diagnosed dissociation on attachment to companion animals and stuffed animals. *Psychological Trauma: Theory, Research, Practice, and Policy* 4(5), 501–506.

Beck, L. and Madresh, E.A. (2008) Romantic partners and four-legged friends: An extension of attachment theory to relationships with pets. *Anthrozoös* 21(1), 43–56.

Bellet, B.W., Jones, P.J., Neimeyer, R.A. and McNally, R.J. (2018) Bereavement outcomes as causal systems: A network analysis of the co-occurrence of complicated grief and posttraumatic growth. *Clinical Psychological Science* 6(6), 797–809.

Brown, B.H., Richards, H.C. and Wilson, C.A. (1996) Pet bonding and pet bereavement among adolescents. *Journal of Counseling & Development* 74(5), 505–509.

Brown, C.M., Shilling, A.A., Young, S.G. and Berrong, L.E. (2015) Acceptance and rejection of pets and parasocial others cause corresponding changes in the self's perceived relational value. *Self and Identity* 14, 233–251.

Cohen, S.P. (2002) Can pets function as family members? *Western Journal of Nursing Research* 24(6), 621–638.

Cordaro, M. (2012) Pet loss and disenfranchised grief: Implications for mental health counseling practice. *Journal of Mental Health Counseling* 34(4), 283–294.

Cowles, K.V. (2016) The death of a pet: Human responses to the breaking of the bond. In: Sussman, M.B. (ed.) *Pets and the Family*. Routledge, New York, NY, pp. 135–148.

Cromer, L.D. and Barlow, M.R. (2013) Factors and convergent validity of the pet attachment and life impact scale (PALS). *Human-Animal Interaction Bulletin* 1(2), 34–56.

Cross, S.E., Gore, J.S. and Morris, M.L. (2003) The relational-interdependent self-construal, self-concept consistency, and well-being. *Journal of Personality and Social Psychology* 85, 933–944.

Davis, H.L. (2011) Death of a companion animal: Understanding human responses to bereavement. In: Blazina, C., Boyra, G. and Shen-Miller, D.S. (eds) *The Psychology of the Human-Animal Bond*. Springer, New York, NY.

Davis, J.L., Green, J.D. and Reed, A. (2009) Interdependence with the environment: Commitment, interconnectedness, and environmental behavior. *Journal of Environmental Psychology* 29(2), 173–180.

Faul, F., Erdfelder, E., Buchner, A. and Lang, A.G. (2009) Statistical power analyses using g*power 3.1: tests for correlation and regression analyses. *Behavior Research Methods* PMID(4), 1149–1160. DOI: 10.3758/BRM.41.4.1149.

Flynn, C.P. (2000) Woman's best friend: Pet abuse and the role of companion animals in the lives of battered women. *Violence Against Women* 6(2), 162–177.

Gabriel, S. and Gardner, W.L. (1999) Are there "his" and "hers" types of interdependence? The implications of gender differences in collective versus relational interdependence for affect, behavior, and cognition. *Journal of Personality and Social Psychology* 77, 642–655.

Gosse, G.H. and Barnes, M.J. (1994) Human grief resulting from the death of a pet. *Anthrozoös* 7(2), 103–112.

Green, J.D., Mathews, M. and Foster, C.A. (2009) Another kind of "interpersonal" relationship: humans, animal companions, and attachment theory. In: Cuyler, E. and Ackhart, M. (eds) *Psychology of Relationships*. Nova Science Press, New York, NY, pp. 87–109.

Green, J.D., Davis, J.L., Luchies, L.B., Coy, A.E., Van Tongeren, D.R. *et al.* (2013) Victims versus perpetrators: Affective and empathic forecasting regarding transgressions in romantic relationships. *Journal of Experimental Social Psychology* 49, 329–333.

Green, J.D., Coy, A.E. and Mathews, M.A. (2018) Attachment anxiety and avoidance influence pet choice and pet-directed behaviors. *Anthrozoös* 31, 475–494.

Griffin, B.J., Moloney, J.M., Green, J.D., Worthington, Jr. E. L., Cork, B. *et al.* (2016) Perpetrators' reactions to perceived interpersonal wrongdoing: The associations of guilt and shame with forgiving, punishing, and excusing oneself. *Self and Identity* 15(6), 650–661.

Handlin, L., Hydbring-Sandberg, E., Nilsson, A., Ejdebäck, M., Jansson, A. *et al.* (2011) Short-term interaction between dogs and their owners: Effects on oxytocin, cortisol, insulin and heart rate—an exploratory study. *Anthrozoös* 24(3), 301–315.

Hayes, A.F. (2012) PROCESS: A versatile computational tool for observed variable mediation, moderation, and conditional PROCESS modeling.

Hess-Holden, C.L., Monaghan, C.L. and Justice, C.A. (2017) Pet bereavement support groups: A guide for mental health professionals. *Journal of Creativity in Mental Health* 12(4), 440–450.

Hunt, M. and Padilla, Y. (2006) Development of the pet bereavement questionnaire. *Anthrozoös* 19, 308–324.

Kaplow, J.B., Howell, K.H. and Layne, C.M. (2014) Do circumstances of the death matter?: Identifying socioenvironmental risks for grief-related psychopathology in bereaved youth. *Journal of Traumatic Stress* 27(1), 42–49.

Kenny, D.A. (2017) MedPower: An interactive tool for the estimation of power in tests of mediation [Computer software]. Available at: https://davidakenny.shinyapps.io/MedPower

Lagoni, L. (2011) Family-present euthanasia: Protocols for planning and preparing clients for the death of a pet. In: Blazina, C., Boyra, G. and Shen-Miller, D.S. (eds) *The Psychology of the Human-Animal Bond*. Springer, New York, NY, USA.

Lobb, E.A., Kristjanson, L.J., Aoun, S.M., Monterosso, L., Halkett, G.K. *et al.* (2010) Predictors of complicated grief: A systematic review of empirical studies. *Death Studies* 34(8), 673–698.

Losada, A., Márquez-González, M., Peñacoba, C. and Romero-Moreno, R. (2010) Development and validation of the caregiver guilt questionnaire. *International Psychogeriatrics* 22, 650–660.

Marschall, D., Sanftner, J. and Tangney, J.P. (1994) *The state shame and guilt scale*. George Mason University, Fairfax, VA.

McConnell, A.R., Lloyd, E.P. and Buchanan, T.M. (2017) Animals as friends: the social psychological implications of human–pet relationships. In: Hojjat, M. and Moyer, A. (eds) *Psychology of Friendship*. Oxford University Press, Oxford, UK, pp. 157–174.

Meehan, M., Massavelli, B. and Pachana, N. (2017) Using attachment theory and social support theory to examine and measure pets as sources of social support and attachment figures. *Anthrozoös* 30(2), 273–289.

Numan, M. and Young, L.J. (2016) Neural mechanisms of mother–infant bonding and pair bonding: Similarities, differences, and broader implications. *Hormones and Behavior* 77, 98–112.

Packman, W., Field, N.P., Carmack, B.J. and Ronen, R. (2011) Continuing bonds and psychosocial adjustment in pet loss. *Journal of Loss and Trauma* 16(4), 341–357.

Paul, E.S., Moore, A., McAinsh, P., Symonds, E., McCune, S. *et al.* (2014) Sociality motivation and anthropomorphic thinking about pets. *Anthrozoös* 27(4), 499–512.

Redmalm, D. (2015) Pet grief: When is non-human life grievable? *The Sociological Review* 63(1), 19–35.

Rémillard, L.W., Meehan, M.P., Kelton, D.F. and Coe, J.B. (2017) Exploring the grief experience among callers to a pet loss support hotline. *Anthrozoös* 30(1), 149–161.

Roach, L., Laidlaw, K., Gillanders, D. and Quinn, K. (2013) Validation of the caregiver guilt questionnaire (CGQ) in a sample of british dementia caregivers. *International Psychogeriatrics* 25, 2001–2010.

Ryan, S. and Ziebland, S. (2015) On interviewing people with pets: Reflections from qualitative research on people with long-term conditions. *Sociology of Health & Illness* 37(1), 67–80.

Spain, B., O'Dwyer, L. and Moston, S. (2019) Pet loss: understanding disenfranchised grief, memorial use, and posttraumatic growth. *Anthrozoös* 32(4), 555–568.

Stoeckel, L.E., Palley, L.S., Gollub, R.L., Niemi, S.M. and Evins, A.E. (2014) Patterns of brain activation when mothers view their own child and dog: an fmri study. *PLoS One* 9(10), e107205.

Tangney, J.P., Miller, R.S., Flicker, L. and Barlow, D.H. (1996) Are shame, guilt, and embarrassment distinct emotions? *Journal of Personality and Social Psychology* 70(6), 1256–1269.

Testoni, I., De Cataldo, L., Ronconi, L. and Zamperini, A. (2017) Pet loss and representations of death, attachment, depression, and euthanasia. *Anthrozoös* 30(1), 135–148.

Trigg, J., Smith, B. and Thompson, K. (2015) Does emotional closeness to pets motivate their inclusion in bushfire survival plans? Implications for emergency communicators. *Australian Journal of Emergency Management, The* 30(2), 24–30.

Trigg, J., Thompson, K., Smith, B. and Bennett, P. (2019) Archetyping relationships with companion animals to understand disaster risk-taking propensity. *Journal of Risk Research* 22(4), 475–496.

Villacieros, M., Serrano, I., Bermejo, J.C., Magaña, M. and Carabias, R. (2014) Social support and psychological well-being as possible predictors of complicated grief in a cross-section of people in mourning. *Anales de Psicología* 30, 944–951.

Vitak, J., Wisniewski, P., Ashktorab, Z. and Badillo-Urquiola, K. (2017) Benefits and drawbacks of using social media to grieve following the loss of pet. In: *Proceedings of the 8th International Conference on Social Media & Society*, ACM.

Weisman, O., Zagoory-Sharon, O. and Feldman, R. (2014) Oxytocin administration, salivary testosterone, and father–infant social behavior. *Progress in Neuro-Psychopharmacology and Biological Psychiatry* 49, 47–52.

Zimet, G.D., Dahlem, N.W., Zimet, S.G. and Farley, G.K. (1988) The multidimensional scale of perceived social support. *Journal of Personality Assessment* 52(1), 30–41.

13 Dealing with Death: The Role of Animal-Themed Literature in Supporting Children with Grief and Loss

Elaine Smit* and Bradley P. Smith
College of Psychology, School of Health, Medical and Applied Sciences, Central Queensland University, Adelaide, Australia

---

Abstract

The way that children deal with, and develop an understanding of death has long-term effects on their development and wellbeing. Mental health practitioners regularly turn to bibliotherapy (the use of books), many of which portray non-human animals as central characters, as a therapeutic tool for bereaved children. However, the extent to which non-human animal characters are used to assist children dealing with loss and dying, nor how and why it is used, particularly in relation to available therapies, is not well understood. To explore this, we conducted an online survey of 47 Australian mental health practitioners (M = 45.55 years of age, SD = 12.81; 80.9% female) who specialise in providing grief counselling to children (average of 13.26 years +/− 10.05 of professional experience). Overall, just over half (60.0%, n = 24/40) of practitioners preferred to use animal-themed death literature. However, it was not the most frequently used, nor considered the most effective therapeutic option across all age groups. There was a clear reduction in perceived usefulness with age. Bibliotherapy with animal characters was considered most effective for children between the ages of 2 and 7, and least effective for those over 12. Thematic analyses of open-ended responses revealed three overarching themes: (1) Animal-themed bibliotherapy was viewed as helpful in creating a bridge to access children's emotions and providing a safe space to share them. (2) Practitioners considered animal-characters helpful for developing accurate death conceptualisation in younger children due to their familiarity with animals. Familiarity helps to encourage children to apply their observations of animal life cycles to human death, children identify with animal-characters, and they generally find animals appealing. (3) Its adoption by a therapist is dependent on children's unique characteristics, practitioners' personal preferences and the availability of appropriate literature. Findings from this study provide insight into practitioner perceptions of the role animal-characters play in children's understanding of death at different ages and help to inform subject-matter choice for bibliotherapy literature. Animal-themed death literature has application as an adjunct therapy tool to assist children experiencing grief related to death and dying, but also more broadly (e.g., teachers and caregivers) to foster a healthy understanding of death in children.

Keywords: animal-themed literature, animal-themed bibliotherapy, animal-characters, death conceptualisation, bibliotherapy

---

*Corresponding author: elaine.smit365@gmail.com

Introduction

Death is an inevitable part of the life cycle (Crosetto and Garcha, 2013). It is important that death and dying is discussed with children (defined here as those under the age of 18 years) honestly because the way children grieve and develop an understanding of death has profound effects on their development, wellbeing and quality of life across the lifespan (Kenyon, 2001; Berns, 2004; Longbottom and Slaughter, 2018). Children are still developing their understanding of life and death and as such, grieve and understand death differently to adults (Carter, 2016). Children's grief reaction to death varies depending on their age, their relationship with the person who has died (Howarth, 2011), how frequently they are exposed to death such as in war zones or natural disasters (Webb, 2010) or countries with a high incidence gun violence (Xu *et al.*, 2019), as well as the how a particular culture and media discuss and deal with death (Park and Pyszczynski, 2016). However, in general, children are less exposed to, and even shielded from death and dying than in previous generations because of their perceived immaturity and their limited capacity to understand death (Willis, 2002; Carter, 2016; Longbottom and Slaughter, 2018). These children may develop inaccurate understandings of death (Longbottom and Slaughter, 2018) and lack the opportunity to discuss their emotions around death and loss (Willis, 2002).

The ability of children to understand the concept of death depends on their developmental age (Speece and Brent, 1984; Slaughter, 2005). A mature conceptualisation of death develops in tandem with cognitive development and life experience (Webb, 2010; Wong, 2010). Early psychoanalysts proposed that children were cognitively and emotionally too immature to understand death (Nagy, 1948; Slaughter, 2005). This early research revealed differences in the understanding of death between young children and adults (Slaughter, 2005). Research in the 1960s and 1970s adopted a Piagetian perspective and focused on children's cognitive understanding of death by tying Piaget's stages of cognitive development to death conceptualisation, postulating that children's general cognitive development mirrored their acquisition of 'death concepts' (Slaughter, 2005). These death concepts were subcomponents of death used to assess and measure the understanding of death (Longbottom and Slaughter, 2018).

A mature conceptualisation of death includes understanding the following death concepts: death is permanent; inevitable; bodily and mental functions cease; and death is caused when the body stops functioning (Speece and Brent, 1984; Kenyon, 2001; Slaughter, 2005; Longbottom and Slaughter, 2018). The developmental age at which children achieve a mature understanding of death is disputed with contemporary researchers revising the traditional Piagetian developmental timeline (Longbottom and Slaughter, 2018). The current consensus is that children can understand death and dying earlier than traditional Piagetian theory proposes (Webb, 2010; Longbottom and Slaughter, 2018). For example, Piagetian theory holds that preschool children aged 2- to 7-years-old do not understand the finality and permanence of death (Webb, 2010), but more contemporary research has shown that children as young as 3-years-old do understand this (Longbottom and Slaughter, 2018). Similarly, an adult understanding of death develops around 11-years-old according to Piagetian theory (Webb, 2010), but contemporary research contends that this develops by 8-years-old (Longbottom and Slaughter, 2018).

Despite attempts by caregivers to shield children from death, it is encountered regularly in their immediate environment through books, film, television and personal experience (Miller *et al.*, 2014). The supportive environment provided by mental health practitioners (hereafter practitioners) can promote positive coping skills and lessen negative impacts on children's development (Wolchik *et al.*, 2009; Bergman *et al.*, 2017). Practitioners use a variety of approaches to support bereaved children including projective play therapy, storytelling, creative writing, memory work, puppets, drawing and bibliotherapy (Berns, 2004; Goldman, 2014).

Bibliotherapy, the use of literature in a therapeutic context (Rusch *et al.*, 2020), is a technique used by practitioners to help children to understand the process of death as well as help them to deal with their grief (Berns, 2004; Heath *et al.*, 2008). In the case of traumatic events such as death, literature provides a powerful tool to help children deal with the trauma by enabling them to cope with their emotions through identifying with the characters, relating to the stories, and coping with complex emotions (Wiseman, 2013). Death-themed literature provides a useful tool to foster conversations about death and assist children to work through their emotions and fears (Arruda-Colli *et al.*, 2017). Little is known about the nature of the literature that is used, nor whether specific types of bibliotherapy may be more useful in helping children conceptualise death.

Of the available death-related storybooks, many appear to depict animal-characters (Heath *et al.*, 2008; Wiseman, 2013; Arruda-Colli *et al.*, 2017). Several theories have been proposed to explain the high rates of animals depicted in such literature. These explanations include that humans are naturally predisposed to turn to animals to understand emotions (Melson, 2001). In this way, animal-characters can be powerfully symbolic for children who may use them as visible examples of their own unseen emotions (Melson, 2001; Melson, 2003). Animal-characters may be comforting when issues relevant to the child's situation are addressed because they function as trusted companions for the child (Suvilehto, 2019). Anthropomorphism (assigning human characteristics to animals) helps children identify with animal-characters (Markowsky, 1975), and creates an emotional distance in which children can safely process painful circumstances (Burke and Copenhaver, 2004). This safe distance may particularly benefit children who have difficulty speaking about death (Heath *et al.*, 2008).

Regular contact with living animals (e.g., as companion animals, exposure to farms, animals on television) in children's day-to-day lives increases their experience with the natural world and helps them make inferences about it (Longbottom and Slaughter, 2016). Longbottom and Slaughter (2018) argue that children's experience with living animals may aid their understanding of death and dying, although this assumption has not been empirically tested. Despite the role of animals generally in a variety of child-related therapies (Chandramouleeswaran and Russell, 2014; Barber *et al.*, 2020), and the presence of animals in death-related literature (Heath *et al.*, 2008; Wiseman, 2013), the role of animal-characters in death-themed bibliotherapy has received little attention in the academic, clinical or grey literature (materials and research produced by organisations outside of commercial or academic publishing). The current literature presents no indication as to how often animal-themed bibliotherapy is used to help children understand death and dying, why animal characters might be preferable for some therapists, and in what contexts might it be effective. To begin addressing these questions, we asked Australian mental health practitioners about their use of animal-themed bibliotherapy with children and adolescents when supporting them during grief and loss.

Method

Recruitment

Australian psychologists, psychotherapists and counsellors were invited to participate in an online survey. Participants were recruited using three advertising strategies. Personalised emails were sent to 1121 practitioners identified as providing services to children around grief and loss through publicly available practitioner lists from the Australian Counselling Association, Australian Psychological Society (APS), Christian Counsellors Association of Australia, Psychotherapy and Counselling Federation of Australia and Psychology Today. The study was advertised on the social media platform Facebook, using Australian practitioners' interest groups with a combined membership of 8853 members. An advertisement was also placed on the APS website and included in their August 2021 newsletter which was emailed to their 27,000 members (APS, 2021).

One of the challenges of researching practitioners is a poor response rate. Despite intensive targeted recruitment strategies, and a sample size higher than comparative studies, the final sample represented a small proportion of practicing therapists in Australia. This is likely to do with survey fatigue and/or a lack of opportunity to complete surveys, particularly the more time consuming qualitative or mixed methods studies such as this one. This survey was conducted during the COVID-19 pandemic when there was a particularly high demand for mental health services. More practically, some practitioners may not have become aware of our survey due to outdated and inaccurate online contact information or fields of expertise; many practitioners worked in multiple practices and their information across practices was inconsistent; and very few websites listed practitioners' direct email addresses so most emails were directed to the reception staff who may not have forwarded them on.

Participants

The sample (n = 47) comprised general psychologists (40.4%), clinical psychologists (12.8%), counselling psychologists (4.3%), psychotherapists (8.5%), counsellors (17.0%) and Other (17.0%). Participants ranged in age from 25 to 70 years-old (M=45.55, SD=12.81) and had between 1 and 40 years of professional experience (M=13.26, SD=10.05). Participants (n = 47) were predominantly female (80.9%) with 19.1% male. Most participants (n = 47) qualified in Australia initially (97.9%,) and were practicing in either Queensland (31.9%), New South Wales (25.5%), Victoria (17.0%) or Western Australia (17.0%).

Design and procedure

The study utilised a mixed-methods approach using quantitative and qualitative data obtained via an online survey. The survey included closed- and open-ended questions and was hosted on the online survey platform Qualtrics between June and August 2021. Demographic information collected included age, gender, geographical area in which practitioners practiced, years of experience and professional registrations, endorsements or memberships held. The complete survey can be found in Supplementary file 1.

A total of 14 closed-response questions were asked to establish the frequency that practitioners provided therapy to children experiencing issues related to death and dying; the therapies they used for each age group were defined according to Piaget's developmental stages (2- to 7-years-old, 7- to 11-years-old, 12-to 18-years-old); and collected demographic information. Three open-ended questions related to: (1) The practitioners' use of bibliotherapy (*From your experience, please describe a time when you used bibliotherapy to support a child or adolescent around death and dying. Was bibliotherapy useful in achieving your therapeutic aims? If yes, how useful was bibliotherapy and why was it useful? If bibliotherapy was not useful, why not?*). (2) Whether they preferred animal-themed characters or not (*If you use books that feature animal-characters, to what extent do you prefer them over books that do not feature animals? Please elaborate on the reasons for your preference*). (3) Their perspective about the influence of animal-characters on children's understanding of death and dying (*In your opinion, in what way do you think animal-characters influence children's understanding of death in terms of understanding its causes and that death is permanent and inevitable?*). These open-ended questions were designed to reflect the literature around bibliotherapy and its use in children's grief and loss, and children's death conceptualisation.

Data analyses

Data were coded, cleaned, and analysed using IBM SPSS Statistics (Version 28). In total, 57 responses were downloaded from Qualtrics, however, incomplete responses (where the open-ended questions were not answered) were removed, resulting in 47 responses in the final data set. Due to the small sample size (n = 47) and exploratory nature of the research, data reflecting close-ended questions were reported using descriptive statistics only. Responses to the open-ended questions were analysed using experiential thematic analysis as outlined by Braun and Clarke (2013). The thematic analysis identifies themes and patterns in a dataset, relative to a research question, by focusing on how participants experience and make sense of the world (Braun and Clarke, 2013). Familiarisation with the data set was achieved by reading entries multiple times and then developing codes that represented the nature of the response. Codes were then organised into initial themes. These initial themes were refined by identifying common patterns which were then grouped together into a final set of themes. To reduce bias as a potential threat to coding reliability, both authors were involved in the coding, and themes were determined through consensus.

The way the open-ended questions were posed meant that there were several opportunities for participants to provide similar answers with different levels of depth. For example, the suitability of animal-themed bibliotherapy for younger rather than older children appeared in all three open-ended questions (bibliotherapy itself, preference for animal-characters and the contribution animal-characters to death conceptualisation). The same was true for animal-characters being 'safe', the normalising of emotions, the individual characteristics of children, the development of death concepts, and how children identify with and relate to animals and animal-characters. This meant that the thematic analysis could not be restricted to responses specific to each of these three open-ended questions separately. Consequently, individual participants' responses across all three questions were consolidated, explored, and coded to generate codes for each participant. Similarities in individual codes were identified and merged into candidate themes which were then reviewed and refined five times until three overarching themes and four sub-themes were identified. A 'thematic map' was used to guide the reporting of the analysis, relating back to the research questions. When reporting results, data excerpts that are quoted as evidence of the validity of the analysis have been amended for clarity (for a full list of responses included in the inductively developed themes, see Supplementary Table 1).

Results and Discussion

Descriptive statistics

Participants were asked to rate a variety of strategies and therapies according to how often they employed them on a scale of 1 ('Never') to 5 ('Always'). The most frequently used therapy was creative writing (93.3%, n = 42/45), followed by storytelling (85.7%, n = 36/42), bibliotherapy without animals (79.5%, n = 35/44) and analysis of drawings (77.8%, n = 35/45). Bibliotherapy with animals (n = 30/43) was used by 41.9% 'sometimes' and by 27.9% about 'half' or' most of the time'. Table 13.1 shows how often practitioners use a range of available therapies for counselling children about death (available options were restricted to this list).

Neither bibliotherapy itself nor death-related literature with animal-characters were the most widely used therapy to support children with death and dying. This is despite the prevalence of animal-characters in bibliotherapy books for grieving children noted by Heath *et al.* (2008), Arruda-Colli *et al.* (2017) and Wiseman (2013), the natural affinity children have for animals (LoBue *et al.*, 2013), and the research showing the effectiveness of bibliotherapy as a therapeutic technique (Mendel *et al.*, 2016).

Table 13.1. The frequency of which a selection of therapies was used by participants to support bereaved children. Therapies ordered by most frequently used.

Therapies	n	Never (%)	Sometimes (%)	About half the time (%)	Most of the time (%)	Always (%)
Creative writing	45	3 (6.7)	12 (26.7)	8 (17.8)	16 (35.6)	6 (13.3)
Storytelling	42	6 (14.3)	11 (26.2)	8 (19.0)	14 (33.3)	3 (7.1)
Bibliotherapy without animals	44	9 (20.5)	20 (45.5)	6 (13.6)	7 (15.9)	2 (4.5)
Analysis of drawings	45	8 (17.8)	19 (42.2)	6 (13.3)	10 (22.2)	2 (4.4)
Projective play with animals	46	16 (34.8)	17 (37.0)	3 (6.5)	9 (19.6)	1 (2.2)
Projective play without animals	47	16 (34.0)	18 (38.3)	6 (12.8)	6 (12.8)	1 (2.1)
Bibliotherapy with animals	43	13 (30.2)	18 (41.9)	5 (11.6)	7 (16.3)	0 (0)

Bibliotherapy (with and without animals) is clearly used, but it is not the preferred therapeutic method. The findings emphasise the need to compare the effectiveness of other therapies with animal-themed bibliotherapy to determine how therapists perceive it.

Participants were then asked to rate the usefulness of each of the various therapies. In the 2- to 7-years-old category, storytelling was rated the most useful, with 50.0% of participants (*n* = 21/42) indicating that it was very or extremely useful. This was followed by bibliotherapy without animals (46.3%, *n* = 19/41) and bibliotherapy with animals (43.6%, *n* = 17/39). In the 7- to 11-year-old category, creative writing was deemed the most useful with 52.3% (*n* = 23/44) rating it very or extremely useful, followed by non-animal-themed bibliotherapy (47.7%, *n* = 20/42), storytelling (47.7%, *n*=21/44) and analysis of drawings (32.6%, *n* = 14/43). Animal-themed bibliotherapy was rated second-last at 19.5% (*n* = 8/41). In the 12–18 year-old category, the usefulness ratings for very or extremely useful were creative writing (75.5%, *n* = 34/45), storytelling (41.3%, *n* = 19/46) and bibliotherapy without animal-characters (40.5%, *n* = 17/42), with bibliotherapy with animals rated least useful (4.8%, *n* = 2/42). A breakdown of therapists' perspectives of various therapies' usefulness is depicted in Table 13.2. The usefulness of animal-themed bibliotherapy decreased as children got older, as shown in Fig. 13.1.

Table 13.2. Practitioners' perspectives on the usefulness of a selection of therapies to support bereaved children, according to the child's developmental age. Therapy approaches are presented in order of perceived usefulness.

Therapy	Age group	n	Not at all or slightly useful (%)	Moderately useful (%)	Very or extremely useful (%)
Creative writing[a]	2–7	42	17 (40.5)	10 (23.8)	15 (35.7)
	7–11	44	6 (13.7)	15 (34.1)	23 (52.3)
	12–18	45	2 (4.4)	9 (20.0)	34 (75.5)
Storytelling	2–7	42	8 (19.1)	13 (31.0)	21 (50.0)
	7–11	44	5 (11.4)	18 (40.9)	21 (47.7)
	12–18	46	14 (30.4)	13 (28.3)	19 (41.3)
Bibliotherapy without animals	2–7	41	10 (24.4)	12 (29.3)	19 (46.3)
	7–11	42	6 (14.3)	16 (38.1)	20 (47.7)
	12–18	42	15 (35.7)	10 (23.8)	17 (40.5)
Analysis of drawings	2–7	42	13 (31.0)	13 (31.0)	16 (38.1)
	7–11	43	10 (23.3)	19 (44.2)	14 (32.6)
	12–18	45	24 (53.3)	13 (28.9)	8 (17.8)
Projective play without animal themes	2–7	41	15 (36.6)	10 (24.4)	16 (39.0)
	7–11	42	19 (45.2)	11 (26.2)	12 (28.6)
	12–18	43	27 (62.8)	9 (20.9)	7 (16.3)
Projective play with animal themes	2–7	40	11 (27.5)	13 (32.5)	16 (40.0)
	7–11	41	19 (46.4)	15 (36.6)	7 (17.0)
	12–18	42	32 (76.2)	7 (16.7)	3 (7.2)
Bibliotherapy with animals	2–7	39	11 (28.2)	11 (28.2)	17 (43.6)
	7–11	41	17 (41.5)	16 (39.0)	8 (19.5)
	12–18	42	34 (81.0)	6 (14.3)	2 (4.8)

[a]Creative writing = poetry, essays, letter writing, feeling journals or projective story writing.

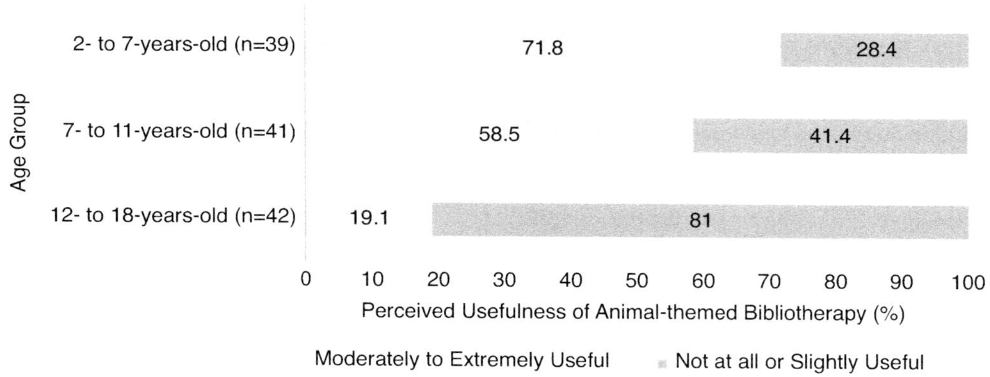

Fig. 13.1. Perceived usefulness of bibliotherapy with animals according to developmental age.

Participants varied in their personal preferences around using bibliotherapy with animals. Overall, just over half (60.0%, n = 24/40) of practitioners preferred to use it, with 30% having no preference, and 10% preferring not to use it altogether. Animal-themed bibliotherapy was not perceived to be more useful than other approaches when supporting children with death and dying, nor considered the most useful strategy in any age-group, especially in children. There was, however, a strong influence of age on those that did rate animal-based bibliotherapy useful. The most effective age group was those aged 2- to 7-years-old and this declined as the children aged. Further investigation is needed to determine the justification for these judgements and the lower rating of usefulness for animal-based bibliotherapy. For example, whether judgements of effectiveness are based on negative personal experience with the technique, or on hearsay from colleagues. Or whether it reflects a lack of knowledge, accessibility or support relating to its use in therapy. What appears clearer, is the contextual or specialist nature of it, and the need or context may not present itself often. A therapist who only sees older children (12-years-old and older) for instance may never use bibliotherapy nor consider it useful for their client base. Indeed, there may be a plethora of contextual uses for animal-themed bibliotherapy that are not relevant to the more general and preferred techniques (such as creative writing, storytelling, and drawing). Some of these questions will be examined in the analysis of the open-ended responses in the following section.

Thematic analysis

Three over-arching themes were extracted from the data corpus. These themes related to the perceived usefulness of animal-characters (themes one and two) and the contexts in which they were used (theme three). The themes were broken down further into sub-themes which will now be discussed in more detail.

Theme one: A means to accessing emotions

The first overarching theme related to the ability of animal-themed bibliotherapy to help children to discuss their feelings and emotions around grief and death. Practitioners believed bibliotherapy provided a way to address grieving children's emotions and feelings by providing a link to engage with the child about their feelings. This is exemplified by one participant who stated that it was "useful as a way to initiate engagement" (Participant 36 [P36], 3 years' experience).

Animal-characters in books were seen to give children the opportunity to ask questions about death and dying, in a safe supported space. This is important because children are often hesitant to ask questions about death when grieving adults are around them. Some participants mentioned that animal-literature made engagement about this topic easier because children easily related to animals. It was also easier for some children to discuss the feelings of the animal-characters than their own feelings. Animal-characters were viewed by some practitioners as an effective way to introduce the concept of grief and loss because children could explore their own emotions alongside the animal-character's emotions. One therapist responded, "We have a number of books featuring animals that are symbolic/ metaphoric of grief...We read...to process grief and provide a space for a child's emotional literacy" (P33, 25 years' experience). Another added:

> The allowance for children to see characters who don't look like them starts the process by which they experience honest and sometimes blunt reactions to the character's emotions. After which we would discuss those emotions, what role (if any) they play in the character's life and what situation they are in (P47, four years' experience).

When death-related literature was animal-themed, practitioners felt a safe space was created for the sharing of emotions. This was because animal-characters were often viewed as less frightening or challenging that human-characters. Animal-characters were consistently perceived as a less confronting way for children to acknowledge and address their emotions because they provided some distance from these emotions and allowed them to be addressed less directly. This is exemplified by the following two extracts:

> I feel animal stories have a gentler way of bridging across death because it is not so close to reality. What I mean is there is a little distance between the child's situation and the characters in the sto-ries...it is similar but not the same as their situation (P28, five years' experience).
>
> And:
>
> [I use] animal-based books to help remove the story a little further away from the child, I believe this enhances their connectivity to the feelings the animal may be experiencing, hence enabling them to feel their own feelings much more (P31, 25 years' experience).

The emotional distance provided by animal-characters can also allow children to be objective about their own emotions and process their own experience with one respondent mentioning that "[Animal-characters] provide space and objective capacity to distance the emotion from self in order to process" (P36, 3 years' experience). Another added that "Animal-characters in books can help reduce the intensity of emotions such that children can use other cognitive resources to understand death" (P37, 12 years' experience).

The ability of bibliotherapy to provide an opportunity for children to explore their feelings has been well discussed in the literature. Berns (2004) argues that stories are interactive catalysts encouraging children to understand and express their emotions. Past research also indicates that books provide a safe distance from experiences that are too overwhelmingly frightening to be faced directly (Burke and Copenhaver, 2004; Mendel *et al.*, 2016). When a story mirrors the same situation that a child is experiencing, the animal-characters are seen as trusted companions that are safe and comforting (Suvilehto, 2019) and a comforting bond is created between them (Dunn, 2011). Burke and Copenhaver (2004) contend that animal-characters create a buffer providing emotional and intellectual distance which protects children's dignity because it allows the animal-characters' emotions to be discussed rather than the child's. Whilst bibliotherapy in general provides a bridge to engage with children about their feelings, animal-themed literature may make this easier because of children's natural affinity for animals and their ability to relate to them easily. It is possible that using bibliotherapy with animals-characters specifically provides a safer and less frightening space for children to do so because of their fondness for animals. This implies that bibliotherapy with animal-characters may be preferable for many children than books without animals in providing a gateway to children's pent-up emotions around death and dying and providing them with a space where it is safe to share these emotions.

Three participants stated that bibliotherapy provided children with the vocabulary to name their experiences and verbalise what they were feeling. This is best emphasised by the following participant, who responded: "Books that deal sensitively with death can be very helpful in providing words to name their experience, and to allow thought and emotion to be named and understood" (P16, 20 years' experience). Past research has also shown that children learn new words through reading or being read to (Zuo and Yan, 2019). As such, these new words give them the language to express and define their emotions and experiences (Berns, 2004; Von Drasek, 2016).

Theme two: The familiarity of animals

Practitioners felt that bibliotherapy with animal-characters made death easier to understand because animals were abundant in children's environments and so were visible and familiar. From lived experience with animals, children are familiar with the fact that animals die. Consequently, children may understand the permanence of death better because they are able to apply this knowledge to human death. In this way, death is also normalised as a common human experience.

This theme was further broken down into two sub-themes. (1) Children were able to extrapolate the biological knowledge they had developed from observing animals to human death and dying. As such, animal-characters helped to normalise death and grief, and (2) Children identified with animal-characters and found them appealing.

Knowledge of animal life cycles can be harnessed. Animals appear frequently in children's everyday environments (Burke and Copenhaver, 2004; Russell, 2017) and in literature to which they are exposed (Burke and Copenhaver, 2004; Geerdts, 2016; Ivanovic, 2017; Suvilehto, 2019). When children recognise the familiarity of a situation depicted in a story, they develop emotional connections to the characters (McCulliss, 2012; De Vries *et al.*, 2017). This allows children to normalise their situation (Mendel *et al.*, 2016) and draw parallels between themselves and the characters (Pardeck, 1990).

Much of children's exposure to live animals includes experiences of animal life cycles that provide valuable representations of death and dying (Berns, 2004). This biological knowledge helps children to understand human death (Corr, 2004; Lee *et al.*, 2009; Geerdts, 2016; Longbottom and Slaughter, 2018) when they connect animal death to human death (Russell, 2017). This biological knowledge was mirrored by many of the participants, who mentioned that children who had regular contact with animals as pets or farm animals, as toys or as characters in stories and on film are usually familiar with the fact that animals die. For example, one believed that: "...lived experience of pets and farm animals dying helps relate this and then apply it to the experience of a human dying" (P18, 13 years' experience). Another suggested that "If a child ... has had or knows of a loved pet that has passed, it is helpful to be able to make sense of the death using the animal analogy" (P26, 13 years' experience).

Within this overarching theme of familiarity with animals, two participants reported using examples of pets and farm animals with children of all developmental ages when discussing death and dying, even if they elected not to use animal-themed bibliotherapy. "... we often would talk about animals dying, death of pets, how [they] coped, what rituals were useful etc" (P27, 15 years' experience). Another wrote, "I do use real life examples of pets and farm animals with all ages" (P37, 12 years' experience).

Participants observed that familiarity with animals meant that children had an opportunity to observe their life cycles which were shorter than human life cycles, and that death was natural and certain. It also made the experience of death more concrete; children understood the permanence of death better due to their exposure to animal deaths. Discussing animal life cycles was a technique employed by participants to introduce death and dying as a process of change. For example, one practitioner wrote "It helps them understand the life cycles concept and that all animals and people eventually die" (P41, 19 years' experience). Another explained that:

> Animals assist because their life cycle is much shorter in general – children can be aware of their birth and passing. This opens up conversation about the cycle of life [and] assists with the under-standing of death, that someone is gone, and they will not return (P2, 9 years' experience).

Practitioners saw bibliotherapy as helping to normalise children's emotional experience of grief by putting it in context as a common life-event. This helped children to realise that there would be a time when they would no longer experience such intense emotions. When these books were animal-themed, familiarity with animals helped to normalise grief as a common life experience. This view is exemplified by the following extracts: "[Books help] to communicate that it is normal to have big feelings when someone isn't still with us... [it] allows the child to learn that feelings and emotions are normal" (P37, 12 years' experience), and "[Animal-characters] help them understand the life cycles concept and that all animals and people eventually die. It makes it seem more natural and normal" (P41, 19 years' experience).

Berns (2004) contends that reading a story echoing a child's personal experience helps them become aware that others are experiencing similar grief in similar situations. Burke and Copenhaver (2004) propose that portraying significant life events in literature helps readers apply the story to their own lives. Since children are familiar and comfortable with animals (Burke and Copenhaver, 2004), it is possible that this normalisation of grief also occurs through the presence of animal-characters in the story.

The implication is that animal-themed bibliotherapy can be useful in helping children conceptualise death because they are already familiar with and drawn to animals. Children's familiarity with animals and their identification with animal-characters may help to normalise both death and grief. Consequently, bibliotherapy with animal-characters may be a more effective choice of subject-matter compared with other types of literature because children have pre-existing positive relationships with animals.

Animal-characters are appealing and identifiable. Children typically have a natural affinity for animals. LoBue *et al.* (2013) concluded that children demonstrate an affinity for animals as early as 7- to 16-months-old, while Melson (2001) contends that children have an innate urge to turn to animals to understand emotions. Additionally, the biophilia hypothesis (Wilson, 1984) argues that humans have an instinctive emotional connection to other living beings, including animals. Practitioners stated that children identified with animal-characters and connected to them easily. This allowed children to explore the concept of death and their own emotions. They were empathetic towards the animal-characters and could then apply this empathy towards themselves. One therapist responded, "Children relate to animals – its natural and holds quick connectedness" (P33, 25 years' experience).

This sub-theme varied in the perspectives of why animal-characters were appealing, with two participants suggesting that children recognised some of the animal-characters' traits in themselves, or in the person who had died. This provided a sense of connection to the deceased person. For example, one commented "For animal literature, it is as if they can portray people in their lives as animals – almost like an externalisation of their feelings, losses and grief" (P24, 6 years' experience). Other responses suggested that animal-characters have particular characteristics that made them interesting and effective such as being entertaining and different. Another commented that "Most children find [animal] characters funny and engaging due to [the] colours, shapes and species" (P47, 4 years' experience). Practitioners felt that the 'otherness' of animal-characters made them appealing because it allowed thought and conversation that was slightly distanced from the child's immediate grief. This encouraged honest reactions to the animal-character's emotions. For example, "[Animal-characters] are similar but not the same as their situation" (P28, 5 years' experience).

Children identify with characters in stories, and this provides opportunities for observing and discussing important concepts (Suvilehto, 2019). Melson (2001) argues that this identification with animals allows an emotional connection to what the animal-character is experiencing in the text. Identification with characters is an important step in the process of bibliotherapy (Goddard, 2011; McCulliss, 2012), and is necessary for emotional connection with the characters (Goddard, 2011).

Children identify more closely with animal-characters than with human-characters (O'Donnell, 1980). When animal-characters display human traits and characteristics, children's identification with them increases (Markowsky, 1975). Animals are also appealing because they have unique features that make them attractive to children such as opening up a fantasy world in which animals speak and depict stereotypical humans (Markowsky, 1975). O'Donnell (1980) suggests that animal-characters appeal to children because they find them impressive, and humorous when they depict familiar people or display human idiosyncrasies. Animal-characters may also be appealing because of their 'otherness' (Selly, 2014). Myers (2007) contends that children recognise the 'otherness' of animals by understanding that animals have agency and affect. Children find the autonomy of animals intriguing and recognise that they have moods and emotions in response to their environment (Myers, 2007). These unique features and characteristics may make animal-characters both more appealing and more effective when selecting death-themed literature for children. The implication is that young children may identify and connect with animal-characters more easily than with human-characters.

Theme three: The complementary and contextual nature of animal-themed bibliotherapy

The third overarching theme was that the use of bibliotherapy with animal-characters depends upon the individual child and/or the practitioner. Responses of this nature were further discussed in terms of either the context or the factors determining its use.

Animal-themed bibliotherapy as a therapeutic tool. Bibliotherapy with animal-characters was used as an integrated part of a whole approach towards therapy. Common strategies used alongside animal books were sand play, drawing, non-directive play, animal puppets, letter writing, and as part of established bereavement support programs. For example, "I have woven bibliotherapy into work with children regarding grief a lot and found this very successful - especially for younger children" (P33, 25 years' experience), and "I have used [bibliotherapy with animal-characters] with sand play and drawing often, used for children to show their experience with the grief" (P22, 5 years' experience).

In addition to this use as an adjunct tool, participants often passed on books to carers, parents, and grandparents to read with the child at home. One participant also provided psychoeducation about the language carers should use when discussing death and dying:

> Family and parents don't know what to say to kids and too often lie to them or don't tell them about death or use silly terms like 'gone to sleep' or using religious concepts that don't make logical sense to the child. Books are helpful for parents to read at home with their child when they are upset (P41, 19 years' experience).

Animal-themed bibliotherapy was used as an adjunct therapy and passed onto other caring adults as a homework task to complete with the child. These results are supported by previous research suggesting that bibliotherapy is used by both skilled practitioners as part of clinical therapy and informally by other caring adults concerned about the emotional wellbeing of the child (Berns, 2004; McCulliss, 2012; Suvilehto *et al.*, 2019). In this context, bibliotherapy can be extremely helpful (Suvilehto *et al.*, 2019). As an adjunct therapy, bibliotherapy allows children to talk about the emotions elicited from reading the story when other therapeutic activities follow the reading of the story (Berns, 2004; Lucas and Soares, 2013; Suvilehto *et al.*, 2019). Additionally, bibliotherapy is more effective when used with other therapies (Berns, 2004; McCulliss, 2012; Lucas and Soares, 2013; Pierce, 2015; Suvilehto *et al.*, 2019). In fact, when bibliotherapy is used for trauma, the recommended use is as an adjunct therapy (Heath *et al.*, 2005; De Vries *et al.*, 2017). As such, therapists should consider adding animal-themed bibliotherapy to other types of therapy routinely as an adjunct tool to help younger children to understand death and grief.

The contextual and preferential nature of animal-themed bibliotherapy

The decision to use animal-themed books depended on the circumstances and preferences of the child and the practitioner. Unique characteristics of the child influencing the choice of subject-matter included their interests, age and the situation at hand. Factors that were practitioner-specific included their personal preferences and the availability of animal literature. These are described in turn.

Child Specific Factors. Many participants selected resources based on the interests of the child presenting for therapy. These included whether the child had a good relationship with books and an interest in animals. One participant found animal-characters to be particularly valuable when the child was having difficulty discussing the death directly. Additionally, the storyline and themes also had to be relevant to the child's situation. "I do have books about animals and also not about animals, depends on what the moment held for us and where the child's attention was drawn at that present time" (P24, 6 years' experience). Another noted, "[The choice is] dependent on the interests of the child or young person and what they find interesting...[The] child chooses what they want to do. Agency is important" (P42, 22 years' experience).

Participants reported animal-characters to be less helpful in certain situations. For example, two participants reported that bibliotherapy with animals was not useful in children with autism spectrum disorder (ASD) because resources had to be very clear and concrete. "I don't generally use books that feature animal-characters to represent what humans are experiencing as my clients will take the literal interpretation more often than not" (P15, 2 years' experience). Previous studies have also shown that using bibliotherapy in children with ASD may be challenging. For example, children with autism have difficulty recognising emotions in others or themselves (theory of mind) (Baron-Cohen, 1999; Brinton and Fujiki, 2017). Both anthropomorphism and theory of mind involve thinking about the intentions of non-human animals (Epley *et al.*, 2007; Atherton and Cross, 2018). The same brain areas activate for the theory of mind and anthropomorphising (Chaminade *et al.*, 2007) such that deficits in one correspond to deficits in the other (Cullen *et al.*, 2014). Consequently, it is possible that these children have difficulty identifying with animal-characters.

Participants also reported the child's age to be a major factor in the decision to use animal-themed bibliotherapy. Most reported using it for younger children but not for older children as these children often considered themselves too mature for animal stories. For example, "I think once the child is about 11[years-old], they would start to view [animal literature] as childish and would be put off by it" (P25, one year's experience).

Within this sub-theme participants varied in their perspective on the upper age limit for using animal-themed bibliotherapy. Opinions varied in 7-, 8-, 10- and 12-years-old as the cut-off age for using animal-themed bibliotherapy. Additionally, while most participants reported using animal-characters with 'younger children', no definitive age range was given. To illustrate, 'It does depend on age, with younger clients preferring animals to older clients' (P18, 13 years' experience).

Many of the practitioners indicated that the effectiveness of animal-themed bibliotherapy decreased with the age of the child. Practitioners reported animal-themed bibliotherapy to be most useful in the 2- to 7-year-old category, with none deeming it appropriate for children over the age of 12 years (also see Fig. 13.1). Animal-themed bibliotherapy is being applied to children well before traditional theories of development consider them to have developed appropriate death concepts. For example, Piagetian developmental theory suggests that a mature understanding of death does not develop until around 11-years-old (Webb, 2010), and an understanding of death's permanency is acquired between 7- and 11-years-old (Slaughter, 2005). Contemporary studies, however, such as by Speece and Brent (1984) and Longbottom and Slaughter (2018) argue that death concepts are acquired as early as 3- to 7-years of age. The fact that therapists we surveyed are utilising animal-themed bibliotherapy with children exclusively under the age of 12 adds weight to the modern development theories that children are able to understand death at these younger ages.

Practitioners agreed that animal-themed bibliotherapy helps with death conceptualisation, suggesting that animal-characters helped younger children to understand death's *permanency*, but they did not state specifically at what age this understanding occurred. This concurs with previous research that young children benefit from the use of animal-themed literature (Burke and Copenhaver, 2004). Children's emotional interest in animals also peaks around 6- to 9-years old (Kellert, 1985). The implications of this are that animal-literature may be most useful during the ages that more contemporary research suggests children develop a mature understanding of death i.e., around 7- to 8-years-old. Also, there may be a specific age-range during which animal-themed bibliotherapy is most effective. Geerdts (2016) for instance, found that anthropomorphism was most beneficial to 5- to 7-year-olds in terms of their learning and cognitive processes.

Age and individual characteristics were thus important considerations in selecting animal-themed bibliotherapy. Most children are interested in animals (LoBue *et al.*, 2013), but there are age differences in the way that children relate to animals (Kellert, 1985) and different types of animal depictions appeal to different age-groups (O'Donnell, 1980). For example, children aged 3- to 7-years-old prefer animal-characters that behave like human-characters, but from around 8- years-old onwards children prefer animal-characters that act like animals. Likewise, for bibliotherapy to be successful, book selection needs to be done with sensitivity towards the individual circumstances of the particular child in their own unique situation (Crosetto and Garcha, 2013; Sevinç, 2019). These include specific needs and interests (Berns, 2004), cultural and religious values, and social relevance (Heath *et al.*, 2008; Suvilehto *et al.*, 2019). And whilst most children love stories (Suvilehto *et al.*, 2019), bibliotherapy is less successful when children do not enjoy reading (Pardeck, 1990; Lucas and Soares, 2013).

Practitioner Specific Factors. The personal preferences of participants also influenced whether bibliotherapy with animal-characters was selected. While most participants preferred books with animals, 12 respondents indicated no preference stating that book choice depended on the relevance of the themes, age-appropriateness, availability of animal-themed books and interests of the child. One participant responded: "It is not a mindful decision to use animal books over books without animals" (P12, 7 years 'experience).

Three participants preferred not to use animal-themed books. The reasons for preferring not to use animal-themed bibliotherapy were clients with ASD, animal-characters being "too fanciful" (P30, 23 years' experience) and the inappropriateness of using animal-characters. One noting for instance: "...not sure if hiding behind [animal] characters rather than people is that appropriate" (P46, 20 years' experience).

The choice of subject matter was also influenced by the availability of resources. Many participants who did not use animal bibliotherapy stated that they used the resources that were available to them or that they were unaware of animal-themed books on the subject. For example: "I think the reason for not using the animal-character books with children will have been because we didn't have any" (P20, 30 years' experience).

The unavailability of literature addressing pertinent topics as well as a lack of knowledge about suitable books hindered the effectiveness of bibliotherapy (Lucas and Soares, 2013). Given the capacity of children to make emotional connections with animal-characters, animal-themed bibliotherapy may be a particularly useful vehicle for discussing emotions. It is important that practitioners be educated on the benefits of animal-themed literature over other literature so that clinical outcomes are maximised.

Conclusion

This research explored perceptions of Australian therapists around animal-themed bibliotherapy in the context of children's grief and understanding of death. Bibliotherapy offers an accessible therapeutic tool for therapists to assist children to navigate their grief, but also for teachers and caregivers for developing and discussing children's general understanding of death. Animal-themed bibliotherapy, particularly, presents children with a safe space in which to express and explore their own emotions around death and loss. This is because, amongst others, children have a natural affinity to animals, are drawn to animal characters, and are exposed to animals and animal life cycles in their everyday life. Animal-themed bibliotherapy was used by many therapists and perceived to assist most children to understand death and dying more easily than non-animal-themed literature. Despite this, animal-themed literature was not a preferred therapeutic option for all age groups when compared to alternative approaches. Bibliotherapy with animal-characters was of greatest benefit for younger children aged between two and seven, and who show an affinity to animals.

Overall, animal-themed bibliotherapy was seen favourably by those who used it, but more so as an adjunct therapy to support young children dealing with death and dying. Given therapists who used it, often viewed it favourably, its lack of general use may be a result of individual therapeutic preferences, a client base in which animal-themed literature is not appropriate, or a lack of awareness or education of the method. In these situations, providing practical suggestions and clinical examples of where animal-themed bibliotherapy can be effectively applied to young children experiencing grief may be beneficial. An audit of death literature for children would be valuable to determine the prevalence of animal characters, and how animals are represented in these books, especially in relation to the developmental age of the intended audience. Publishers and therapists should work together to create age-appropriate and effective death-themed literature. Resources aimed at health practitioners in utilising animal-themed death literature may foster a greater understanding of its merits and delivery, and thus its adoption.

Conflict of Interest

The authors have no conflicts of interest to declare.

Funding

The authors received no financial support for the research, authorship and publication of this article.

Ethics Statement

The authors confirm that the research meets any required ethical guidelines, including adherence to the legal requirements of the study country. All research presented here was approved by the Human Research Ethics Committee of CQ University (approval number 2021-039). Written informed consent was obtained from all participants.

Author Contributions

Both E.S. and B.S. contributed to the development of the study and preparation of the manuscript. Data were collected by E.S. and analysed by E.S. and B.S.

References

Arruda-Colli, M.N., Weaver, M.S. and Wiener, L. (2017) Communication about dying, death, and bereavement: A systematic review of children's literature. *Journal of Palliative Medicine* 20(5), 548–559. DOI: 10.1089/jpm.2016.0494.

Atherton, G. and Cross, L. (2018) Seeing more than human: Autism and anthropomorphic theory of mind. *Frontiers in Psychology* 9, 528. DOI: 10.3389/fpsyg.2018.00528.

Australian Psychological Society (2021) About the APS. Available at: https://psychology.org.au/about-us/who-we-are/about-the-aps

Barber, O., Somogyi, E., McBride, A.E. and Proops, L. (2020) Children's evaluations of a therapy dog and biomimetic robot: Influences of animistic beliefs and social interaction. *International Journal of Social Robotics* 13(6), 1–15. DOI: 10.1007/s12369-020-00722-0.

Baron-Cohen, S. (1999) *The Evolution of a Theory of Mind*. Oxford University Press, Cambridge, UK.

Bergman, A.-S., Axberg, U. and Hanson, E. (2017) When a parent dies: A systematic review of the effects of support programs for parentally bereaved children and their caregivers. *BMC Palliative Care* 16(1), 1–15. DOI: 10.1186/s12904-017-0223-y.

Berns, C.F. (2004) Bibliotherapy: Using books to help bereaved children. *Omega: Journal of Death and Dying* 48(4), 321–336. DOI: 10.2190/361d-jhd8-rnjt-ryjv.

Braun, V. and Clarke, V. (2013) *Successful Qualitative Research: A Practical Guide for Beginners*. Sage Publications, London.

Brinton, B. and Fujiki, M. (2017) The power of stories: Facilitating social communication in children with limited language abilities. *School Psychology International* 38(5), 523–540. DOI: 10.1177/0143034317713348.

Burke, C.L. and Copenhaver, J.G. (2004) Animals as people in children's literature. *Language Arts* 81(3), 205–213.

Carter, M. (2016) *Helping Children and Adolescents Think about Death, Dying and Bereavement*. Jessica Kingsley Publishers, London.

Chaminade, T., Hodgins, J. and Kawato, M. (2007) Anthropomorphism influences perception of computer-animated characters' actions. *Social Cognitive and Affective Neuroscience* 2(3), 206–216. DOI: 10.1093/scan/nsm017.

Chandramouleeswaran, S. and Russell, P.S. (2014) Complementary psychosocial interventions in child and adolescent psychiatry: Pet assisted therapy. *Indian Journal of Psychological Medicine* 36(1), 4–8. DOI: 10.4103/0253-7176.127240.

Corr, C.A. (2004) Pet loss in death-related literature for children. *Omega: Journal of Death and Dying* 48(4), 399–414. DOI: 10.2190/HXQY-DU5D-YC39-XKJ9.

Crosetto, A. and Garcha, R. (2013) *Death, Loss, and Grief in Literature for Youth: A Selective Annotated Bibliography for K-12*. Scarecrow Press, Plymouth, UK.

Cullen, H., Kanai, R., Bahrami, B. and Rees, G. (2014) Individual differences in anthropomorphic attributions and human brain structure. *Social Cognitive and Affective Neuroscience* 9(9), 1276–1280. DOI: 10.1093/scan/nst109.

De Vries, D., Brennan, Z., Lankin, M., Morse, R., Rix, B. *et al*. (2017) Healing with books: A literature review of bibliotherapy used with children and youth who have experienced trauma. *Therapeutic Recreation Journal* 51(1), 48–74. DOI: 10.18666/TRJ-2017-V51-I1-7652.

Dunn, E.A. (2011) Talking animals: A literature review of anthropomorphism in children's books. [Unpublished masters' thesis], University of North Carolina, Chapel Hill, NC.

Epley, N., Waytz, A. and Cacioppo, J.T. (2007) On seeing human: A three-factor theory of anthropomorphism. *Psychological Review* 114(4), 864–886. DOI: 10.1037/0033-295X.114.4.864.

Geerdts, M.S. (2016) (Un)real animals: Anthropomorphism and early learning about animals. *Child Development Perspectives* 10(1), 10–14. DOI: 10.1111/cdep.12153.

Goddard, A.T. (2011) Children's books for use in bibliotherapy. *Journal of Pediatric Health Care* 25(1), 57–61. DOI: 10.1016/j.pedhc.2010.08.006.

Goldman, L. (2014) *Life and Loss: A Guide to Helping Grieving Children*. Routledge, New York.

Heath, M.A., Sheen, D., Leavy, D., Young, E. and Money, K. (2005) Bibliotherapy: A resource to facilitate emotional healing and growth. *School Psychology International* 26(5), 563–580. DOI: 10.1177/0143034305060792.

Heath, M.A., Leavy, D., Hansen, K., Ryan, K., Lawrence, L. *et al*. (2008) Coping with grief: Guidelines and resources for assisting children. *Intervention in School and Clinic* 43(5), 259–269. DOI: 10.1177/1053451208314493.

Howarth, R.A. (2011) Promoting the adjustment of parentally bereaved children. *Journal of Mental Health Counseling* 33(1), 21–32. DOI: 10.17744/mehc.33.1.a2m06x0835352741.

Ivanovic, C. (2017) Talking animals and politics of world literature. *Comparative Literature Studies* 54(4), 702–730. DOI: 10.5325/complitstudies.54.4.0702.

Kellert, S.R. (1985) Attitudes toward animals: Age-related development among children. *Journal of Environmental Education* 16(3), 29–39. DOI: 10.1080/00958964.1985.9942709.

Kenyon, B.L. (2001) Current research in children's conceptions of death: A critical review. *Omega: Journal of Death and Dying* 43(1), 63–91. DOI: 10.2190/0x2b-b1n9-a579-dvk1.

Lee, J.O., Lee, J. and Moon, S.S. (2009) Exploring children's understanding of death concepts. *Asia Pacific Journal of Education* 29(2), 251–264. DOI: 10.1080/02188790902859020.

LoBue, V., Pickard, M.B., Sherman, K., Axford, C. and DeLoache, J.S. (2013) Young children's interest in live animals. *British Journal of Developmental Psychology* 31(1), 57–69. DOI: 10.1111/j.2044-835x.2012.02078.x.

Longbottom, S. and Slaughter, V. (2018) Sources of children's knowledge about death and dying. *Philosophical Transactions of the Royal Society B: Biological Sciences* 373(1754), 20170267. DOI: 10.1098/rstb.2017.0267.

Longbottom, S.E. and Slaughter, V. (2016) Direct experience with nature and the development of biological knowledge. *Early Education and Development* 27(8), 1145–1158. DOI: 10.1080/10409289.2016.1169822.

Lucas, C.V. and Soares, L. (2013) Bibliotherapy: A tool to promote children's psychological well-being. *Journal of Poetry Therapy* 26(3), 137–147. DOI: 10.1080/08893675.2013.823310.

Markowsky, J.K. (1975) Why anthropomorphism in children's literature? *Elementary English* 52(4), 460–466.

McCulliss, D. (2012) Bibliotherapy: Historical and research perspectives. *Journal of Poetry Therapy* 25(1), 23–38. DOI: 10.1080/08893675.2012.654944.

Melson, G.F. (2001) *Why the Wild Things Are: Animals in the Lives of Children*. Harvard University Press, Cambridge MA and London.

Melson, G.F. (2003) Child development and the human-companion animal bond. *The American Behavioral Scientist* 47(1), 31–39. DOI: 10.1177/0002764203255210.

Mendel, M.R., Harris, J. and Carson, N. (2016) Bringing bibliotherapy for children to clinical practice. *Journal of the American Academy of Child & Adolescent Psychiatry* 55(7), 535–537. DOI: 10.1016/j.jaac.2016.05.008.

Miller, P.J., Rosengren, K.S. and Gutiérrez, I.T. (2014) Children's understanding of death: Toward a contextualized and integrated account I. Introduction. *Monographs of the Society for Research in Child Development* 79(1), 1–18. DOI: 10.1111/mono.12076.

Myers, O.G. (2007) *The Significance of Children and Animals: Social Development and Our Connections to Other Species*. Purdue University Press, West Lafayette, IN.

Nagy, M. (1948) The child's theories concerning death. *The Pedagogical Seminary and Journal of Genetic Psychology* 73(1), 3–27. DOI: 10.1080/08856559.1948.10533458.

O'Donnell, H. (1980) ERIC/RCS report: Animals in literature. *Language Arts* 57(4), 451–454.

Pardeck, J.T. (1990) Using bibliotherapy in clinical practice with children. *Psychological Reports* 67(3), 1043–1049. DOI: 10.2466/pr0.67.7.1043-1049.

Park, Y.C. and Pyszczynski, T. (2016) Cultural universals and differences in dealing with death. In: Harvell, L.A. and Nisbett, G.S. (eds) *Denying Death: An Interdisciplinary Approach to Terror Management Theory*. Routledge, New York, pp. 193–213.

Pierce, L.M. (2015) The use of bibliotherapy with adolescents and their families. *Journal of Family Psychotherapy* 26(4), 323–330. DOI: 10.1080/08975353.2015.1097294.

Rusch, R., Greenman, J., Scanlon, C., Horne, K. and Jonas, D.F. (2020) Bibliotherapy and bereavement: Harnessing the power of reading to enhance family coping in pediatric palliative care. *Journal of Social Work in End-of-Life & Palliative Care* 16(2), 85–98. DOI: 10.1080/15524256.2020.1745728.

Russell, J. (2017) "Everything has to die one day": Children's explorations of the meanings of death in human-animal-nature relationships. *Environmental Education Research* 23(1), 75–90. DOI: 10.1080/13504622.2016.1144175.

Selly, P.B. (2014) *Connecting Animals and Children in Early Childhood*. Redleaf Press, St Paul, MN.

Sevinç, G. (2019) Healing mental health through reading: Bibliotherapy. *Psikiyatride Güncel Yaklaşimlar* 11(4), 483–495. DOI: 10.18863/pgy.474083.

Slaughter, V. (2005) Young children's understanding of death. *Australian Psychologist* 40(3), 179–186. DOI: 10.1080/00050060500243426.

Speece, M.W. and Brent, S.B. (1984) Children's understanding of death: A review of three components of a death concept. *Child Development* 55(5), 1671–1686. DOI: 10.2307/1129915.

Suvilehto, P. (2019) A study of animal characters as representations of humans: the animality/bibliotherapy test. *Journal of Poetry Therapy* 32(2), 95–108. DOI: 10.1080/08893675.2019.1583414.

Suvilehto, P., Kerry-Morgan, K. and Aerila, J.-A. (2019) Supporting children's social and emotional growth through developmental bibliotherapy. In: Kerry-Morgan, K. and Aerila, J.-A. (eds) *Story in Children's Lives: Contributions of the Narrative Mode to Early Childhood Development, Literacy, and Learning*. Springer, Cham, Switzerland, pp. 299–314.

Von Drasek, L. (2016) Grief in picturebooks: An evaluative rubric. *Children and Libraries* 14(4), 25–31. DOI: 10.5860/cal.14n4.25.

Webb, N.B. (2010) *The child and death*. In: Webb, N.B. (ed.) *Helping Bereaved Children: A Handbook for Practitioners*. Guilford Publications, New York, pp. 3–21.

Willis, C. (2002) The grieving process in children: Strategies for understanding, educating, and reconciling children's perceptions of death. *Early Childhood Education Journal* 29(4), 221–226. DOI: 10.1023/A:1015125422643.

Wilson, E.O. (1984) *Biophilia: The Human Bond with Other Species*. Harvard University Press, Cambridge MA and London.

Wiseman, A.M. (2013) Summer's end and sad goodbyes: Children's picture books about death and dying. *Children's Literature in Education* 44(1), 1–14. DOI: 10.1007/s10583-012-9174-3.

Wolchik, S.A., Coxe, S., Tein, J.Y., Sandler, I.N. and Ayers, T.S. (2009) Six-year longitudinal predictors of posttraumatic growth in parentally bereaved adolescents and young adults. *Omega: Journal of Death and Dying* 58(2), 107–128. DOI: 10.2190/om.58.2.b.

Wong, M. (2010) Chinese children's understanding of death. *Australasian Journal of Early Childhood* 35(2), 63–71. DOI: 10.1177/183693911003500209.

Xu, J., Murphy, S.L., Kochanek, K.D. and Arias, E. (2019) Deaths: Final data for 2019. *National Vital Statistics Reports* 70(8). Available at: https://www.cdc.gov/nchs/data/nvsr/nvsr70/nvsr70-08-508.pdf

Zuo, F. and Yan, X. (2019) Incidental english vocabulary acquisition through reading: A review in the last two decades. *English Language Teaching* 12(12), 39–45. DOI: 10.5539/elt.v12n12p39.

14 How to Care for the Caregiver: The Power of Ritual

Loretta Truman*
Argus Institute, Colorado State University, Veterinary Teaching Hospital, Fort Collins, CO, USA

Abstract
Now more than ever, we understand the depth and power of the human–animal bond. With this increased awareness comes increased responsibility to more fully educate and support families of veterinary patients for end-of-life care. This author is a licensed clinical social worker (LCSW), holding an Animal-Assisted Social Work specialty certification, who works within a veterinary teaching hospital. In the LCSW role, this author partners closely with veterinary medical teams to offer support and counseling to the human family members of pets coming in for care. This support takes a wide variety of shapes and forms, but one consistent theme is caring for the caregiver as they navigate a terminal illness and subsequent loss of their animal. How do we support people who are caring for their ill pet? How do we help prepare them for what is to come, make decisions in line with their values and goals, and mitigate potential regrets as much as possible? One of the most beneficial tools this author has found that significantly helps families minimize regret, make the most out of their time with their pets, and move through the grieving journey post-loss is the incorporation of mindful, thoughtfully chosen rituals into their lives. This topic will be explored through the lens of a couple of case frameworks to illuminate key points and demonstrate how this tool can be used in practice (names and identifying details have been changed to protect confidentiality).

Keywords: human–animal bond, pet grief and loss, anticipatory grief, mourning, ritual

Introduction

Throughout history, we see rituals and customs surrounding death in every culture and society worldwide. How we honor people we love who have died, what actions we take in remembrance of them, and the ways in which we choose to memorialize those lost, exist and vary widely across a vast spectrum attuned to our corner of the world, our culture, and our personal belief system. Historically, rituals around death and dying often stem from religious or spiritual sources, and yet rituals can also be completely secular. So what makes a ritual a ritual? Rituals are embodied actions that hold a specific protocol or structure, differ from ordinary or everyday routines, and must be enacted or executed in a specific manner (Wojtkowiak *et al.*, 2021). The most important component is the meaning we derive and attach to the ritual itself; this meaning is what transforms the actions into an emotionally impactful and consequential experience.

*Corresponding author: Loretta.truman@colostate.edu

It can be helpful to consider the subtle yet distinct difference between grief and mourning and how this distinction intersects with ritual. Grief embodies the "constellation of internal thoughts and feelings we have when someone we love dies"; it is the personal meaning we attach to the experience of the loss (Wolfelt, 2004, p. 3). Mourning requires you to "take the grief you have on the inside and express it outside of yourself" (Wolfelt, 2004, p. 3). Mourning takes the internal experience of grief and transforms it into an action, into how you choose to actively engage with your grief to start to process and move through it. Identifying, creating, and then engaging with rituals requires you to actively engage with your grief, to turn it outward, to mourn. Wolfelt (2004) notes that "to mourn is to heal" (p. 3).

Just as we can grieve following the loss of a loved one, we can and often do also grieve in anticipation of such a loss. Anticipatory grief can manifest with all the same physical and emotional expressions of what is considered a "normal" or "typical" grief response following a death (Laing and Maylea, 2018). Laing and Maylea (2018) also note the high likelihood that pet owners will experience anticipatory grief at some time during their pet ownership, due to the shorter lifespan of their animal family members. Grief is an experience often characterized by chaotic, overwhelming emotions that can feel disorienting and all-consuming. Rituals provide a structure, with boundaries drawn around the focus, the planned order of actions, and the time allotted for the ritual, which allows one to channel those chaotic emotions and feel a little more in control (Castle and Phillips, 2003; Rando, 1985; Romanoff and Terenzio, 1998; Sas and Coman, 2016). Rituals offer a safe outlet for creating mindful, protected time to address our emotional needs and take care of ourselves.

Rituals in Grief

In a qualitative systematic review of studies exploring the psychosocial impact of bereavement and pet grief and loss, Cleary *et al.* (2021) found that "an important part of the grief process for many was the instigation of rituals." The key missing component for many people when attempting to move through the grief process for a pet is the lack of formalized customs and ceremonies that we have in place when we mourn human loss. Typically, losing a pet does not prompt the start of the automatic processes of official burial arrangements and funereal ceremonies, which are often expected and commonplace following the loss of a human (Cleary *et al.*, 2021). This lack of structure, the missing piece of how to honor our deceased animal family member, can leave one feeling lost and adrift in grief, with no clear direction forward. It can also create a feeling that the loss of the pet is not or should not be as significant as the loss of a human, attributing the lack of commemoration to mean that this loss is not as important or meaningful (Cleary *et al.*, 2021). Grieving pet families often experience this form of disenfranchised grief – when our grief is not as supported, as validated or publicly acknowledged as real and true – within our larger society or culture. Giving ourselves permission to grieve fully, take up space with the depth of our true emotion, and engage in meaningful rituals around our loss can help empower us to move through our grieving journey in a healthy way, rather than having us shut down, feel shame around the intensity of our experience, or hide or attempt to stifle our honest grief to try to fit in with cultural norms.

The goal, what we hope to achieve out of participating in these rituals, will differ depending on where we are in the trajectory of our pet's illness or aging journey – whether we are engaging in ritual pre-loss or post-loss. Many clients, shortly after receiving a serious diagnosis for their pet, become so overcome with fear and sadness that they struggle to cope and manage daily activities. Many share feeling consumed by racing thoughts, catastrophizing worst-case scenarios, and ruminating on what the end will look like, the frightening stretch of time that will exist beyond their pet's death, unable to ground in the present or enjoy the time they have with their pets while their pets are doing well. In this author's experience, introducing rituals during this stage can be an incredibly helpful tool for slowing down and grounding in the present moment. It can also introduce the practice of mindfulness, which holds many benefits for physical and emotional health, especially during times of increased stress. Mindfulness consists of "being fully aware of whatever is happening in the present moment, and can be brought to any situation"; it embodies "cultivating awareness of the mind and body and living in the here and now" (Stahl and Goldstein, 2019, p. 17). For example, when we walk our dog, are we fully present in that activity and that activity alone: feeling the breeze on our face, smelling the neighborhood foliage, hearing the tip-tap of our dog's feet on the pavement, noticing the vibrant or muted colors around us, enjoying observing our dog find joy in sniffing every blade of grass? Or are we running through the ever-present mental to do list, what are we going to make for dinner tonight, the conversation from earlier that is still bothering us, that situation at work that is causing stress? For many people, without active practice, it is the latter. The walk is then over, and we may find that we do not actually remember much of it, as our brain was elsewhere. Clients in anticipatory grief have a finite length of time left with their precious pet, and this can be a beneficial time for reflection on what they would like to share with their pet during this season of life. In these situations, the introduction of mindfulness and ritual can be helpful for creating intentional, meaningful, shared experiences. An important reminder is that rituals do not have to involve big, grand gestures (although you can do that too if you wish). A bucket list does not have to mean driving to the Grand Canyon on an epic road trip. A bucket list can consist of the smallest of rituals: mindful movie nights on the couch, where we put our phones away, make a special human and pet-friendly snack, snuggle up with our coziest blankets next to our pet, and enjoy the snug and warm evening of shared time together. Pre-loss rituals are about honoring the bond, sharing mindful time together, and creating meaningful memories that will bring comfort when our pet is no longer physically with us.

These goals shift when we transition to post-loss rituals. The goals of engaging in post-loss rituals often include maintaining a connection with our lost loved one, allowing for the evolution of how we continue that special bond as it takes new shapes, as well as taking time, space, and meaningful action to honor the life of the lost family member (Wojtkowiak *et al.*, 2021). Additionally, these rituals serve to take care of ourselves and help us mourn and heal through our journey of grief. For many, they can also help make meaning out of the loss, which can be a cathartic component of healing through significant loss. Klass, Silverman, & Nickman (1996) found that the pet families who engaged in rituals considered them "as a form of a continuing bond, whereby the bereaved adapt by developing new memories, feelings, and actions that help maintain a sense of connection to the deceased" (as cited in Cleary *et al.*, 2021).

Case Example One

This author met Juniper and her mom, Miranda, when Juniper was diagnosed with lymphoma. Juniper was a 10-year-old female golden retriever, who was the light of her mom's life. Miranda felt completely shaken, emotional, and overwhelmed by what this diagnosis would mean for Juniper and their little family of two. Juniper's medical oncology team facilitated an introduction between Miranda and this author, an LCSW, in the hope of offering more comprehensive support for Juniper's human. At the beginning of Juniper's cancer treatment, Miranda struggled with anxiety and anticipatory grief. This author began working with Miranda to identify what would be helpful during this time and to create a plan to build in some supportive structure, outlining two categories: self-care grounding rituals to manage anxiety during Juniper's treatment and rituals for shared time with Juniper, to meaningfully engage and make the most of the time they had with one other. Self-care rituals included a short daily guided meditation for anxiety (5 to 10 min) utilizing a free app, twice-weekly yoga practice, journaling, and an evening wind-down comfort ritual that could be used as needed (softest pajama set, hot mug of tea, candle lit, and watching a comfort show – in this case, Parks and Recreation). Shared rituals with Juniper included a daily walk around their neighborhood – ambling along at Juniper's pace, stopping for sniffs whenever Juniper desired – playing fetch in their backyard, lying in the soft grass in the garden and looking up at the stars in the evenings (Juniper liked to lie on her back, tummy up for belly rubs), leisurely drives up mountain roads where Juniper could pop her head out the window, and a whole host of holiday-specific plans that became cherished memories. For Halloween that fall, Juniper dressed up as a fairy princess and helped hand out candy to children. For Thanksgiving, Miranda invited Juniper's puppy friends over, along with their humans, to watch the National Dog Show, replete with a special dog-friendly holiday meal (turkey and mashed pumpkin with whipped cream for dessert). For the Christmas season, Miranda baked home-made themed dog treats, ordered a new ornament with a favorite Juniper photo of the year, and made a small donation in Juniper's name to an animal cancer research fund. Following the loss of Juniper, the knowledge of all the meaningful time and thoughtful activities Miranda shared with Juniper during her last year brought Miranda an immense amount of comfort, even during the heaviest moments of her grief.

A few months later, in the early days of grief and mourning, Miranda shared that she was struggling to remember or focus on anything outside of the painful end. She kept replaying saying goodbye: the sudden decline, the morning she made the decision, and the euthanasia appointment, all playing on a constant loop in her head. In grief counseling, the idea of ritual was revisited and how this tool could be adapted, or how new practices could be established, during this time to support her in her grief. The idea of a guided journaling practice was introduced, with a focus on gratitude and favorite memories. Miranda had already been journaling throughout Juniper's illness, so she was just tweaking an already-existing practice. She began to journal one item each day that she was thankful for related to Juniper or one happy or silly memory. This ritual supported her brain in seeking out the positive, the treasure trove of years of shared experiences, instead of hyper-focusing on the end. As humans can have a tendency toward a negativity bias, practices such as these can be helpful in balancing the scales. Of course, this practice did not erase Miranda's pain or suddenly press a fast-forward button through the worst of the grief. It simply introduced more gratitude, more warm and positive memories, to co-exist alongside the more painful memories. Miranda would sometimes bring her journal to counseling sessions and she would laugh through her tears, recounting tales of Juniper defying odds to make it on the highest kitchen countertop to steal the laid out BBQ, Juniper leaving trails of tennis balls in the unlikeliest of places for Miranda to discover later: in a shoe, in the bathtub, under the leaf of a houseplant. Additional rituals Miranda would engage with in time include setting up a memorial space in her garden for Juniper, with a personalized engraved stone and other markers honoring her in that space she loved so much, so that the seasonal rituals of tending to the garden always created a tug of energy where Miranda felt connected with Juniper. Every Christmas, Miranda would go shopping and deliver a donation of supplies to her local animal shelter, in Juniper's name. Then she would come home, light a candle, and hang Juniper's special ornament on her tree. These rituals helped to create space and air for the depth of Miranda's grief. This gave her an outlet, a way to engage with her grief that was tangible and real. Finally, it allowed her to feel an ongoing and evolving connection with Juniper. Juniper is no longer physically with her, but Miranda honors her continued spirit and presence in her life through these rituals.

Case Example Two

In the following case, Jackson and Emma sought to connect with this author for additional support when their dog, Finn, was diagnosed with a nasal sarcoma at 11 years of age. Finn was the happiest boy, a Labrador (lab) who would come bounding into every appointment, his tail and entire back-end wagging, as he was so excited to see his friends in oncology. His disease progressed faster than expected, despite radiation treatment. When Finn's parents discussed what they wanted to share with Finn before he was gone, hoping to mitigate any potential regrets in the future, one topic kept coming up: the beach. Finn was a quintessential lab; he positively adored water. They had always dreamed of taking him to the beach someday but had never gotten around to it. Jackson and Emma decided that it was time; it was helpful that Finn also loved a good car ride. They packed up and hit the road with Finn, heading to the west coast. When they arrived, they could not stop snapping photos, taking videos, capturing Finn: ecstatic, splashing in the water, swimming, leaping with joy, and running circles in the sand. This family trip, culminating in Finn's first and only coastal beach experience, held the significance and meaning of a sacred ceremony. A celebration of Finn, the carving out of shared family time, a path chosen as Finn neared the end-of-life transition to send him off with joy and love.

Emma and Jackson had time during Finn's illness to start thinking about what they might want to do to honor him following his passing. After Finn died, they decided on three things: writing him a letter, creating a photobook, and eventually embarking on a farewell road trip back to the same beach where they would hold an intimate celebration of life ceremony. There were a few things weighing heavily on their minds, regrets they were holding from how things unfolded during the trajectory of Finn's disease progression. In grief counseling, they were gently encouraged to consider what it might feel like to set that weight down and to share everything weighing on them with Finn. They wrote a letter addressed to Finn, unfurling everything on their minds and in their hearts: their regret, their guilt, the immeasurable depth of their love, and how every decision they made was with his best interest at heart. They poured out what they fervently hoped Finn felt and knew to be true: how much they loved him and how deeply they wanted to do right by him. They combed through digital catalogs of years of photos, selected their favorites for printing, and created a photo album. Jackson wrote detailed captions, capturing what was happening in each photo, while Emma painstakingly organized the order and placement of pictures. This labor of love gifted them a journey down memory lane, bringing to the surface forgotten misadventures, laughs, and treasured memories of years of family exploits. They worked on these projects as they planned ahead for their road trip. Their schedules allowed them to next take time off work and prepare for a weeklong trip about a year after Finn passed. Jackson and Emma returned to the same beach and held a small ceremony, just the two of them, to honor Finn's life. They had a bonfire, read aloud the letter they wrote to Finn, and then burned it, symbolizing letting it go. They also took turns sharing their favorite stories and reading a couple of poems. They ate a peanut butter banana dessert (two of his favorite things) as they watched the flames crackle.

Emma shared that she was initially hesitant to do any of the above. She worried, would people think she was silly or weird for holding a funeral service for a dog? Who does that? After giving herself permission to identify and then carry through with the plans she felt in her heart were what she needed, regardless of societal expectations, she felt immense relief and liberation from those constraints. She realized if it worked for her and it felt meaningful and healing, what did it matter if a colleague or family member may think it's a little over the top or different? Humans are such a diverse species; how could one possibly expect every person to need or want the same things, especially in grief? If it is true and right for you, that is all it needs to be. Giving yourself permission to explore and personalize your rituals, your self-care, and what you need through a season of caregiving or season of grief, is an incredibly kind and radical act of self-compassion.

Discussion

This author has had the honor of working with many pet families and remains in awe of their resilience and creativity. One family organized a final weekend on the boat at the lake, their dog's favorite place where she could feel the wind and spray on her face one more time; another went on a final hike on their favorite usual route with his dog strapped to his back and a playlist going of their favorite tunes (the playlist was 100% Led Zeppelin). One family gave each of their two children the opportunity to choose a bucket list party to help them celebrate and say goodbye to their dog, leading up to euthanasia. One chose a pancake party with whipped cream, and one chose a hamburger party, complete with hamburger party hats. One woman, whose cat's favorite thing in the world was being a complete menace at Christmas, climbing and playing all over the tree, put up a Christmas tree in June, so her cat could enjoy a final cherished play. Another cat parent's go-to ritual was getting their cat out in a stroller to chase sun patches, as lying in sunny spots was always his favorite activity. One person chose to have his priest perform a blessing ritual for his dog prior to proceeding with euthanasia. Another family requested time, space, and privacy to perform a bathing ritual of the body after their pet died, in line with Hindu tradition. Working alongside the veterinary team, the social worker made sure the family had everything they needed to perform this sacred ritual, to make space for and honor their cultural and religious values during this time of loss. This author has helped clients arrange for special, significant items to be cremated alongside their pet's body, items carefully chosen in line with the client's spiritual belief system, to help the pet's spirit through the next phase of its journey. Some families put together elaborate goodbye picnics enjoyed outside, celebration of life events while their animal was still alive with a giant ice cream cake and all the pet's favorite humans coming together to share time, final meals of steak and potatoes or chicken nuggets and ice cream. It feels important to acknowledge that not every family gets the luxury of a thoughtful, time-rich goodbye, and of course, not every animal is still interested in food or more taxing activity closer to the end. There are a myriad of ways to honor and share time, to engage with rituals, across the diversity of experiences and limitations. And when one is fortunate enough to have some time with which to get creative, it is this author's sincere hope that people are not afraid to think outside the box.

Conclusion

Navigating a terminal illness or decline due to advanced age with one's pet can be an incredibly challenging and emotionally exhausting experience. Those working in the veterinary field with families approaching end-of-life care for their animals hold an important responsibility to educate and prepare families on how to best support their pet and themselves through their care journey. Minimizing potential regrets, making the most out of the time they have left, sharing meaningful, connected moments with their beloved animal, and engaging in healthy grief processing following a loss are all areas in which we can offer more comprehensive support by encouraging families to consider building in mindful, thoughtfully curated rituals into their routines. These rituals can help ground us in the present moment, share special time with our animals while they are still with us, and help us honor our grief once they have passed. The field of human–animal bond research would benefit from additional study focused on best practices for anticipatory grief support for pet families and the effects of rituals as assigned interventions for grief support. Advancing our understanding of these topics will allow us to better care for the caregiver, a crucial component of holistic support for the entire family system – pet and human.

Conflict of Interest

The author has no conflicts of interest to declare.

Funding

The author has no funders to declare.

Ethics Statement

The author confirms that the research met any required ethical guidelines, including adherence to the legal requirements of the study country

Author Contributions

The author is solely responsible for the research, writing, and finalization of this work.

Data Availability

No data applicable.

References

Castle, J. and Phillips, W.L. (2003). Grief rituals: Aspects that facilitate adjustment to bereavement. *Journal of Loss and Trauma* 8(1), 41–71. DOI: 10.1080/15325020305876.

Cleary, M., West, S., Thapa, D.K., Westman, M., Vesk, K. *et al*. (2021) Grieving the loss of a pet: A qualitative systematic review. *Death Studies* 46(9), 2167–2178. DOI: 10.1080/07481187.2021.1901799.

Klass, D., Silverman, P.R. and Nickman, S.L. (1996). *Continuing Bonds: New Understandings of Grief*. Routledge, New York, NY. https://doi.org/10.4324/9781315800790

Laing, M. and Maylea, C. (2018) They burn brightly, but only for a short time": The role of social workers in companion animal grief and loss. *Anthrozoös* 31(2), 221–232. DOI: 10.1080/08927936.2018.1434062.

Rando, T.A. (1985). *Bereavement, Dying, and Death: Clinical Interventions for Caregivers*. Research Press,Champaign, IL.

Romanoff, B.D. and Terenzio, M. (1998) Rituals and the grieving process. *Death Studies* 22(8), 697–711.

Sas, C. and Coman, A. (2016) Designing personal grief rituals: An analysis of symbolic objects and actions. *Death Studies* 40(9), 558–569. DOI: 10.1080/07481187.2016.1188868.

Stahl, B. and Goldstein, E. (2019) A mindfulness-based stress reduction workbook.

Wojtkowiak, J., Lind, J. and Smid, G.E. (2021) Ritual in therapy for prolonged grief: A scoping review of ritual elements in evidence-informed grief interventions. *Frontiers in Psychiatry* 11, 623835. DOI: 10.3389/fpsyt.2020.623835.

Wolfelt, A.D. (2004) *When Your Pet Dies: A Guide to Mourning, Remembering, and Healing*. Companion Press, Fort Collins, CO.

15 Supporting Clients Through Loss: A Qualitative Review of Current Practices of Accredited Assistance Dog Organizations

Dena DeSantis[1]* and Janet Hoy Gerlach[2]

[1]The University of Alabama, Tuscaloosa, AL, USA; [2]Director of Veterinary Social Work, Open Door Veterinary Collective, Grand Rapids, OH, USA

Abstract

This qualitative study aims to empirically identify, and document current practices employed by United States-based assistance dog organizations accredited by Assistance Dogs International (N = 21) to support clients in preparing for and coping with the loss of their assistance dogs. The target population was identified using the Assistance Dogs International Membership List. Representatives from each organization were invited to participate in semi-structured interviews. The interview protocol was developed based on extant literature on the end of the partner-assistance dog relationship, with additional input from professionals affiliated with the Association of Pet Loss and Bereavement, assistance dog advocacy, and individual assistance dog partners who had experienced such a loss. A thematic analysis of the interviews was conducted to identify recurring themes and practices. The findings demonstrate that assistance dog organizations offer a range of support strategies for clients grieving the loss of their dogs, from low-cost, informal methods to more structured, high-cost programs. These strategies align with the Dual Process Model and Continuing Bonds Theory, addressing both emotional needs and ongoing connections to the dog. Strong relationships with assistance dog organizations were identified as key protective factors in mitigating grief. Effective strategies to encourage emotional healing include fostering community connections, preparing clients for the eventual loss, and facilitating opportunities to maintain a meaningful connection with the dog after its passing or retirement. By helping clients through this difficult transition, assistance dog organizations can promote healthier grief processing and support clients in adjusting to the loss of a dog that played such a vital role in their lives.

Keywords: assistance dog, service dog, guide dog, grief, loss, death, retirement, bereavement

Introduction

The World Health Organization estimates that 1 in 6 people globally live with a disability (World Health Organization, 2020). In the United States, up to 500,000 individuals partner with assistance dogs to enhance their independence (Trainer, 2016). Assistance Dogs International (ADI) reports that in 2022, 206 accredited organizations worldwide supported over 28,000 active teams with a primary presence in North America, Europe, and Oceania (Assistance Dogs International, n.d.-a). International research consistently shows that assistance dogs enhance

*Corresponding author: ddesantis@crimson.ua.edu

their partners' self-confidence, social participation, and activity levels (Audrestch *et al.*, 2015; Rodriguez *et al.*, 2020; Currin-McCulloch *et al.*, 2021; Gibson *et al.*, 2022; Singleton, 2023). For example, a study in the United Kingdom found that 73% of partners reported making new friends since being partnered with their assistance and 92% experienced increased community inclusion (Lane *et al.*, 1998). Relatedly, a study by South African researchers described blind individuals' partnerships with guide dogs as having a "life-altering effect" on the partner (Wiggett-Barnard and Steel, 2008). The growing body of evidence about the impact of assistance dogs has helped support the global enactment of laws granting public access rights to assistance dog teams (Assistance Dogs International, n.d.-b).

Canadian researchers Kwong and Bartholomew (2011) found the relationship between partners and assistance dogs to be deeply interdependent, cultivated through time spent together fulfilling functional tasks and fostering social connections. Assistance dogs are often considered integral family members, providing both functional and emotional support (Ng and Fine, 2019a; Yamamoto and Hart, 2019; Singleton, 2023). The loss of this bond can lead to complex disenfranchised grief, which is often unrecognized by society (Packman *et al.*, 2011; Spain *et al.*, 2019). The Dual Process Model and Continuing Bonds Theory offer valuable insights into how individuals navigate this loss, highlighting the need for tailored support to help assistance dog partners process and adopt (Klass *et al.*, 1996; Stroebe and Schut, 1999).

The global assistance dog industry lacks universal guidelines to prepare clients for or support them through the eventual loss of their assistance dogs. Existing scholarship on how individual organizations address this need is sparse (Miller, 2019; Yamamoto and Hart, 2019; Currin-McCulloch *et al.*, 2021; Kogan *et al.*, 2021; Gibson *et al.*, 2022). Further research into the preparatory practices and supports offered by assistance dog organizations is necessary to identify existing practices and gaps in support services. Gaining this understanding is essential to better meet the needs of assistance dog partners coping with the loss of their dogs.

Grief support for assistance dog partners: A review of current literature

Across the world, recent investigations conducted into the impact of death or retirement of the assistance dog on the human partner found that grief support is crucial and that assistance dog organizations are uniquely positioned to offer such services (Nicholson *et al.*, 1995; Miller, 2019; Yamamoto and Hart, 2019; Currin-McCulloch *et al.*, 2021; Kogan *et al.*, 2021; Gibson *et al.*, 2022). Miller (2019) and Yamamoto and Hart (2019) discussed the importance of the relationship between the partner and the assistance dog organization citing that the strength of the relationship can be a mediating factor in the partner accessing available support from the organization, such as seeking guidance, consultation, networking with other assistance dog partners who have experienced loss, or identifying external resources (e.g., professional counseling). Additionally, Miller (2019) found that expressions of support through phone calls, e-mails, in-person follow-up visits, sending condolence cards, and working collaboratively with partners to explore interest and readiness for a successor dog were grief support strategies that could be used by assistance dog organizations to benefit clients.

Currin-McCulloch *et al.*'s (2021) research detailed how one assistance dog organization actively prepares assistance dog partners for the eventual death or retirement of their assistance dog: first through psychoeducation and later through discussions on retirement planning and preparing for end-of-life decision making. Similar strategies for educating clients on these processes as well as sharing expectations for the unique experiences of grief following the loss of the assistance dog relationship were also identified as key responsibilities of assistance dog organizations by Miller (2019), Yamamoto and Hart (2019), Kogan *et al.* (2021), and Gibson *et al.* (2022). Further, the development of psychoeducational materials that accurately portrayed pre-loss and bereavement using personal stories and lived experiences was suggested to normalize and validate the partner's grief experience (Kogan *et al.*, 2021).

Building on the findings of Currin-McCulloch *et al.* (2021), researchers and scholars discussed the availability of proactive supports for partners before, during, and after the loss of an assistance dog as critical resources for assistance dog organizations to supply to bereaved partners (Miller, 2019; Yamamoto and Hart, 2019; Kogan *et al.*, 2021; Gibson *et al.*, 2022). Gibson *et al.*'s (2022) qualitative research with Canadian military veterans uncovered the importance of assistance dog organizations having conversations with partners about how to develop and express continuing bonds with their assistance dogs, including ways to memorialize the assistance dogs and commemorate their relationship. Kogan *et al.* (2021) found similar themes around supporting the development of continuing bonds and suggested assistance dog organizations provide opportunities for bereaved assistance dog partners to engage in narrative constructivist therapy, directed journaling activities, and create epitaphs or life imprints detailing the significance of their relationship with their assistance dogs.

While the literature identifies and suggests various strategies for providing grief support to bereaved assistance dog partners (Miller, 2019; Yamamoto and Hart, 2019; Currin-McCulloch *et al.*, 2021; Kogan *et al.*, 2021; Gibson *et al.*, 2022), there is no systematic knowledge about current practices employed by assistance dog organizations and anecdotal evidence reveals a significant gap in the support offered. Although ADI accreditation standards require organizations to extend support to the assistance dog team throughout the lifetime of the working relationship, there is currently no language in the accreditation standards around the provision of grief support (Assistance Dogs International, n.d.-c). Thus, how individual organizations understand and operationalize the 'lifetime support' standard varies significantly across organizations.

Informal conversations with individuals who have been paired with assistance dogs through multiple assistance dog organizations indicate that preparation and support for the death or retirement of an assistance dog are not uniformly or consistently provided. Human partners discussed their perceptions of feeling unprepared for the loss of their assistance dog and needing additional support to buttress the grief they experienced at the end of their relationship with their assistance dog. The variability in the organizational provision and partner perception of grief support services highlights the need to explore how ADI-accredited assistance dog organizations provide grief support to bereaved clients. The current lack of specific standards from ADI regarding grief and loss further underscores the importance of identifying current practices and establishing a knowledge base that enables organizations to enhance their support for clients grieving the loss of their assistance dogs. This research aims to systematically explore and record current practices used by assistance dog organizations accredited by Assistance Dogs International to help clients navigate the preparation for and adjustment to the loss of their assistance dog.

Methods

Qualitative research is appropriate for this study as it allows for an in-depth exploration of the best practices used by assistance dog organizations to support clients through grief and loss, providing insight into organizational strategies, policies, and approaches that may not be captured through quantitative methods (Rubin and Rubin, 2012; Tracy, 2019).

The researchers acknowledge their positionality in this study. One researcher has personally witnessed the profound impact of assistance dog loss through friends who experienced this grief, feeling that the support offered by their organizations did not meet their needs. This firsthand exposure underscored the importance of exploring how organizations can better assist clients through this difficult transition. The other researcher brings extensive knowledge and a well-established publication record in the human–animal bond space, providing a strong foundation for examining practices in grief support within assistance dog organizations. Together, their perspectives inform a balanced and insightful approach to this study.

Study sample

Inclusionary criteria for this study required that assistance dog organizations (1) are based in the United States, (2) have been in operation for more than 10 years, and (3) have earned accreditation by ADI. As a result of achieving ADI-accredited status, organizations have recognized credibility in the assistance dog industry and are considered to operate under gold-standard benchmarks for all aspects of service delivery. ADI accreditation standards do not mandate a fixed retirement age for assistance dogs (Assistance Dogs International, n.d.-b). However, recent scholarship by renowned researchers Ng and Fine (2019a) cited an 8-year average working life for an assistance dog, which served as a useful guideline for establishing the minimum organizational life inclusion criteria benchmark for this study.

A review of the ADI website identified 81 accredited assistance dog organizations in the United States (Assistance Dogs International, n.d.-d). The ADI-accredited member list was used to develop a target population of participant organizations, after which purposive sampling was used to recruit representatives from the target population of assistance dog organizations. Recruitment entailed a multi-pronged approach. An e-mail introducing the study was sent to each organization in the target population along with a flyer describing the study. The flyer encouraged participation by inviting organizations to share their expertise and strategies for supporting clients. Concurrently, the Principal Investigator (PI) conducted a member search on the professional networking platform LinkedIn to identify organizational employees who were active on this platform and requested a professional connection. When the professional connection request was accepted, the PI contacted the organizational representative through the LinkedIn platform, introducing the study and sharing the flyer describing the study. Two attempts at follow-up contact were made either through e-mail or LinkedIn if no response was received from the organizational representative within 3–6 weeks of the prior outreach attempt. Interested representatives from organizations within the target population ("participants"), utilized a link contained on the flyer to complete a brief Qualtrics survey which captured demographic information, verified inclusionary criteria, and provided informed consent for participation in the study. After completing these steps, the participant was able to schedule an interview with the PI through the Calendly scheduling platform.

Representatives from 21 assistance dog organizations consented to participate in semi-structured interviews discussing how that individual assistance dog organization supports clients around assistance dog loss. A total of 20 organizations were represented by one individual and one organization was represented by two individuals. Participating organizations varied in size, ranging from organizations placing fewer than a dozen assistance dogs per year to organizations placing over 300 assistance dogs per year. The length of organizational life ranged from 11 to 82 years with an average of 27.04 years (Table 15.1). Participating organizations predominantly serve adults with a variety of disabling conditions such as vision loss, hearing loss, post-traumatic stress disorder, seizure disorder, and autism. Participants and organizations received no incentive for their participation in this study, which was approved by the University of Alabama Institutional Review Board #24-03-7425.

Data collection

Representatives from assistance dog organizations who consented to participate in a recorded, semi-structured, technology-mediated

Table 15.1. Description of organizational characteristics.

Statistic	Number of assistance dogs placed annually	Length of organizational life (Years)
Mean	43.14	27.048
Median	12	20
Mode	6	16
Standard deviation	83.289	17.122
Standard deviation of the mean	18.175	3.736
Range	4–340	11–82

interview did so with the PI between May and September 2024. Although participants had the option to decline recording, no participant elected to do so. Interviews lasting between 30 and 90 min were conducted and recorded using Zoom, a video conferencing software platform. The closed captioning feature was enabled to aid in interview transcription. The PI reviewed the interview transcripts to ensure accuracy and manually anonymized the transcripts by redacting identifying information during the verification process.

The semi-structured interview protocol was formulated based on the extant literature related to the end of a partner's relationship with their assistance dog (Ng and Fine, 2019b; Currin-McCulloch *et al.*, 2021; Kogan *et al.*, 2021; Bussolari *et al.*, 2022; Gibson *et al.*, 2022). In addition, questions were also guided by personal communication with professionals affiliated with the Association for Pet Loss and Bereavement and a nationally renowned expert specializing in assistance dog advocacy and education, as well as individual partners who lost their assistance dog to death or retired their assistance dog. The 18-question interview protocol gathered background and demographic information about the participants and organizations, along with an in-depth overview of clients' bereavement experiences and the organization's response to their needs.

Data analysis

Inductive thematic analysis of interview transcripts was completed on an ongoing basis throughout the interview process to identify common themes, patterns, similarities, and differences in the data set and facilitated an in-depth accounting of how assistance dog organizations help prepare clients for and support clients through the loss of their assistance dog (Braun and Clarke, 2012). This research employed a multi-case study approach, using a blend of deductive codes based on the Dual Process Model and Continuing Bonds Theory, as these conceptual frameworks are consistently found in scholarly literature addressing assistance dog loss (Currin-McCulloch *et al.*, 2021; Kogan *et al.*, 2021; Gibson *et al.*, 2022), as well as inductive codes that emerged directly from the data. The PI reviewed and coded the transcripts to conduct a primary thematic analysis. This process involved sorting line-by-line codes into broader categories, followed by the development of high-level codes and prominent themes. A second-level review of the data, codes, and themes was then conducted by the collaborating researcher to further enhance the trustworthiness and validity of the analysis and ensure that a comprehensive review of the data was completed (Tracy, 2019). The authors held debriefing sessions to discuss and align emerging themes and confirm data saturation. Inter-coder reliability was enhanced by reaching consensus on research objectives, data collection methods, coding procedures, and interpretations of the data (Rubin and Rubin, 2012; Tracy, 2019).

After agreeing upon themes and findings, the results were shared with interview participants via e-mail for member checking. Member checking, a process by which the data results are verified as accurate by participants, has been shown to enhance the credibility of research findings (Birt *et al.*, 2016) by placing participants in the role of experts of their lived experiences (Knapik, 2006). Member checking also increases the likelihood that research findings accurately represent participants' perspectives (Knapik, 2006; McKim, 2023) and objectively mirror their participation and experience (Rubin and Rubin, 2012; Tracy, 2019).

Results

Study participants universally acknowledged the critical need to support clients through the loss of their assistance dog, whether the loss was due to the dog's death or retirement. Participants reported that their organizations employ a wide range of approaches, offering both formal and informal support systems to assist grieving clients.

The strategies implemented vary significantly in terms of complexity and resource allocation, from low-cost interventions requiring a modest investment of staff time to more structured programs that entail substantial financial investment and human capital. This spectrum of support reflects each organization's capacity to balance available resources with the essential task of addressing clients' emotional and practical needs during a period of profound transition following the death or retirement of their assistance dogs. Organizational theory suggests that an organization's size, resources, and structure play a key role in shaping its ability to implement and sustain such support services (Cappellaro *et al.*, 2023), which is evident in the varied approaches observed across organizations in this study.

Participants' responses reflected the Dual Process Model in their approach to offering ongoing support tailored to each client's unique grief needs, balancing mourning with adaptation. Similarly, the Continuing Bonds Theory was evident in strategies that helped clients honor their bond with their assistance dog, such as retaining the dog's equipment as a tangible connection to their shared relationship.

Current practices offered by organizations

The current practices for grief support identified by study participants from ADI-accredited assistance dog organizations encompass a range of cost points, providing flexible options for organizations with varying financial resources. Acknowledging that these current practices require human capital, which must be balanced with other responsibilities, these practices accentuate the importance of understanding and addressing clients' individual emotional needs.

By incorporating multiple interventions such as direct staff involvement, peer support, education, and personalized care, organizations help clients navigate the emotionally complex process of losing their assistance dog. Additionally, by giving consideration to retirement planning, the potential for successor dogs, and the grieving process, organizations ensure clients feel supported every step of the way during this challenging transition.

Low-cost options for client support

To support clients facing the loss of their assistance dog, organizations can provide a variety of low-cost resources and guidance (Table 15.2). The most widely discussed low-cost option for client support identified by participants was placing an intention focus on building a trusting relationship with and between clients. Participants consistently pointed to these relationships as crucial components of fostering open communication, enabling individuals to feel safe sharing their experiences and needs and organizations to respond to those needs.

Participants also stressed the importance of psychoeducation on topics such as retirement, successor dogs, anticipatory grief, and disenfranchised grief can be shared via podcasts, newsletters, or virtual seminars, allowing clients to prepare for their dogs' life cycle in a supportive and informative way. During key interactions such as the application and training process, annual visits, or recertifications, organizations can introduce clients to these concepts and provide practical information on retirement and the signs of aging in senior dogs.

For ongoing support, some organizations offer 24/7 access to staff as well as regular check-ins by phone, text, or virtual meetings, adjusting frequency based on each client's needs. Regular communication with clients, including acknowledgment of the loss in addition to check-ins and empathetic conversations, helps clients navigate their grief. One participant explained that within their organization, the staff makes a directed outreach to the client to offer support, "We know this just happened and that there's going to be a period of adjustment, but please know that we are here and available to help, available to provide resources."

For clients with dogs facing terminal illnesses, assistance provided by the organization can include consultations with the organization's veterinarian to translate medical terminology and provide guidance during end-of-life care and euthanasia discussions. Following the passing of an assistance dog, the organization can reach out with condolences, provide a "Certificate of Service," share a tribute on social media (with permission), or invite clients to campus to spend time with training puppies, creating a compassionate environment that honors both grief and healing.

Organizations can also encourage clients to connect with their own support networks,

Table 15.2. Low-cost current practices.

Support strategies	Description	Timing/format
Psychoeducation	Offers key topics on grief, retirement, and successor dogs.	Newsletter, podcast, or seminar
• Retirement • Successor dogs • Grief (normalizing, anticipatory, disenfranchised)	Overview of planning for retirement. Discussing the decision and process of applying for a successor dog. Educating on grief stages, emphasizing that all grief is valid.	Newsletter, seminar Application process, training Training, annual recertification
Application process support	Overview of life cycle expectations for assistance dog partnership.	During application process
Training stage support	Lectures and articles that introduce retirement planning, senior dog care.	Initial training
Annual recertification process for assistance dog teams	Open conversations on retirement and provide video on senior dog care and end-of-life planning.	Annual recertification
Individual conversations	Personal discussions with staff on retirement, euthanasia, pet insurance.	As needed, often at retirement
Resource page	One-page resource sheet with grief support, euthanasia, and cremation/ burial options.	Provided to all clients
Staff support	Staff available via check-ins or 24/7 support for certain clients.	Phone, text, email, virtual meetings
Encouraging use of the client's personal network	Encourages connection with family, friends, or providers.	Ongoing
Peer support	One-on-one mentor support, peer-led groups, and private social media groups for alumni.	Ongoing, virtual or in-person
Continuing bonds activities	Suggests commemorative activities for ongoing connection with retired or deceased dogs.	In-person and virtual opportunities
Support during illness	Offers guidance with canine health and decision-making support.	As needed
End-of-life support	Staff attendance and guidance at vet or euthanasia appointments.	Euthanasia appointment, if possible
Post-loss support	Acknowledgment card, campus visit, puppy therapy session.	Post-passing
Graduation/Alumni events	Tribute opportunities, such as video collages or remembrance moments for clients' dogs.	Graduations, retreats, reunions
Successor dog training support	Retraining events offer tribute to retired or deceased dogs.	During retraining

peer mentors, or alumni groups for shared experiences and mutual support. Participants frequently spoke of the particular importance of peer-to-peer support, as peers who have experienced the loss of an assistance dog can offer a unique level of understanding that professionals or friends may not. This peer support is especially vital because the grief associated with losing an assistance dog is often disenfranchised, meaning that it may not be recognized or understood by those unfamiliar with the bond between an assistance dog and its partner.

Moderate-cost options for client support

Current practices within the moderate cost price range emphasize personalized remembrance efforts that assistance dog organizations provide to help clients honor their relationships with their assistance dogs (Table 15.3). Mementos such as framed photos, care packages, and memorial gifts serve as tangible acknowledgments of the client's loss, allowing them to maintain continuing bonds with their assistance dogs as part of a healthy grieving process. These personalized items enable clients to commemorate their dogs in meaningful ways. One participant illustrated this approach, stating, "We always send something. That's the immediate, 'This has happened; we're acknowledging it.'" Additionally, educational events like "lunch and learns," which include a light meal, support clients by proactively addressing topics such as retirement planning and grief, equipping them with the knowledge to better navigate these experiences. Virtual memory walls on an organization's website provide a platform for community members to extend their support and condolences, while some organizations also offer mental health resources for more structured grieving opportunities. This resource can be particularly impactful when the mental health professional also has lived experience with assistance dog loss, creating a unique and valuable perspective that can resonate deeply with clients. One participant, who is also an assistance dog partner, explained that having an experienced peer as a resource is helpful for clients. "They appreciate being able to have a conversation with me, who's a fellow handler, who's been through the process."

High-cost options for client support

Assistance dog organizations with greater financial resources often invest in long-term commemorative initiatives and memorialization, in addition to traveling to clients to provide support and offering monetary assistance for veterinary bills and final expenses (Table 15.4). These strategies include creating physical spaces for reflection or hosting remembrance events where clients can gather as a community to honor their deceased or retired dogs. Permanent memorials, such as plaques or engraved pavers, serve as enduring symbols of the bond between

Table 15.3. Moderate-cost current practices.

Support type	Description	Suggestions
Send gift or memento	Send a thoughtful gift to commemorate the client's relationship with their retired or deceased assistance dog.	• Shadowbox with assistance dog memorabilia • Chocolates • Framed photo of the assistance dog team • Windchimes • Flowers • Individualize care package
Host lunch and learn	Provide an educational gathering to discuss relevant topics related to assistance dog partnerships.	Topics: • Normalization of grief • Retirement planning
Construct virtual memory wall	Create a dedicated page on the organization's website as a virtual memory wall for clients to honor their assistance dogs.	• Client photos can be included • Clients can write an epitaph about their assistance dog
Offer structured counseling or therapeutic support	Provide additional support with a mental health staff person, if available, for clients needing more structured grief support.	• Counseling sessions • Therapeutic support tailored to the client's grieving process

Table 15.4. High-cost current practices.

Support type	Description	Suggestions
Campus reflection space	Create a designated quiet space on campus for clients to reflect or meditate in memory of their dogs.	• Reflection or meditation area on campus
Annual remembrance event	Host an annual event to honor and remember retired or deceased assistance dogs and handlers.	• Event designed specifically for remembrance, allowing clients to gather and share memories
Continuing bonds memento on campus	Install a dedicated memento on campus to commemorate each team.	• Photos of teams • Personalized bricks, pavers, or plaques
In-person support for clients	Provide on-site support to clients in need, regardless of their geographic location.	• Staff or representatives available for in-person support as needed
Organizational funding for veterinary and final arrangements	Financial support for veterinary care or final arrangements related to the assistance dog's passing.	• Funding options for veterinary expenses • Coverage of final arrangements such as cremation or burial

the client and assistance dog, further reinforcing the principles of continuing bonds by allowing clients to maintain a sense of connection to their dogs even after their passing. Additionally, financial support for veterinary care and end-of-life arrangements can alleviate the practical burdens clients face, providing a more holistic approach to supporting them through grief.

Discussion

This research represents the first qualitative study examining how accredited assistance dog organizations support bereaved clients following the loss of their assistance dogs. The study's findings reflect an overall organizational awareness of the profound impact that the loss of an assistance dog has on clients and the need to meaningfully support grieving individuals. Each organization operationalizes this support differently based on several factors, including the perceived client need, availability of staff resources, and funding to support grief programming. Organizations resoundingly stressed the importance of the relationship between the partner and the assistance dog organization, citing that the strength of this relationship can be a moderating factor in the partner accessing available support from the organization, such as seeking guidance, consultation, networking with other assistance dog partners who have experienced loss, or availing themselves of external resources (e.g., professional counseling). This finding aligns with Yamamoto and Hart's (2019) assertion that the relationship between the organization and the client can positively impact the client's experience of grief. Additionally, organizations reported that strong relationships with clients facilitated individualized expressions of support, such as phone calls, emails, in-person follow-up visits, sending condolence cards, and collaborating with partners to assess interest in and readiness for a successor dog. This is consistent with Miller's (2019) findings, which emphasize the importance of personalized support in enhancing clients' emotional well-being during the grieving process.

While participants noted that many relationship-driven supports were implemented informally, an analysis of the data also revealed the existence of formalized proactive supports within organizations. Some organizations reported conducting structured psychoeducational activities focused on retirement planning and end-of-life decision making during the application phase of acquiring an assistance dog, whereas others chose to address these sensitive topics later in the team's working relationship. Regardless of the timeline, each organization agreed that it was a fundamental responsibility to educate clients about these processes and communicate expectations regarding the unique experiences of grief following the loss of an assistance dog. This approach reflects the principles of the Dual Process Model, which stresses the importance of addressing both loss and restoration-oriented aspects of grief, consistent with recent research (Miller, 2019; Yamamoto and Hart, 2019; Currin-McCulloch *et al.*, 2021; Kogan *et al.*, 2021; Gibson *et al.*, 2022). Many organizations identified that they support clients by formally and informally helping them develop and express continuing bonds with their assistance dogs. Examples of formal supports mentioned by participants included providing clients with a memento of their relationship with the assistance dog or encouraging them to create a "legacy piece," a written tribute to their assistance dog reflecting on the significance of their relationship, for posting on social media or the organization's website. Participants also described how they engaged clients in informal conversations that provided opportunities to exercise continuing bonds with their assistance dogs by commemorating their relationships. These discussions were encouraged as a means to facilitate emotional expression and remembrance, while also providing an opportunity for organizations to educate clients about and/or suggest other means of developing continuing bonds and normalizing their grief experience, approaches consistent with the grief support strategies suggested by Kogan *et al.* (2021) and Gibson *et al.* (2022).

This research underscores the essential role of assistance dog organizations in helping clients manage grief through a multifaceted approach that includes acknowledging the centrality of the loss, fostering supportive relationships with and among clients, community-building, and proactive planning for both dog retirement and successor partnerships. Recognizing a client's loss plays a key role in the bereavement process by validating their grief and providing a supportive environment that promotes emotional healing. Strong relationships between organizations and clients enable clients to access a range of grief support resources from informal conversations to formal programs that offer emotional support and continuity in the bond shared with their assistance dogs. Community-building efforts, such as alumni networks, in-person events, and virtual meetings, provide clients with peer support that validates shared experiences and offers an additional layer of encouragement during challenging times. Additionally, the identified practices in proactive retirement and successor planning help prepare clients for their assistance dog's end-of-life stage, furthering a sense of readiness and control. Equally important is recognizing that the bond between the client and their dog holds significant emotional value, not just functional tasks, and supporting this connection while encouraging clients to consider their own well-being and future functioning is essential.

Organizational factors, such as length of time in operation, size, and staff expertise, affect the scope of available grief support, with larger and/or longer-established organizations generally offering more structured programs. However, even smaller organizations with fewer resources aim to provide meaningful support by implementing personalized and adaptable services. The findings of this study provide a comprehensive body of knowledge that organizations can leverage to enhance their services for grieving clients. By engaging in meaningful dialogue and promoting program adaptation, organizations can effectively tailor their grief support strategies to most effectively address the unique needs of their clients.

Strengths

This is the first known research study to focus on how assistance dog organizations support clients through the death or retirement of their assistance dog. The findings of this study illuminate available practices to support bereaved clients that are taking place within assistance dog organizations of varying sizes located in the United States accredited by Assistance Dogs International (ADI). This knowledge can facilitate conversations that allow enhanced services to be offered to grieving clients across the assistance dog industry at all levels. Many of the practices identified through this research have the potential for practical implementation by assistance dog organizations with minimal financial costs outside the allocation of staff time, which is a significant, valuable, and limited resource.

Limitations

This study captured information from representatives of a portion of assistance dog organizations accredited by ADI that voluntarily agreed to participate in semi-structured interviews. These interviews focused on how the organization supports clients through the loss of their relationship with their assistance dogs. The study participants reflect a small sample of assistance dog organizations with the resources to pursue accreditation through ADI. Organizational accreditation through ADI was selected as an inclusionary criterion due to the required adherence to rigorous standards that are the global benchmark of excellence within the assistance dog industry. Organizations that have chosen not to pursue or have not yet earned accreditation through ADI were not eligible for inclusion in this study. Such organizations may also provide support to clients around the loss of their assistance dogs. The use of a convenience sample of participants who consented to an interview may skew the findings of this study as the findings may not adequately represent the broader population, which can affect the generalizability of the results. Representatives from eligible organizations that do not offer grief support to clients may have declined to be interviewed.

Another limitation of the study is that it primarily reports the perceived impact of loss from the perspective of individuals working with the organization, rather than those who have directly experienced the loss. Few participants had lived experience as assistance dog partners who have navigated the grief process. This absence of lived experience raises a key question about who is best equipped to describe the grief of clients. While participants shared narrative accounts of how clients expressed the centrality of their loss to the organization, the perspective remains filtered through those working with the clients.

An additional limitation of this study is the absence of data on demographic diversity within each organization's client base, such as race, age, gender, socio-economic status, and geographic location. While represented organizations serve clients throughout the United States, the study did not address how demographic factors may shape clients' perceived needs and the grief support services offered. This lack of specificity may limit insights into how diverse client backgrounds influence the support provided by assistance dog organizations.

Directions for future research

Avenues for future research into the impact of assistance dog loss are limitless. Future studies could expand the target population to include non-ADI-accredited organizations to further explore the full range of supports and programming available to aid clients who are experiencing the loss of their assistance dogs. Another way to expand upon this study would be to engage international assistance dog organizations to discuss how grieving clients are supported by their organization with attention to the impact of cultural and societal norms. Understanding that different cultures may hold varying perspectives on the role and significance of assistance dogs and the grief around the loss of this pivotal relationship is essential in providing culturally sensitive support, as these views can shape not only the scope of available support but also how individuals perceive the benefits and acceptance of such services.

Aside from novel considerations of how the greater assistance dog industry is impacted by grief and loss and the end of the relationship, there are myriad opportunities for research to explore other facets of the assistance dog community. Scholarship contributing to a greater understanding of the impact of assistance dogs on their human partners may include case studies that allow for in-depth consideration of the benefits and drawbacks of having an assistance dog partner, societal attitudes related to the use of assistance dogs, and exploration into partners' lived experience regarding the loss of their assistance dog. Future studies may also address veterinary professionals' training and experiences in working with assistance dogs and their human partners. Future research may also build upon the seminal work taking place at the University of Arizona, where the O'Haire lab continues to investigate different aspects of how assistance dogs are improving the lives of veterans and their families as well as the work of independent researchers such as Dr. Lori Kogan, who has spearheaded multiple qualitative and quantitative studies on how human partners are impacted by the retirement or death of their assistance dogs.

Future research into the assistance dog industry can provide invaluable data that will drive service provision and could meaningfully contribute to decreasing disparities between people requiring an assistance dog to mitigate a disability and other facets of the population.

Conclusions and Implications

The findings of this study illuminate the multifaceted impact of assistance dog loss, addressing practical, ethical, cultural, and economic dimensions. Practically, the research informs assistance dog organizations about innovative programs employed by others in the field, providing avenues to adapt or replicate successful models. This exchange of information encourages organizations to brainstorm new strategies, thereby enhancing existing services and ultimately improving their capacity to meet the unique needs of clients. Ethically, the study emphasizes the necessity of supporting individuals with disabilities, a marginalized community that heavily relies on assistance dogs. By minimizing the negative impacts of grief associated with the loss of these vital relationships, assistance dog organizations can promote inclusivity and equity within the industry.

Culturally, the findings foster meaningful dialogue among assistance dog organizations, encouraging the sharing of current practices to collaboratively enhance the quality of care provided to clients. This collective effort cultivates a culture of continuous improvement, ensuring organizations remain responsive to the evolving needs of those they serve. Economically, this study underscores the importance of strategic resource allocation to enhance grief support services. By investing in these areas, organizations can optimize compassionate care and improve client outcomes. Furthermore, the findings have significant implications for social work and ancillary professionals who support individuals with disabilities. The study equips practitioners with insights to tailor interventions, develop effective support systems, and create evidence-based programs by identifying current practices for assisting clients through the loss of assistance dogs. Ultimately, these advancements can lead to improved care and outcomes for clients navigating the complexities of assistance dog loss.

Acknowledgements

The authors would like to acknowledge the support of Drs. Leah Cheatham and Lori Kogan along with the representatives of the assistance dog organizations who participated in interviews, shared expertise, and offered feedback to enhance the quality of the research findings.

Funding

This research project was funded by the Primary Investigator with in-kind support (i.e. technology resources) provided by the University of Alabama.

Conflict of Interest

The authors have no conflict of interest to declare.

Author Contributions

The first author served as the Primary Investigator. The second author participated in data analysis and manuscript development.

Ethics Statement

The study received approval from the Institutional Review Board at the University of Alabama #24-03-7425.

Data Availability

The data that support the findings of this study are available from the corresponding author, DD, upon request.

References

Assistance Dogs International (n.d.-a) ADI Member Program Statistics. Available at: https://assistancedogsinternational.org/members/adi-member-program-statistics/ (accessed August 2024).

Assistance Dogs International (n.d.-b) Public Access Laws. Available at: https://assistancedogsinternational.org/resources/public-access-laws/ (accessed 14 August 2024).

Assistance Dogs International (n.d.-c) Summary of Standards. Available at: https://assistancedogsinternational.org/standards/summary-of-standards/ (accessed 14 August 2024).

Assistance Dogs International (n.d.-d) Member search. Available at: https://assistancedogsinternational.org/member-search/?query=%28Region.eq.ADINA%29 (accessed 14 August 2024).

Audrestch, H.M., Whelan, C.T., Grice, D., Asher, L., England, G.C. *et al.* (2015) Recognizing the value of assistance dogs in society. *Disability and Health Journal* 8(4), 469–474. DOI: 10.1016/j.dhjo.2015.07.001.

Birt, L., Scott, S.E., Cavers, D., Campbell, C. and Walter, F.M. (2016) Member checking. *Qualitative Health Research* 26(13), 1802–1811. DOI: 10.1177/10497323.

Braun, V. and Clarke, V. (2012) Thematic Analysis. Research Gate. Available at: https://www.researchgate.net (accessed 14 August 2024).

Bussolari, C., Currin-McCulloch, J., Packman, W., Kogan, L.R. and Erdman, P. (2022) The loss of a service dog through death: Experiences of partners. *Illness, Crisis and Loss* 32(1), 80–94. DOI: 10.1177/10541373221113336.

Cappellaro, G., Compagni, A. and Vaara, E. (2023) Ambiguity in organization theory. DOI: 10.1017/9781009358460.

Currin-McCulloch, J., Bussolari, C., Packman, W., Kogan, L. and Erdman, P. (2021) The loss of a service dog through retirement: Experiences and impact on human partners. *Human-Animal Interaction Bulletin* 11(3), 39–53. DOI: 10.1079/hai.2022.0017.

Gibson, M., Chalmers, D. and Ru, S. (2022) "My lifeline is gone": An exploration of the experiences of veterans following the loss of their psychiatric service dog(s). *Human-Animal Interaction Bulletin* 11(3), 54–74. DOI: 10.1079/hai.2022.

Klass, D., Silverman, P.R. and Nickman, S. (eds) (1996) *Continuing Bonds: New Understandings of Grief.* Taylor and Francis, London.

Knapik, M. (2006) The qualitative research interview: Participants' responsive participation in knowledge making. *International Journal of Qualitative Methods* 5(3), 77–93. Available at: https://sites.ualberta.ca/~iiqm/backissues/5_3/HTML/knapik.htm (accessed 14 August 2024).

Kogan, L.R., Packman, W., Currin-McCulloch, J., Bussolari, C. and Erdman, P. (2021) The loss of a service dog through death or retirement: Experiences and impact on partners. *Illness, Crisis and Loss* 105413732110541, 80–94. DOI: 10.1177/10541373211054168.

Kwong, M.J. and Bartholomew, K. (2011) "Not just a dog": An attachment perspective on relationships with assistance dogs. *Attachment and Human Development* 13(5), 421–436. DOI: 10.1080/14616734.2011.584410.

Lane, D.R., McNicholas, J. and Collis, G. (1998) Dogs for the disabled: Benefits to recipients and welfare of the dog. *Applied Animal Behaviour Science* 59(1–3), 49–60. DOI: 10.1016/s0168-1591(98)00120-8.

McKim, C. (2023) Meaningful member-checking: A structured approach to member-checking [journal-article]. *American Journal of Qualitative Research* 2, 41–52. DOI: 10.29333/ajqr/12973mehc.34.4.41q024845.

Miller, C.A. (2019) Supporting bereaved clients after the death of an assistance dog. In: Kogan, L. and Erdman, P. (eds) *Pet Loss, Grief, and Therapeutic Interventions*. Routledge, New York, pp. 209–235. DOI: 10.4324/9780429505201-14.

Ng, Z. and Fine, A. (2019a) Paving the path toward retirement for assistance animals: Transitioning lives. *Frontiers in Veterinary Science* 6, 1–10. DOI: 10.3389/fvets.2019.00039.

Ng, Z. and Fine, A.H. (2019b) Considerations for the retirement of therapy animals. *Animals* 9(12), 1100. DOI: 10.3390/ani9121100.

Nicholson, J., Kemp-Wheeler, S. and Griffiths, D. (1995) Distress arising from the end of a guide dog partnership. *Anthrozoös* 8(2), 100–110. DOI: 10.2752/089279395787156419.

Packman, W., Field, N.P., Carmack, B.J. and Ronen, R. (2011) Continuing bonds and psychosocial adjustment in pet loss. *Journal of Loss and Trauma* 16(4), 341–357. DOI: 10.1080/15325024.2011.572046.

Rodriguez, K.E., Greer, J., Yatcilla, J.K., Beck, A.M. and O'Haire, M.E. (2020) The effects of assistance dogs on psychosocial health and wellbeing: A systematic literature review. *PLoS One* 15(12), e0243302. DOI: 10.1371/journal.pone.0243302.

Rubin, H.J. and Rubin, I.S. (2012) *Qualitative Interviewing: The Art of Hearing Data*. 3rd edn, SAGE Publications, Thousand Oaks, CA.

Singleton, J.K. (2023) Benefits of being teamed with a service dog for individuals living with visible and invisible disabilities. *Health* 11(22), 2987. DOI: 10.3390/healthcare11222987.

Spain, B., O'Dwyer, L. and Moston, S. (2019) Pet loss: Understanding disenfranchised grief, memorial use, and posttraumatic growth. *Anthrozoös* 32(4), 555–568. DOI: 10.1080/08927936.2019.1621545.

Stroebe, M. and Schut, H. (1999) The dual process model of coping with bereavement: Rationale and description. *Death Studies* 23(3), 197–224. DOI: 10.1080/074811899201046.

Tracy, S.J. (2019) *Qualitative Research methods: Collecting Evidence, Crafting Analysis, Communicating Impact*, 2nd edn. John Wiley and Sons, Hoboken, NJ.

Trainer, M. (2016) Service Dogs Save Lives. Share America. Available at: https://share.america.gov/service-dogs-save-lives/ (accessed 14 August 2024).

Wiggett-Barnard, C. and Steel, H. (2008) The experience of owning a guide dog. *Disability and Rehabilitation* 30(14), 1014–1026. DOI: 10.1080/09638280701466517.

World Health Organization (2020) Disability. Available at: https://www.who.int/health-topics/disability#tab=tab_1 (accessed 14 August 2024).

Yamamoto, M. and Hart, L.A. (2019) Separation from assistance dogs: The complicated psychological burden during loss of the relationship. In: Kogan, L. and Erdman, P. (eds) *Pet Loss, Grief, and Therapeutic Interventions*. Routledge, New York, pp. 188–208. DOI: 10.4324/9780429505201-13.

16 The Loss of a Service Dog Through Retirement: Experiences and Impact on Human Partners

Jennifer Currin-McCulloch[1]*, Cori Bussolari[2], Wendy Packman[3], Lori R. Kogan[4] and Phyllis Erdman[5]

[1]Colorado State University, School of Social Work, Fort Collins, CO, USA; [2]University of San Francisco, Department of Clinical Psychology, San Francisco, CA, USA; [3]Professor Emerita, Palo Alto University, Department of Psychology, Palo Alto, CA, USA; [4]Colorado State University, College of Veterinary Medicine and Biomedical Sciences, Department of Clinical Sciences, Fort Collins, CO, USA; [5]Washington State University, College of Education, Pullman, WA, USA

Abstract

This study describes the experiences of service dog partners (N=22) whose service dog had retired within the previous five years. The participants were service dog partners who participated in a larger quantitative study (N=56) and agreed to a follow up interview. Guided by bereavement and human–animal bond theories and prior research, researchers coded the interviews using directed content analysis to identify prevalent themes. Findings underscore that the retirement of a service dog is poorly understood by others, and often results in disenfranchised grief about this ambiguous loss. The retirement process is difficult and often partners struggled with the need to quickly acquire another service dog and the subsequent impact this had on their ability to grieve. These results suggest that, given the unique nature of service dogs and the relationship between dog and partner, it is important that service dog organizations, mental health counselors and veterinarians are aware of the challenges and losses associated with the retirement of a service dog and offer appropriate tools and support to their clients during this challenging time.

Keywords: service dog partners, retirement, ambiguous loss, continuing bonds

Introduction

Approximately 25% of adults in the United States live with some form of disability (Bureau, n.d.) and over 80 million of these individuals have a service dog (American Kennel Club, 2022). Service dogs offer a myriad of benefits including social support and an increased sense of independence and well-being (Winkle *et al.*, 2012; Walther *et al.*, 2017; Ng and Fine, 2019). The loss of a service dog through death or retirement, therefore, places the partner in a physically, vocationally, and socially vulnerable position (Herlache-Pretzer *et al.*, 2017; Rodriguez *et al.*, 2020a; Kogan *et al.*, 2021) that often leads to

*Corresponding author: Jen.Currin-McCulloch@colostate.edu

unique physical and psychological stressors (Yamamoto and Hart, 2019). Yet, despite the expanded use of service dogs, there remains a paucity of research about the impact of the loss of these partnerships.

Relationship Between Service Dogs and Their Partners

The Americans with Disabilities Act of 1990 (Bureau, n.d.) describes service dogs as dogs individually trained to perform specific tasks for a person with a physical, psychiatric, intellectual, sensory, or mental disability (U.S. Department of Justice, 2021). This status offers service animals legal access to almost all public places (U.S. Department of Justice, 2021). Service animals include guide dogs for the visually or hearing impaired, as well as psychiatric or medical alert animals such as seizure detection dogs. Each service animal receives individualized training to perform complex tasks to support their partner's independence and well-being. For example, a service dog might receive training to alert their partner to a phone call or an emerging medical emergency such as a seizure or insulin response. These dogs can also support their partners in psychiatric crises and interrupt self-injurious behaviors (Yamamoto and Hart, 2019; Rodriguez *et al.*, 2020b). Service dogs also can be trained to retrieve objects, open doors, or pull wheelchairs. Due to the unique support each partner requires, each service dog's training period takes about two years and includes a substantial financial investment by the service dog training organization (Gravrok *et al.*, 2020).

The bond between a service dog and partner is a unique, supportive, and independence-enhancing relationship (Stewart, 2006). Studies have identified numerous ways in which service dogs positively impact people with disabilities, including the ability to foster opportunities for socialization and community participation (Rodriguez *et al.*, 2020a). Service dogs can increase people's locus of control, confidence, and self-concept; provide emotional support and security; contribute to an increased sense of independence and mobility; and can help soften feelings of stigmatization (Sanders, 2000; Wiggett-Barnard and Steel, 2008; Rintala *et al.*, 2008; Walther *et al.*, 2017; Fairman and Huebner, 2021).

Transition Into Retirement

Decision-making process

While the decision-making process related to retirement may occasionally happen in an acute or traumatic manner, most assistance partners spend significant time pondering when and how to transition their service dog into retirement. In her personal narrative describing her own transitions with three guide dogs, Schneider (2005) portrayed the grueling decision-making process surrounding the "the three good-byes:" the initial decision to say goodbye, the end of the working relationship, and the final goodbye at death. Transitions commonly begin when the dog approaches old age or when the partner notices changes in the dog's ability to carry out physical activities or respond to behavioral requests (Caron-Lormier *et al.*, 2016).

Retirement decision-making processes are often fraught with emotional distress, guilt, and remorse – in addition to the profound grief caused from losing a canine partner with whom they could trust to meet their physical and emotional needs (Schneider, 2005; Yamamoto and Hart, 2019; Ng and Fine, 2019). Instrumental in the decision-making process is the partner's desire to provide a conducive environment in which their dog can smoothly transition into the role of pet (Ng and Fine, 2019). Once a service partner enters the decision-making process around their dog's retirement, they face multiple options for how and where their dog can retire. Each option comes with logistical and emotional consequences.

Options for retirement include (a) keeping the dog in the home, (b) rehoming the dog to a trusted person (e.g., family member, friend, puppy raiser), or (c) rehoming the dog to a stranger (the least common option). If the need to retire stems from a service dog's progressive illness, partners may also face the challenge of physically caring for an ailing dog, tasks which may not be possible due to their own physical or financial limitations (Yamamoto and Hart, 2019). Even without these additional challenges, partners must still help their service dogs transition into their new role as a pet. Given service dogs' training and mentality, most will continue to try and meet their partner's needs, regardless of their capabilities. This can be especially challenging for all involved when a successor dog enters the home and assumes the retired dog's former role (Miller, 2019).

Service dog partners' grief response to ambiguous loss

Inevitably, through death or retirement, the time will come when a service dog's working role ends. In the case of retirement, there is a major loss as the relationship shifts from service dog to pet dog. Given the overall disenfranchised nature of companion animal loss (Doka, 2008), partners experiencing the retirement of their service dog may also lack the benefit of an understanding and supportive community. Findings from our larger quantitative study found that the death of a service dog can have a profound impact, with partners' grief scores comparable to those reported by pet guardians (Kogan *et al.*, 2021). For those suffering a loss due to retirement, the added ambiguity of this type of loss can exacerbate feelings of disenfranchised grief and decrease the likelihood that they will have an adequate social support system with whom to share their grief. While the service dog community may recognize the meaning of this type of loss, partners may still encounter challenges in talking about the loss with family members, colleagues, and friends (Chur-Hansen, 2010).

The term "ambiguous loss," first coined by Boss (1977), is defined as a situation in which a person does not know if their loved one is alive or dead, present or absent. There are two categories of ambiguous loss: family members who are psychologically absent but remain physically present, and members who are physically absent but remain psychologically present (Boss and Yeats, 2014). Examples of the former may be a parent dealing with a substance use disorder who, although can be literally present at family gatherings, is figuratively absent in terms of their limited ability to reprise the family roles they once assumed (Boss, 2006; Brumett, 2022). In most cases of a retired service dog, there is a loss of relational roles - the dog is still living, but he/she is not there in the same way.

The grief process in ambiguous loss is often forestalled, remaining in a "frozen" state when one can never be certain of what has been lost (Boss, 2006). According to Boss, the paradox inherent in ambiguous loss produces the most stressful, immobilizing form of grief (Boss, 2006). An ambiguous loss challenges a person's existing coping strategies and the bereaved may not be able to participate in rituals that typically surround a death. The lack of traditions, communication, and social support around ambiguous losses are coupled with the inherent perceptual and emotional dissonance created by uncertainty (Brumett, 2022). Because of these conditions, those experiencing ambiguous loss are more likely to develop complicated grief symptoms (Boss, 2006). In the case of a retired service dog, support is needed to understand the nuances of this kind of loss.

While many factors that impact companion animal grief have been studied, to our knowledge, there is little research that has explored grief in relation to service dogs. The purpose of this study was to gain a better understanding of how service dog partners experience the decline and subsequent retirement of their service dog in order to make clinically meaningful suggestions for service dog partners, service dog organizations, and veterinarians.

Method

Study sample

The research team partnered with Canine Companions (CC) (https://canine.org/), a national service dog training organization founded in 1975, to recruit current and former service dog partners via CC's internal emails and newsletters. Interested partners were invited to visit an online Qualtrics study information page to learn about the study. Following informed consent, the participants could choose to complete an anonymous survey (Kogan *et al.*, 2021).

At the end of the survey, participants could elect to be contacted for an optional individual interview. Twenty-two individuals volunteered to participate in an individual interview, the sample evenly split between males and females. The 22 interviews are the focus of this manuscript. The research was approved by [redacted name's] Institutional Review Board. Participants received a $50 gift card for participation in the interview. Funding for these incentives was made possible through a grant from Human Animal Bond in Colorado.

Data Collection

Participants who indicated interest in an individual interview as part of a larger quantitative study (Kogan *et al.*, 2021) were contacted by the research team to discover whether their loss was due to their service dog's death or retirement. Those who experienced a retirement loss completed an individual semi-structured interview between October -November 2021. Interviews, conducted by counseling graduate students who received interview training, lasted between 30–90 min, and took place by Zoom or telephone. The interviews centered around the events leading up to the service dogs' retirement, the impact of these associated losses, the partners' potential transition to a successor dog, and their grief process. Each interview was recorded, transcribed, and reviewed by the research team to verify accuracy of data. The transcribed Microsoft Word documents were uploaded into MAXQDA, a software program that supports the systematic organization of qualitative data such as coding, and the analysis of qualitative data. Of note, MAXQDA supports the organization of qualitative data but does not perform data analysis.

Data Analysis

The first three authors performed the data analysis. They each have had extensive experience as both clinicians and researchers in the fields of human grief and loss as they relate to the death of both humans and animals. We used directed content analysis, a qualitative method that is guided by theory or prior research (Potter and Levine-Donnerstein, 1999) to analyze participants' responses to the interview. This method aims to validate or extend a theoretical framework (Hsieh and Shannon, 2005) and utilizes a more structured, rather than conventional, content analysis (Hickey and Kipping, 1996). We initially read through each transcript and identified key concepts as initial coding categories (Potter and Levine-Donnerstein, 1999). Next, formal theories from bereavement and continuing bonds frameworks supported operational definitions for each coding category, including bereavement and continuing bonds theories (Doka, 2008; Field *et al.*, 2009), as well as prior research on pet loss (Carmack, 2003; Orsini, 2005; Packman *et al.*, 2011; Habarth *et al.*, 2017). Data that could not be coded were identified and analyzed later to determine if they represented a salient theme or subcategory of an existing category.

Participants' responses were first independently coded and then reviewed together by the study's first three authors until consensus was reached. The creation of theoretical and analytic memos captured code definitions, themes, and patterns within the data. The team tracked progress towards code and meaning saturation (Hennink *et al.*, 2017) and determined that code saturation was achieved at interview nine. The authors reviewed all interviews until they reached meaning saturation (interview 12) in which interview data no longer elucidated nuanced meanings.

The transcribed interviews were uploaded into Relative Insight, a comparative text analysis tool that provides a systematic approach to analysis of qualitative data (Relative Insight Ltd, 2021). Using Relative Insight, we compared the language of the responses between partners whose service dogs had retired and partners whose service dogs had died. This form of natural language processing detects the topics, words, phrases, grammar and emotion more likely to be seen in one set of words compared to another. It is important to point out that Relative Insight does not provide an actual analysis of data; rather, similar to MAXQDA, it is an organizational tool that assists with qualitative analysis.

Results

Liminal state - complexities of decision-making

From the initial days that they meet their service dog at the training facility, partners who receive dogs through Canine Companions receive psychoeducation to prepare them for the inevitable retirement or death of their service dog. They are guided throughout their dog's aging process and instructed in how to talk with veterinarians about their dog's health status. In addition, as the dog ages, Canine Companions helps partners evaluate the service dog's continued ability to carry out their roles, and their physical and cognitive well-being. One partner described this incremental transitional process:

> And they go over [retirement] very specifically in team training. They explain, you know, you're going to have this dog for a number of years. And at some point in the future, the dogs are gonna retire. And except for unusual circumstances, for illness or, or death, those instances are pre planned. And so, you have time emotionally, to get your mind around that concept. And it's not like a sudden thing (P01, male).

Partners shared how Canine Companions also initiates dialogue with them about how they would like to retire their dog. Options include the dog remaining in the partner's home transitioning the dog into a companion role, or rehoming the dog to someone else (e.g., family member, their dog's puppy raiser, a friend, or a vetted stranger). The complex decision-making process regarding where the dog would retire was based on numerous factors including available support at home to care for the aging dog's health needs; the existence of a strong attachment between the dog and other people living in the partner's home; and having close friends or their puppy raiser willing to care for their dog until his/her end of life. Another essential facet of the retirement plan includes a discussion of whether the partner would like to initiate the process for a successor dog. Once the partner sets their dog's retirement plan, they share this information with Canine Companions and the official retirement process begins. To denote the official day of retirement, the training organization provides the partners an official retirement document. Upon the receipt of this document, the transition from working dog to pet dog begins, as does the process of rehoming, if this is the choice of the partner.

As service dogs entered old age, their partners became intimately aware of the magnitude of approaching retirement decisions. Partners began to watch for changes for physical or cognitive declines that signal the approaching end to their dog's working role. The partners who had lost dogs through death and other dogs through retirement shared that when dogs have health crises or life-limiting illnesses, as partners, they have less time to make decisions and often, the only option is for euthanasia. With retirement, partners frequently had time to perseverate on the instrumental and emotional aspects of a pending retirement plan. Those who relied on their dog to interact in society (e.g., shopping, work, volunteering, socializing, etc.), faced a difficult struggle. Their independence and identity, enabled and enhanced by their service dog, became blurred as they began to reframe their dog's role. As the service dogs' health declined, partners became more vulnerable to losing integral facets of their identity and connection to the world. An active partner shared:

> So, you kind of worry about that, you know, and the things that he's done with me and the places we work together. I do a lot of volunteer work. And so, I was looking at eliminating that which, you know, wasn't an easy call (P02, male).

In addition to their own identity changes, partners also had to prepare their service dog for the transition from a working role into that of a companion animal. If they are planning on rehoming their dog, partners have the additional emotional and instrumental planning and challenges that surrounds letting their dog physically go to another person. As service dogs transitioned into pets, they also lost their ability to participate in activities that gave their life meaning and joy. Partners reported feeling that since their dog's identities were wrapped up in their working role, when this role is lost, their dogs struggled and appeared sad, perhaps projecting their own emotions onto their dogs. These feelings and observations became even more heightened if a new service dog entered the home.

This period of retirement transition forced partners into a liminal state, characterized by living between two worlds – that of having the dog still alive and working, while also bracing for transition into retired life. This ambiguous emotional space left partners feeling immense grief for what was currently happening and what was going to happen; thus, setting the stage for emotional distress. Compounding the grief associated with these ambiguous losses was the lack of support many partners felt since so few people understand the complexity and magnitude of their unique grief.

To better understand the specific semantics of retirement loss, we used Relative Insight to compare responses between partners whose dogs had died (Currin-McCullouch *et al.*, 2022) and partners whose dogs had been retired. The partners whose service dogs had retired expressed more anxiety, worry, and grief, suggesting a "stressful, immobilizing form of grief" consistent with ambiguous loss (Boss, 2006).

Waiting for the shoe to drop: Partner's vigilance of their dog's behavioral decline

Either personally driven, or through the impetus of Canine Companions or their veterinarians, partners faced the ultimate decision about when and how their dog would retire. As shared by one partner, this control and planning offered comfort: "I appreciated being able to have the choices of what was going on and feeling like I had control rather than kind of being told what to do and dictated on stuff" (P05, female). Yet, the multiple options for retirement and their desire to provide the best possible final days for their dog magnified the partner's decision-making stress.

Commonly, partners shared that the most distressing decision centered on the timing of when to relinquish their dog's working role. As their dog's behaviors started to change, feelings of dread began to arise: "So when I call him to wake up, I don't know if he has, you know, hearing issues, but he doesn't respond right away. And I'm thinking, 'Oh, boy, you know, is this the day?'" (P03, female). For many, the decision was a long, gradual process with a sequence of grief reactions that led up to the final day of retirement:

> I always tell people, I don't know which is worse. Is it completing the application? Is it the phone call when it comes in? Because now you know that you have a finite amount of time with your dog? Or is it the day you hand over the leash the final time and take off the vest? It's all horrible. And it's heartbreaking. And it feels like death (P12, male).

From the timing of the initial thought about retirement to the official day of signing their dog's retirement papers, partners encountered a plethora of losses. Unlike the concrete losses associated with death, retirement brought gradual and ambiguous losses. Most striking about the ambiguity was the fact that their dog was still alive and often still present in the home, yet not there in its service dog role. A partner shared the complexities of their loss:

> And yes, I mean, there was an awful lot of loss other than the loss of them. Being able to do things with me and not being able to take him, and you can see in his face that he wants to go on. So, I mean, that's the hardest thing is that, like, I take him for short walks and several long walks, because he still has the drive stuff, but he can't physically do things for me (P05, female).

These nebulous transitions resulted in partners feeling challenged as they attempted to psychologically separate from their dog. With time and multiple transitions between service dogs, the concrete tasks around the retirement plan became easier; however, the grief always appeared. The retirement of each dog brought different types of losses, most commonly based on the ability of each dog to perform tasks to promote their partner's independence and ease in carrying out activities of daily living. Echoing throughout partners' responses was a stronger grief response surrounding the retirement of their first service dog, as well as dogs who had an ability to anticipate and support their partner's unique needs.

Amidst their grief, partners reported finding some meaning in being able to reciprocate the caregiving role for their dogs. Whether it was providing in-home nurturing, or creating a loving rehoming environment, partners found comfort in knowing that their dog would have the highest quality end of life possible. Many verbalized the "promises" that they made to their dogs to keep them safe and comfortable. A partner who retained their service dog and cared for him in his declining health explained:

> I was able to give to him the emotional support. Because like when he had the surgery, I mean, I was sitting there. I kept him on a leash at night. And I had him right beside me so that if he was moving around, I could feel him and see if he needed anything. So, I kind of fell into this [caregiving] role for a bit so I didn't have some of those [relationship] lines [that I did when he was in a working dog role]. And it did make a difference for me when not being able to have him go out and to do things for me (P05, female).

Partners commonly shared how the ability to care for their dog's physical needs provided them an opportunity to repay the love and kindness that their dogs unconditionally shared with them. When partners lacked resources or the physical ability to keep their dogs at home with them, rehoming to puppy raisers appeared to be a viable option. Placement with puppy raisers offered mutual benefit for the dog, the partner, and the raiser as it provided a full circle of healing and options for continuing bonds. A partner who was no longer physically able to care for her dog shared about their continued connection to her retired dog that their puppy raiser was able to offer:

> She's been very proactive and kept me involved in [her life] and we started a habit of bringing [my service dog] to visit me about once a month... She came to visit often and we would go for a walk to a restaurant and then there's a park that's nearby and we would let the girls off leash and let them play for a while (P11, female).

When they placed their dog with another person, they had limited control over their retired dog's care. When placing their dogs with a vested stranger, they had concerns about whether those caring for their dog would make the best decisions for their dog's well-being. On most accounts, partners reported having positive rehoming stories to share. However, one partner shared a traumatic experience surrounding their dog's end of life:

> I would have let him go way earlier than she did, and I felt like he lost his dignity. Last time I saw him, because I am intuitive, I knew that he pleaded with me to please let him go. And I tried, and I could not get her to do it. So, he hung on for two more months before she finally said it's time. She never let me know until after [he died] so I could not be there with him (P10, male).

This partner shared immense emotional turmoil about this decision and was still grappling with the aftereffects years later.

Integration of successor dogs

Another key decision-making element around retirement centers on whether to pursue a successor service dog. Factors that can impact the decision to apply for a successor dog include concerns that new dogs would not be able to meet the partner's needs; they might not be a good personality fit for the partner; or the partner may have limited energy or desire to navigate the dynamics of integrating a new service dog with their retired dog. Due to service dogs' short lifespan and the physical demands of their work, partners frequently had several service dogs over their lifetime. They shared stories of how they integrated successor dogs in their home and frequently made comparisons between their different dogs' skills and personalities. Partners proclaimed that these comparisons often created challenges in bonding with the successor dog.

The notion of having a successor dog brought mixed emotions for many partners, including feelings of hope. For those who had to wait for a new dog, they often felt a sense of anticipation and excitement in having a new companion who could open opportunities for increased independence:

> There is a degree of sadness because you've been so close to this dog for, you know, eight or nine years. But for me, at the same time, because I knew I was going to immediately get another dog, there's a sense of anticipation. You know, what's this new dog going to be like? What's its personality? What are its quirks? What are the specific things that come out in their personality? And so, there's that level of anticipation, that kind of doesn't make the sadness aspect as bad (P01, male).

Many partners held hope for their future yet also worried that the new dog might not be able to live up to their expectations. Of note, not all partners desired to immediately pursue a successor dog. Some partners chose to take time to grieve the losses associated with their service dog's retirement or rehoming prior to seeking a successor dog.

When the time came to transition to a successor service dog, blurred boundaries and identities emerged as partners attempted to integrate a new service dog into the home. If their retired dog has been rehomed or died, partners often grieved and held closely memories of their dog. When their retired service dog still lived in the home, difficulties often emerged in integrating the successor dog with the retired dog. Due to their training, retired service dogs struggled to understand how to let go of their daily tasks and simply provide companionship. Thus, issues arose when the retired dog attempted to carry out their usual tasks while their successor was trying to learn their duties. A partner explained: "Having two dogs is difficult. It's a lot more work. I mean, I take [my successor dog] for a walk, and then [my former service dog] pushes into the door to get his walk' (P03, female). Balancing the needs of two dogs often left partners feeling sad that they could never quite meet the needs of either dog. A partner portrayed this struggle:

> So, he goes to the back door because he knows that I'm leaving the home. And he's used to just going every place with me and it's sad for me to tell him that I'll be back soon. But you can go and I just have to keep leaving and not look back at his eyes. So that's very sad. He's my buddy and it's very difficult for me to leave him behind (P11, female).

With support from Canine Companions, fellow service dog partners, or their dog's puppy raiser, partners were able to gather insights into how to transition their retired dog more successfully into a companion role and move their successor dog into its new working role. An example of a smooth integration and win-win for both dogs appears as follows:

> It's gotten better because I have another dog that does the actual things for me and helps me get dressed and things like that. And it doesn't put the demand on [my retired dog]. I actually think he's starting to enjoy it because I think he gets this little smirk and it's cute to see that (P03, female).

After partners successfully negotiated the process of integrating a new dog into the home, they described taking a deep breath, hoping that they would have several years to cultivate a bond with their new dog while also sharing love and gratitude for their retired dog.

Partners' challenges in accessing social support

As partners approached the retirement of their service dog, they reached out to people they trusted to talk through their decisions. Commonly, partners drew on Canine Companions, their family members, friends, and puppy raisers for emotional and practical support as their dogs' health declined. Yet, despite having supportive people in their lives, partners shared feeling alone in their grief and isolated in their decision making. Few partners had strong connections to their peers or someone who they felt truly understood the layers of ambiguous loss they encountered. Therefore, many partners excluded family members or friends from their decision-making process because they weren't prepared for the possible responses. For example:

> The last time I ever took his vest off of him, almost killed me. He was by far my heart [most loved] dog. I did not tell a soul I was [applying for another dog] because I knew people would try to talk me out of it. And I knew I was doing what was best for him. He was slowing down. He didn't really have any health issues. But I knew if I kept pushing him, there's no way [his health decline] wasn't going to start. My mom was living with me at the time and I didn't even tell her until she heard my voicemail. And I had it on speaker and my mom heard CC say we sent the application out to you. My mom was like, 'What are you doing'? I said, 'I'm putting in for my next dog'. And she said, 'But he's not ready' (P12, male).

Unlike humans' transitions into retirement, few rituals existed around service dogs' retirement to offer partners the ability to process their grief. This only seemed to exacerbate the partners' sense of isolation and created grief that frequently felt disenfranchised. A partner described their initial days after retiring their dog:

> I felt extraordinarily lonely. Not only lonely, but alone. I told my caregiver that I was going to eat lunch out. And then I was meeting my friend who is a puppy raiser. She said, 'Don't go out to eat. Let me make you something here'. And I said, 'No, no. Really, I need to get out of the house. I don't think sitting here will be good for me'. And she said, 'If that's what you want, okay'. I went down to [a fast-food restaurant] by myself, ordered my food, got to the table and looked down to talk to [my retired dog] under the table and realized he's not there. And I lost it in the middle of [a fast-food restaurant]. It couldn't stop crying for 20 min (P12, male).

This quote highlights the social constraints partners encountered in coping with their retirement-associated losses. Even though many had support, they didn't feel that others could fully grasp their grief.

Discussion

This is one of the few qualitative research studies to address the experiences of service dog partners following the retirement of their dog (Schneider, 2005; Yamamoto and Hart, 2019; Ng and Fine, 2019). This study's results illuminate the ambiguous losses that partners have to navigate over the course of the anticipated and actual retirement of their service dog. This most prominently occurs when a new service dog is introduced and the older service dog is either still in the house (but not working) or has been rehomed. It seems clear from our interviews that the retirement of a service animal, while not a physical death, can be viewed as the death of their relationship, and as such, is fraught with transitional challenges and intense grief. Numerous studies have highlighted the strong attachments we have with our companion animals (Kurdek, 2008, 2009; Kwong and Bartholomew, 2011). This has been evidenced historically through humans' tendency to anthropomorphize their animals (Mithen, 1996). The current study also portrays the close connections human partners have with their service animals. In a companion qualitative study (Currin-McCullouch *et al.*, 2022), we found that the death of a service dog has profound impacts on partners. The grief scores of partners whose service dog had died were comparable to previous companion animal loss studies (Kogan *et al.*, 2021) and slightly higher than the grief scores for those whose dog had been retired. Yet, consistent with ambiguous loss theory (Boss, 2006), partners whose dog had retired expressed higher levels of on-going worry than partners whose dogs had died. The retirement of a service dog places individuals at increased risk for additionally experiencing disenfranchised grief – a loss that involves limited social recognition and a lack of ritualized support (Doka, 1999).

Partners whose service dogs had retired also experienced high levels of social constraints (Kogan *et al.*, 2021), indicating that they did not feel that they were able to share their experiences with their support system. Retirement is not a well-understood type of loss – partners encounter few people who fully understand the complexity of this ambiguous loss. Furthermore, when considering that service dog partners typically retire several dogs, the magnitude of this type of loss has the potential to grow exponentially over their lifetime (Wenthold and Savage, 2007; Yamamoto and Hart, 2019). Retirement transitions occur in rapid succession and leave service dog partners limited time to process the magnitude of their loss. Having to build a bond with and train a new service dog while a retired service dog is still alive is a source of distress and profoundly difficult to navigate.

Strengths, Limitations, and Future Research

While many factors that impact companion animal grief have been studied, there is little research that has explored grief in relation to service dogs. Importantly, this is one of the only studies to assess the lived experiences of service dog partners' surrounding the retirement of their dog. Findings from this study provide practical clinical implications for service dog organizations to provide as examples, anticipatory grief psychoeducation, specific suggestions regarding the transitional process in getting a successor dog, and the disenfranchised nature of their ambiguous loss. A few limitations also bear mentioning. The study was conducted during the initial months of the COVID-19 pandemic when access to veterinary care, successor dogs, and psychosocial support services were limited; thus, these reported experiences may not reflect partners' experiences outside this moment in time. Understanding the retrospective nature of data collection, participants' memories of how events occurred may be skewed. From the sample of individuals who participated in the parent quantitative survey, those experiencing emotional distress may have been less likely to participate in the follow-up interview. The sample comes from one service dog organization in the United States; thus, the findings might not be generalizable to other organizations or in other countries. Lastly, the participants in this study specifically included mobility or hearing impairments only. Future research is needed to explore the experiences of service dog partners who receive dogs from other training organizations and for those who receive a service dog for other disabilities (visual, psychiatric, etc.). Based on findings from secondary analysis utilizing Relative Insights that analyzes participants' chosen phrasing, additional studies may want to investigate the role of partners' "anxiety" surrounding pivotal moments during their service dog's retirement transitions.

Conclusions and Implications

Novel insights about service dog partners' ambiguous and disenfranchised losses experienced throughout the transition to retirement lead to several implications for counselors, veterinarians, and service dog training organizations. Given partners' nuanced experiences, having access to peers who have been through the retirement process may promote opportunities to talk through their decisions and receive validation of their grief responses. Some options partners suggested were one-on-one peer mentors and having virtual monthly retirement transition support group meetings. Partners frequently felt that their dog's retirement snuck up on them emotionally and as such, requested having a concrete transitional plan that would guide them through steps to take each month. They shared that having ways to help the transition become more realistic would improve their grief response and potentially promote a smoother process for the dogs to relinquish their roles, especially for partners who bring a successor into the home. There may also be activities that partners could explore with their retired dogs that are less physically taxing such as nose work (i.e., the scent training of dogs is designed to tap into their sense of smell to explore the focus and fun activity of scent detection") or volunteering at schools where children can read to the dog.

Many partners shared the fact that there are few socially sanctioned rituals around key transitions in a service dog's retirement. Incorporating a ceremony at the time of retirement with close friends and families, their puppy raiser, or members of their training organization may provide a socially sanctioned opportunity to process and document the loss. Therapy could benefit partners throughout their transitional service dog retirement journey to help them create meaning through rituals/memorials and engage in comforting continuing bonds expressions (Neimeyer *et al.*, 2006; Packman *et al.*, 2011). Counselors can also help teach clients to directly communicate their needs to their support system and work through feelings of isolation. Overall, a team approach can be helpful in mitigating partners' negative feelings related to the transition. In summary, service dog partners who experience the retirement of their service dog undergo a unique, seldomly understood series of losses that must be better recognized, validated, and supported.

References

American Kennel Club (2022) Service dogs 101: Everything you need to know. Available at: https://www.akc.org/expert-advice/training/service-dog-training-101/

Boss, P. (1977) A clarification of the concept of psychological father presence in families experiencing ambiguity of boundary. *Journal of Marriage & the Family* 39(1), 141–151. Available at: https://psycnet.apa.org/doi/10.2307/351070

Boss, P. (2006) *Loss, trauma, and resilience*. Norton.

Boss, P. and Yeats, J. (2014) Ambiguous loss: A complicated type of grief when loved ones disappear. *Bereavement Care* 33(2), 63–69. DOI: 10.1080/02682621.2014.933573.

Brumett, A. (2022) When a pet goes missing: An exploratory study on ambiguous pet loss. [Doctoral dissertation, Palo Alto University].

Bureau, U.C. (n.d.) Americans with Disabilities: 2014. The United States Census Bureau. Available at: https://www/census.gov/library/publications/2018/demo/p70-152.html

Carmack, B.J. (2003) *Grieving the Death of a Pet*. Augsburg Books.

Caron-Lormier, G., England, G.C., Green, M.J. and Asher, L. (2016) Using the incidence and impact of health conditions in guide dogs to investigate healthy ageing in working dogs. *The Veterinary Journal* 207, 124–130. DOI: 10.1016/j.tvjl.2015.10.046.

Chur-Hansen, A. (2010) Grief and bereavement issues and the loss of a companion animal: People living with a companion animal, owners of livestock, and animal support workers. *Clinical Psychologist* 14(1), 14–21. DOI: 10.1080/13284201003662800.

Currin-McCullouch, J., Bussolari, C., Packman, W., Kogan, L.R. and Erdman, P. (2022) Loss of a service dog through retirement: Experiences and impact on partners. *Human-Animal Interaction Bulletin* 11(3), 39–53. DOI: 10.1079/hai.2022.001.

Doka, K.J. (1999) Disenfranchised grief. *Bereavement Care* 18(3), 37–39.

Doka, K.J. (2008) Disenfranchised grief in historical and cultural perspective. In: Stroebe, M.S., Hansson, R.O., Schut, H. and Stroebe, W. (eds) *Handbook of Bereavement Research and Practice: Advances in Theory and Intervention*. American Psychological Association, pp. 223–240.

Fairman, S.K. and Huebner, R.A. (2021) Service dogs: A compensatory resource to improve function. *Occupational Therapy Health Care* 12(2), 41–52. DOI: 10.1080/j003v13n02_03.

Field, N.P., Orsini, L., Gavish, R. and Packman, W. (2009) Role of attachment in response to pet loss. *Death Studies* 33, 332–355. DOI: 10.1080/07481180802705783.

Gravrok, J., Howell, T., Bendrups, D. and Bennett, P. (2020) Thriving through relationships: Assistance dogs' and companion dogs' perceived ability to contribute to thriving in individuals with and without a disability. *Disability and Rehabilitation: Assistive Technology* 15(1), 45–53. DOI: 10.1080/17483107.2018.1513574.

Habarth, J., Bussolari, C., Gomez, R., Carmack, B.J., Ronen, R. *et al.* (2017) Continuing bonds and psychosocial functioning in a recently bereaved pet loss sample. *Anthrozoös* 30(4), 651–670. DOI: 10.1080/08927936.2017.1370242.

Hennink, M.M., Kaiser, B.N. and Marconi, V.C. (2017) Code saturation versus meaning saturation: How many interviews are enough. *Qualitative Health Research* 27(4), 591–608. DOI: 10.1177/1049732316665344.

Herlache-Pretzer, E., Winkle, M.Y., Csatari, R., Kolanowski, A., Londry, A. *et al.* (2017) The impact of service dogs on engagement in occupation among females with mobility impairments: A qualitative descriptive study. *International Journal of Environmental Research and Public Health* 14(6), E649. DOI: 10.3390/ijerph14060649.

Hickey, G. and Kipping, C. (1996) A multi-stage approach to the coding of data from open-ended questions. *Nurse Researcher* 4(1), 81–91. DOI: 10.7748/nr.4.1.81.s9.

Hsieh, H.F. and Shannon, S.E. (2005) Three approaches to content analysis. *Qualitative Health Research* 15(9), 1277–1288. DOI: 10.1177/1049732305276687.

Kogan, L., Packman, W., Currin-McCulloch, J., Bussolari, C. and Erdman, P. (2021) The loss of a service dog through death or retirement: Experiences and impact on partners. *Illness, Crisis & Loss*. DOI: 10.1177/10541373211054168.

Kurdek, L.A. (2008) Pet dogs as attachment figures. *Journal of Social and Personal Relationships* 25, 247–266. DOI: 10.1177/0265407507087958.

Kurdek, L.A. (2009) Pet dogs as attachment figures for adult owners. *Journal of Family Psychology* 23, 409–446. Available at: https://psycnet.apa.org/doi/10.1037/a0014979

Kwong, M.J. and Bartholomew, K. (2011) Not just a dog": An attachment perspective on relationships with assistance dogs. *Attachment and Human Development* 13, 421–436. DOI: 10.1080/14616734.2011.584410.

Miller, C.A. (2019) Supporting bereaved clients after the death of an assistance dog. In: Kogan, L. and Erdman, P. (eds) *Pet Loss, Grief, and Therapeutic Interventions: Practitioners Navigating the Human-Animal Bond*. Routledge.

Mithen, S. (1996) *The Prehistory of the Mind: The Cognitive Origins of Art, Religion and Science*. Thames & Hudson.

Neimeyer, R., Baldwin, S. and Gillies, J. (2006) Continuing bonds and reconstructing meaning: Mitigating complications in bereavement. *Death Studies* 30, 715–738. DOI: 10.1080/07481180600848322.

Ng, Z. and Fine, A. (2019) Paving the path toward retirement for assistance animals: Transitioning lives. *Frontiers in Veterinary Science* 6, 39. DOI: 10.3389/fvets.

Orsini, L.M. (2005) Attachment styles and pet bereavement discussed in the context of attachment theory. [Unpublished Doctoral Dissertation, Pacific Graduate School of Psychology]. Available at: https://www.proquest.com/openview/0ecf941d302cdac77fa32bd511df58c2/1?pq-origsite=gscholar&cbl=18750&diss=y

Packman, W., Field, N.P., Carmack, B.J. and Ronen, R. (2011) Continuing bonds and psychosocial adjustment in pet loss. *Journal of Loss and Trauma* 16(4), 341–357. DOI: 10.1080/15325024.2011.572046.

Potter, W.J. and Levine-Donnerstein, D. (1999) Rethinking validity and reliability in content analysis. *Journal of Applied Communication Research* 27(3), 258–284. DOI: 10.1080/00909889909365539.

Relative Insight Ltd (2021) Text analysis software.

Rintala, D.H., Matamoros, R. and Seitz, L.L. (2008) Effects of assistance dogs on persons with mobility or hearing impairments: A pilot study. *Journal of Rehabilitation Research and Development* 45(4), 489–503. DOI: 10.1682/jrrd.2007.06.0094.

Rodriguez, K.E., Bibbo, J. and O'Haire, M.E. (2020a) The effects of service dogs on psychosocial health and wellbeing for individuals with physical disabilities or chronic conditions. *Disability and Rehabilitation* 42(10), 1350–1358. DOI: 10.1080/09638288.2018.1524520.

Rodriguez, K.E., LaFollette, M.R., Hediger, K., Ogata, N. and O'Haire, M.E. (2020b) Defining the PTSD service dog intervention: Perceived importance, usage, and symptom specificity of psychiatric service dogs for military veterans. *Frontiers in Psychology* 11, 1638. DOI: 10.3389/fpsyg.2020.01638.

Sanders, C.R. (2000) The impact of guide dogs on the identity of people with visual impairments. *Anthrozoös* 13(3), 131–139. DOI: 10.2752/089279300786999815.

Schneider, K.S. (2005) Practice report: The winding valley of grief: when a dog guide retires or dies. *Journal of Visual Impairment & Blindness* 99(6), 368–370. Available at: https://files.eric.ed.gov/fulltext/EJ718713.pdf

Stewart, D. (2006) Investigating the relationship between assistance dogs and their owners with physical disabilities: Complex affection or simple attachment? [Thesis, Simon Fraser University]. Available at: https://summit.sfu.ca/item/2305

U.S. Department of Justice (2021) ADA 2010 revised requirements: Service animals. U.S. Department of Justice Civil Rights Division Disability Rights Section. Available at: https://www.ada.gov/service_animals_2010.htm

Walther, S., Yamamoto, M., Thigpen, A.P., Garcia, A., Willits, N.H. *et al*. (2017) Assistance dogs: Historic patterns and roles of dogs placed by ADI or IGDF accredited facilities and by non-accredited US facilities. *Frontiers in Veterinary Science* 4(2), 1. DOI: 10.3389/fvets.2017.00001.

Wenthold, N. and Savage, T.A. (2007) Ethical issues with service animals. *Topics in Stroke Rehabilitation* 14(2), 68–74. DOI: 10.1310/tsr1402-68.

Wiggett-Barnard, C. and Steel, H. (2008) The experience of owning a guide dog. *Disability and Rehabilitation: An International, Multidisciplinary Journal* 30(14), 1014–1026. DOI: 10.1080/09638280701466517.

Winkle, M., Crowe, T.K. and Hendrix, I. (2012) Service dogs and people with physical disabilities partnerships: A systematic review. *Occupational Therapy International* 19(1), 54–66. DOI: 10.1002/oti.323.

Yamamoto, M. and Hart, L.A. (2019) Separation from assistance dogs. In: Kogan, L. and Erdman, P. (eds) *Pet Loss, Grief, and Therapeutic Interventions: Practitioners Navigating the Human-Animal Bond*. Routledge, pp. 108–208.

17 "My Lifeline is Gone": An Exploration of the Experiences of Veterans Following the Loss of their Psychiatric Service Dog(s)

Maryellen Gibson[1], Darlene Chalmers[2*] and Siyu Ru[1]
[1]Department of Sociology, University of Saskatchewan, Canada; [2]Faculty of Social Work, University of Regina, Saskatchewan, Canada

Abstract

Canadian veterans with PTSD are increasingly accessing psychiatric service dogs (PSDs) as a complementary treatment for their symptoms. Due to the short life span of dogs, however, it is inevitable that these veterans will experience the loss of their PSD either through death, retirement, or relinquishment. This exploratory qualitative study shares the findings from interviews with four veterans who had experienced grief at the loss of a PSD. The themes that emerged suggest that participants experienced a grief cycle: building of a bond with their PSD, a grief response after the loss of their PSD, healing and coping, and a transitional stage when introducing a new PSD into their lives. Recommendations are made for health care professionals working with veterans with psychiatric service dogs and for service dog providers and organizations to better prepare and support their clients leading up to and after the loss of their service dog.

Introduction

The Human-Animal Bond (HAB) refers to the mutually beneficial relationship between animals and people and can be essential to the health and well-being of both parties in many ways including but not limited to: emotional, psychological, and physical benefits (Fine, 2019; Human Animal Bond Research Institute, 2021). In many cases, humans consider their pets or companion animals as members of their family unit due to their close loving reciprocal relationship (Risley-Curtiss *et al.*, 2011; Laing and Maylea, 2018; Volsche, 2019; Menna *et al.*, 2019). The relationship with a pet can be especially important in circumstances in which a person feels either physically or psychologically unable to connect with others, due to stressful or traumatic experiences (Sharkin and Knox, 2003). One relationship where this may be seen is between a military veteran and their psychiatric service dog (PSD).

Military veterans' careers may lead to traumatic exposures which can contribute to Operational Stress Injury (OSI); the psychological struggles resulting from operational duties, with Post-Traumatic Stress Disorder (PTSD) being the most common form. Veterans with Operational Stress Injuries such as PTSD (Veterans Affairs Canada [VAC], 2019b) are a

*Corresponding author: Darlene.chalmers@uregina.ca

population increasingly accessing PSDs. Reported rates of PTSD among Canadian veterans range from 8 to 20% (Jin, 2017), and up to 67% (Sterniczuk and Whelan, 2016) which is generally found to be higher than among the general population (Veterans Affairs Canada [VAC], 2019a). Recently, there is emerging research indicating the benefits a PSD can bring to the lives of military veterans in Canada (Husband *et al.*, 2019; Williamson *et al.*, 2021aWilliamson *et al.*, 2021bWilliamson *et al.*, 2021b) and elsewhere (Yarborough *et al.*, 2017; McCall *et al.*, 2020).

Psychiatric service dogs (PSDs) are highly skilled dogs trained to perform specific tasks (e.g., sensing medical emergencies, waking from nightmares) for people with physical, psychiatric, sensory, or intellectual disabilities (Americans with Disabilities Act, 2010; Assistance Dogs International, n.d.; LaFollette *et al.*, 2019; Williamson *et al.*, 2021a). While these tasks are important, traditionally less attention has been paid to the importance of the human–animal bond in relation to PSDs (Dell *et al.*, 2017). The PSDs' connection with the veteran can lead to increased psychological, emotional, physical, and social benefits (Dell *et al.*, 2017; Husband *et al.*, 2019; Williamson *et al.*, 2021aWilliamson *et al.*, 2021bWilliamson *et al.*, 2021b). A study by Williamson *et al.* (2021a) explored Canadian veterans' health impacts when paired with a PSD. The authors found the veterans and their PSD experienced a strong bond that can lead to strengthening feelings of companionship, increased sense of purpose and daily routine; and perception of having someone (their PSD) who understood them, cared about them, comforted them, made them laugh, and had their back (Williamson *et al.*, 2021a).

The Government of Canada supports the accessibility of PSDs on national transportation structures (Accessible Transportation for Persons with Disabilities Regulations, 2022), but no national standards or a legal definition of PSDs exist in Canada to provide a set of agreed-upon rules, guidelines, or characteristics for the PSD industry (Canadian Foundation for Animal Assisted Support Services (CFAASS), 2020). The PSD industry in Canada varies greatly between organizations with some utilizing a for-profit business model while others are designed as non-profits or registered charities (Canadian Foundation for Animal Assisted Support Services (CFAASS), 2020). Provincially, there is variation in laws and regulations with some provinces not having any Service-Dog specific policies. For example, within existing provincial laws, requirements may include that a PSD is sourced from a recognized service dog provider or the dog has undergone evaluation for certification while other provincial laws require documentation from a medical professional outlining a person's disability (Prinold, 2021).

Ensuring animal welfare is vital to the relationship between a PSD and handler. The welfare of service dogs not only impacts the dog's well-being but also influences the quality of the human–animal bond (Glenk, 2017). PSD organizations and handlers may often face the tension between engaging PSD to achieve handlers' goals while enhancing PSD welfare (Wenthold and Savage, 2007). A number of strategies have been proposed that can enhance dog welfare and the relationship between the dog and handler such as using positive reward reinforcement in training service dogs (Hiby *et al.*, 2004); spending time bonding through grooming, practicing commands, and having off-duty activities together (Wenthold and Savage, 2007); and maintaining awareness of the dog's stress-associated behaviours and environmental factors which may trigger stress-associated behaviours (Glenk, 2017; Ng, 2021). Animal welfare also includes the importance of ongoing veterinary care where veterinarians can be an important resource especially with the preparation of an animal's retirement or death (Shubert, 2012). Preparation should also include evaluation of the welfare of the dog by the PSD organization or veterinarian as well as the handler to determine when it is time for retirement or letting go (Ng, 2021). Finally, the handler is also recommended to be prepared for the separation from the dog through retirement or death. However, limited attention has been given to the experience of the handler when arranging for or unexpectedly faced with their service dog's retirement or death.

While this study does not focus on veterans' PTSD and PTSD symptoms specifically, it does highlight that this population is increasingly accessing PSDs often for the benefits that come from dogs that are task trained to meet a veteran's unique needs. Deep and enduring bonds may form between service dog team members that may prove difficult when the bond is severed with the loss of the service dog due to death. The loss of the service dog may be exacerbated further given the utility of the dog in the day to day functioning of the veteran (Schneider, 2005). Because PSDs can provide impactful social, psychological, emotional and physical benefits (Yarborough *et al.*, 2017; Husband *et al.*, 2019; Williamson *et al.*, 2021a), there is likewise a need to understand the challenges a veteran may experience when their PSD retires or dies. Yet a significant dearth of literature exists on the grief experiences of veterans related to the loss of their PSDs.

Grief and Loss

Grief has be defined as the internal, subjective experience of the loss whereas mourning represents the outward expression of this grief through public actions (PDQ Supportive and Palliative Care Editorial Board, 2020). When grief moves from a natural painful response to a more complex experience with long term challenges around intrusive negative thoughts and significant negative health effects, a person may experience complicated grief, otherwise known as prolonged grief (Cohen and Clark, 2019; Messam and Hart, 2019).

Given the reality that animal lives are shorter than human lives, it is inevitable that one will lose a pet and may grieve this loss. Although some researchers have frequently stressed that there are significant differences in grief at the loss of a human companion when compared to the loss of animals, the grief experienced by the latter cannot be discounted, and for some, may be more distressing than the loss of a family member (Weisman, 1995; Morley and Fook, 2005; Field *et al.*, 2009; Laing and Maylea, 2018; Lavorgna and Hutton, 2019). The limited literature on grief associated with the loss of an assistant animal has focused on the grief experienced at the loss of a Guide Dog for the visually impaired (Nicholson *et al.*, 1995; Schneider, 2005; Fischler, 2014) and service dogs for people with physical or hearing disabilities (Kogan *et al.*, 2021) and has not explored the loss of a PSD. When it comes to the loss of assistance dogs, such as a Guide Dog, it is recognized that the loss of the dog is not just the loss of a companion. Losing an assistance animal is also the loss of a caregiver-bond because not only does the human care for the dog, but the dog must care for the human's functional needs and thus is integral to their day-to-day functioning (Kwong and Bartholomew, 2011; Cohen and Clark, 2019).

Literature on the loss of a companion and assistance animals frequently acknowledges the concept of disenfranchised grief (Chur-Hansen, 2010; Huggard, 2014; Packman *et al.*, 2014; Spain *et al.*, 2019). Disenfranchised grief refers to grief that cannot be openly acknowledged due to social constraints by the person's social group or wider society (Doka, 1989; Huggard, 2014; Thomas, 2014). Such grief is particularly pronounced in individuals who have lost an animal as some in society consider animal-human relationships to be of lesser value in comparison to human relations; therefore, grief for such a loss is illegitimate and may even be ridiculed (Cohen and Clark, 2019; Spain *et al.*, 2019). Literature on grief also includes the concept of anticipatory or premature grief. This form of grief can be experienced by those who lose an animal marked by the gradual letting go due to progressive illness or the need for euthanasia and may include feelings of guilt if euthanasia is utilized (Thomas, 2014; Laing and Maylea, 2018; Cohen and Clark, 2019). In some cases, anticipatory grief and disenfranchised grief may be simultaneously experienced by an individual.

Although more research is needed in the area of grief after the loss of a PSD, grief experienced by individuals who have lost an animal cannot be discounted and can have lasting impacts on the health and well-being of those affected (Cohen and Clark, 2019; Fine, 2019). Veterans with PSDs are often connected to a variety of service providers such as service dog organizations or mental health professionals. The role of these providers will be important in the recovery process from grief associated with the loss of a PSD. It is crucial that these providers understand the realities of grief from this type of loss, legitimize the emotions felt by their patients, and offer sufficient support for their healing journey (Risley-Curtiss *et al.*, 2011; Cordaro, 2012; Morris, 2016; Fine, 2019; Kogan *et al.*, 2021).

This exploratory qualitative study focused on the unique relationship between veterans with PTSD and their PSDs and the grief (including anticipatory and disenfranchised) experienced due to the loss of their PSD. Grief may be experienced when a PSD is lost through retirement, return of the dog to the issuing service dog organization, or through anticipated or unanticipated death. The study is significant as understanding the grief experience among potentially vulnerable populations such as veterans living with PTSD will contribute to the consideration and future development of practices and policies for service dog organizations and health care providers in the provision of appropriate mental health supports following such an event.

Methods

The purpose of this study was to highlight the impact of PSDs' loss and the accompanying experiences of grief that can impact on veterans' functioning and wellbeing, and the importance of this understanding for PSD organizations, mental health care providers, and veterans themselves. The aims of the study were to understand how grief was experienced by the participants including how the loss of the animal impacted their daily functioning and willingness to consider a PSD in the future.

Given the dearth of literature in this area, a qualitative approach was used for the purpose of gathering rich descriptive data where little is known about an area of study (Braun and Clarke, 2013). This approach is useful in documenting first-hand accounts in the voice of those with lived experience of a phenomenon through one-on-one, individual interviews (Creswell and Poth, 2018). Approval for the study was obtained from the University of Regina Research Ethics Board. Although animal research ethics was not required, this study adhered to the Canadian Council on Animal Care guidelines and principles for humane animal use.

Data Collection

Participants were recruited through two gatekeepers located in Saskatchewan and Ontario. The two gatekeepers, both veterans, were directly involved with a Canadian veteran-run service dog organization. The organization has contacts and relationships with veteran personnel across Canada. The participant inclusion criteria included: currently or previously serving in the military; experienced the loss of their service dog in the past five years prior to the start of the study; connected with mental health supports in their community; and willing to voluntarily participate in the study. Given the potential risk of psychological or emotional harm or discomfort due to the topic, gatekeepers were well known to the participants and also agreed to provide a support role following the interview, if needed. Gatekeepers were emailed a poster regarding the study and were asked to share this information with potential participants. Interested participants were advised to contact Chalmers directly either by phone or email. Study information was shared, including their role, consent, and withdrawal procedures, and then a time was scheduled for an individual interview via telephone, in person, or Skype.

Participants were emailed a consent form prior to the interview. The consent form was reviewed again with the participants at the time of the interview. Four participants (2 women and 2 men) agreed to participate. An open-ended semi-structured interview guide was used to complete the interviews which were audio-recorded lasting between 45 and 90 min. Participants were given a $50.00 honorarium for their involvement. All interviews were completed by Chalmers between June and November, 2018.

Data Analysis

A professional transcriptionist transcribed the interviews and de-identified the transcripts to protect the confidentiality of the participants. Data analysis was completed manually by Ru using inductive thematic analysis based on the guidelines of Braun and Clarke (2013) where the coder first familiarized themselves with the data by reading through all the transcripts, determined initial codes, searched and then reviewed themes. Tables were used to sort, manage and store segments of text and the identification of preliminary themes. A second level of coding was done independently by Gibson and Ru that provided further distillation of the codes and refinement of emerging themes. Both coders then reviewed the data and reached consensus in the analysis of the final themes. Gibson, Chalmers, and Ru reviewed the themes and their descriptions and all contributed to the development of the grief cycle model. Member checking was completed with two participants who validated the summary of the findings and the grief cycle model.

A total of four themes emerged with eleven corresponding sub-themes. The themes are: development of a bond with a PSD; grief response following the loss of the PSD; stage of coping and healing; and a transitional period. These themes and their accompanying sub-themes are described in detail in the findings section.

Participants

Four veterans (n=2 women; n=2 men) who had lost their PSD were interviewed on their bond and relationship with their PSD and how the loss impacted them. All participants had lost at least one PSD. One participant had lost two PSDs to death while another participant who had lost two PSDs had experienced grief when one died but also when they had to return another dog back to the service dog organization. In total, six dogs were discussed (see Table 17.1). Of the six dogs, four had died from euthanasia, one in a traumatic incident, and one was returned to the service dog organization due to behavioural issues. The length of time spent with their PSD before the loss varied between participants from one year to up to ten years.

Each participant began working with a PSD to help manage their PTSD symptoms, and other physical conditions (e.g. cardiovascular conditions, musculoskeletal injury). Participants reported PTSD symptoms that included depression, nightmares and flashbacks, anxiety, panic attacks, and self-isolation (barely leaving home). Participant 2 and Participant 3 reported medication dependence, and Participant 3 also had a history of excessive alcohol use. The impact of their medical conditions on their quality of life was described to be debilitating and therefore prompted the veterans to partner with their PSDs.

Results

The participant interviews yielded four themes which underscore the veterans' experiences and the impacts of their grief at the loss of their PSD. The first theme, *bond with a psychiatric service dog* is described as the bond participants established with their PSD and which led to increased health benefits and quality of life for the veteran. Unfortunately, this bond and its benefits were interrupted by the loss of the PSD. The second theme, *grief response following the loss of a PSD*, was shared by all participants and captures the impact of the grief on the veterans' lives, the impact the loss had on their functioning, and the grief experienced throughout the

Table 17.1. Participant information and psychiatric service dog relationships.

Participant number & gender	Service dog	When PSD was acquired	Type of loss	Age of the PSD when loss happened	Reason for PSD loss
1 Woman	Dog A	2010	Death	6 years old	Untreatable tumor leading to euthanasia
2 Man	Dog B	–	Death	–	Traumatic accident
	Dog C	2007	Death	10 years old	Untreatable injury, euthanasia
3 Woman	Dog D	2014	Returned to Org	–	Aggressive behaviour
	Dog E	2015	Death	3.5 years old	Cancer causing death
4 Man	Dog F	2015	Death	Approximately 5 years old	Untreatable medical condition leading to euthanasia

euthanasia process. Theme three reflects the stage of coping and healing experienced by the veterans as they navigated grief and the healing process after the loss. The fourth theme, *transitional period*, captures how all participants in this study integrated and navigated the reality of a new PSD in their lives following their previous loss. The experiences of the participants' loss and grief are best described as evolving through a recursive cyclical process and represented by a constituent element stated as: 'my lifeline is gone'.

An overarching thread woven throughout this study was that participants experienced the loss of their lifeline. Because their PSDs played such an integral role in their daily functioning, their grief reflected the loss of a family pet and was further exacerbated by the sudden loss of instrumental support they previously received from their PSD. Not only were they grieving the loss of a close companion, but the veterans also experienced reduced quality of life in some domains which the PSD provided. From the participants stories a holistic model was developed that best represents their shared experiences of the loss of their PSD and how they coped and moved through their grief. The multidimensionality and complexity of their relationship with their PSD is untangled and depicted in Fig. 17.1 as a grief cycle.

The participants described how they first met their PSD and developed a bond over time. At some point thereafter, the veteran lost their PSD due to death or relinquishment, resulting in a grief response which varied between individuals in characteristics as well as duration. Over time, they began to cope and heal from the grief. The four participants all received a new PSD after the loss of their first, leading to a transitional period where they were hesitant to get the new PSD and tentative to build a bond given the grief they recently experienced. The cycle was described as fluid and interconnected and an individual could move between the stages of this model in a back-and-forth manner. The time for someone to move through the stages of this cycle is also

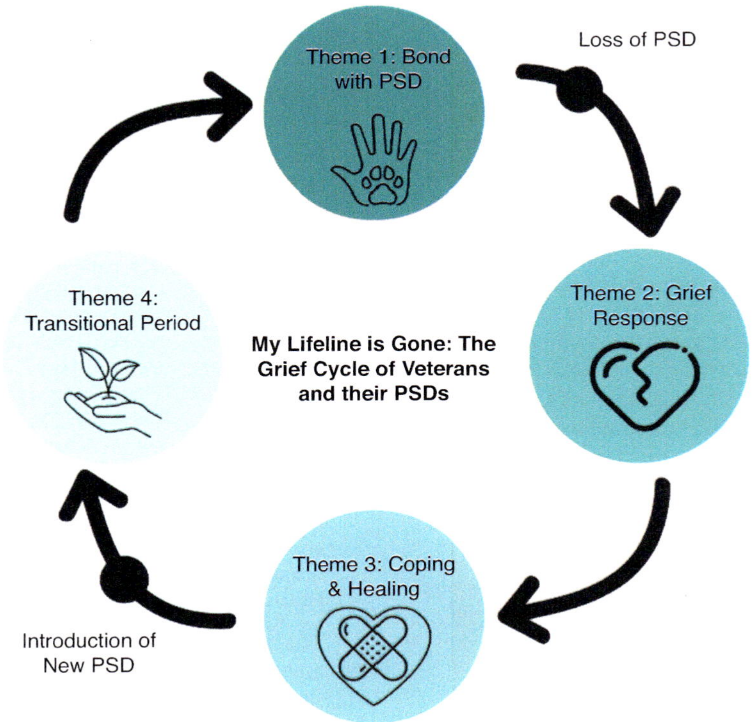

Fig. 17.1. Grief Cycle of Veterans with their PSDs and Themes

highly variable. Given the short life span of a PSD, a veteran may enter this cycle multiple times dependent on how many PSDs they have. The themes and sub-themes are explored in detail below.

Theme 1: Bond with the Psychiatric Service Dog

The first theme expressed by the veteran participants was the depth and breadth of the bond they built with their PSD. This bond took time to develop but was integral to their health and wellbeing. They shared their experiences of enhanced quality of life which they deemed due to the PSD in their life. The participants also noted that this bond was unlike other connections in their lives given the functional as well as emotional support offered by the PSD.

Sub-Theme 1: Veteran experiences of enhanced quality of life due to PSD

Living with the PSD was highly impactful for all of the participants when it came to helping them manage their PTSD symptoms and find companionship. The participants reported that they developed a close connection with their PSD and experienced benefits from having the PSD in their lives. PSDs provided functional assistance and emotional support to the veterans. As Participant 2 commented, "[Dog C] allowed me to function semi-normal." The participants spoke about how their PSD encouraged them to go outdoors and socialize, interrupted bad dreams and flashbacks, blocked other people from getting too physically close to them, provided a sense of security, and offered companionship and comfort.

> I was in a really bad dream... and [Dog A] started to push on my face. He had this thing he would push at my face, and push his tongue in and almost like French-kissing, licking my tongue, so he started to do that, and I kinda like, sat up and held him again. ... He didn't totally, like wake me up as he does, but he woke me up by doing these little, on my face, and I knew who he was and I just cuddled back to sleep. (Participant 1)

Dog C reportedly supported the veteran by alerting him to forthcoming anxiety and panic attacks before negative side effects occurred:

> He knew it was gonna happen before me. And with diabetes and all that they can do blood smell when the sugars are up, they will react. But with PTSD, there is no way you can train a dog, that the dog knows, you know I don't know how they do it. I can't explain it. But [Dog C] would go, and he would tell me when I start to get anxious. (Participant 2)

The participants all noted that their PSD increased their quality of life and helped in coping with their PTSD symptoms. In this way, the PSDs acted as companion animals but also brought a level of functionality to the lives of the veterans.

Sub-Theme 2: A unique bond

PSDs brought positive changes to the veterans' lives, and the bond between the veterans and their PSDs appeared to be strong and unique compared to other animal bonds in their lives. Participant 4 shared the traumatic past of [Dog F], and they had a connection based on "a similar shared life experience".

> So based on that I understood her trauma and she understood mine and this is my heart speaking. [Previous dog] was my primary service dog, absolutely, but the connection of the dog to the person like 100% there for me and me for her was [Dog F]. Each time I had an episode, each time I was depressed, one time I even went and put a hammock in the backwoods that is like their run, the only dog that stayed with me for hours in the rain, laying down beside me on the ground with her. All the others [Dog name], [Dog name], all of them were, it is raining you know, and covered up. [Dog F] was there looking at me and I was talking to her and she was looking at me like she was listening and that is one moment if you want. It was like all the time, each time I was crying, I had a moment, an episode if she was there she was there for me. (Participant 4)

The bond was often so deep between the PSD and the veteran that the PSD was treated as a family member or a child:

> This is the kind of bond I had with [Dog C]. To me, I say [I'm his] dad, because he's one of

> my kids. He's as important to me as one of my children. (Participant 2)

Participant 2 believed that it was because of the deep bond that Dog C could sense his anxiety and panic attacks. The bond between Participant 2 and Dog C was reportedly so deep that Participant 2 felt he could not live without Dog C:

> The bond became such that, and don't ask me how, the bond became such a way that with my problem, my condition, or disease whatever you want to call it, he knew it was gonna happen before me.... So, my bond with the dog, became to a point where, I will be honest, I can't live without him. It's such a strong bond that like, you don't want to be back the way I used to be. And without the dog, I know that's what would what happen to me. (Participant 2)

The veterans acknowledged that their deep bond with their PSDs made their loss more devastating and they were impacted significantly. The next section will explore participants' experiences of loss, including their grief responses, length of grief, as well as overall impact on their well-being.

Theme 2: Grief Responses After the Loss of PSD

The second theme from the interviews reflected the grief the participants felt when their PSD passed away or was relinquished. The participants provided insight into how they experienced grief and the pain associated with the loss of their PSD. Further, the loss of their PSD led to reduced daily functioning given the PSD provided many functional benefits to the participants. Finally, some of the participants described a unique grief experience given their decision to euthanize their PSDs.

Sub-Theme 1: Impact of grief

All participants described their grief over the loss of their PSD as intense and highly impactful on their day-to-day lives. Participants' grief responses included being sad, upset, anxious, a loss of interest in activities, numbness, as well as a sense of uncertainty, fear, and pain. The first PSD of Participant 3 was returned to the service dog organization due to unmanageable aggressive behaviors. After the dog was relinquished, Participant 3 "cried, freaked out" and it felt like "the end of the world".

Participant 4 was still processing the loss of [Dog F], and he tried to avoid looking at photos of them which aroused sadness. Participant 4 compared the loss of his dog with the loss of a friend.

> Well, you are getting to know me. I am a hardcore soldier and I know I have feelings right now, but I am containing a lot because you are not supposed to show feelings, right, and especially with special forces. So I am a great container and I contain my emotions. But yes no joke, I was crying like a baby, like incontrollable cry for a few days so at least that got out but I am still processing.... It was the same loss as losing a friend that committed suicide or I lost in combat. (Participant 4)

As the veterans relied on their PSD for daily functioning, loss of the dog evoked a sense of uncertainty and fear of the future.

> [T]here's grief but there's also the, what's gonna happen now? ... Definitely, a lot of fear, because what is gonna happen? The first thing I think of, they gonna put me on, you know this medicine again. And then the other thing, I think, of is, I'm gonna lose my wife over this. And then the other thing is, I'm gonna lose my friends over this. (Participant 2)

During the interviews, all the participants became emotional (e.g., crying, difficulty speaking, etc.) when talking about their lost PSDs, which signified the intensity of grief and deep connection between participants and their PSDs. This emotional response indicated a loss of a companion but also seemed to represent the loss of the accustomed day to day living the veteran had experienced with their PSD.

Sub-Theme 2: Loss of PSD's influence on functioning

Participants not only experienced grief over the loss of their PSD, as many companion animal owners do, but their functioning and everyday life were also impacted by the loss.

> I haven't slept normal nights since I lost [Dog E]. When I would start having a nightmare or a flashback, I would be lying down, and [Dog E] would lick me and wake me up so I would fall back asleep. But since [Dog E] passed, I just had to have meds adjusted last Saturday because I have a lot of issues with flashbacks and nightmares at night. So that was a big one the fact that I could sleep with her I was not as likely to get depressed and less conflicted with it. (Participant 3)

The impact of the loss of their PSD was devastating for the participants not only because they lost a friend but also a key support in their life that allowed them to function day to day. For the participants, not having their PSD impacted their ability to go out in public, access other supports, and maintain a routine. As Participant 2 shared, "It's your, that family member, that child of yours, I know it's a dog but it's your child, and your lifeline is gone." The participants shared the immense impact the loss of their PSD had on their emotional state and also their ability to manage their PTSD symptoms. The loss of the PSD reflects the loss of a companion animal and the accompanying grief was also experienced with the fear of the potential resurgence of PTSD symptoms related to the loss of their PSD.

Sub-Theme 3: Grief and euthanasia

Among the six PSDs, dogs A, C, and F were diagnosed with untreatable painful illnesses. Participants, therefore, had to make a decision on euthanasia and seemed to experience grief leading up to and after the loss of their PSD.

> So, everything combined, especially the aggression and ramping up because of the pain, irritability and all that stuff, so I said that is it. So we took an appointment and four days later she was gone. So, I had Friday, Saturday, Sunday, Monday with her and I cried those whole four days and I spent a lot of time with her. (Participant 4)

Given all the assistance the PSDs provided to the veterans and their bond, the participants shared that they cared deeply about their PSD's quality of life. The care of the dogs' general well-being and worry about dogs feeling pain played a crucial role in making a decision on euthanasia.

> I said to my wife and son, 'you guys take [Dog C] into the vet, and I wanna know what the vet says, and if he's in pain which I know he is, you put him down. And they took him into the vet, and my wife said, the first thing she said was your dog is in tremendous pain. And then [spouse] said put him down. And that was, you know, there was no more to it. (Participant 2)

When asked if Participant 4 felt guilty to euthanize [Dog F], Participant 4 answered, "No," and further explained, "because I knew she was suffering because of the infection and because I could hear it in her voice or the way she was vocalizing. I could see it in her demeanor and physical aspects so I knew it was the right time." These participant experiences highlight the unique bond held between the veterans and their PSD. The PSDs represent more than a treatment tool and act also as a companion in the lives of the veterans.

Theme 3: Coping and Healing

After experiencing loss, the participants utilized many strategies to cope with their grief and begin to heal. A key strategy was recalling fond memories and reminiscing about the PSD and their bond. Beyond this, participants highlighted the impacts of the supports of family and friends as they grieved, but ultimately felt there was a significant lack of formal supports for them to support their healing process.

Sub-Theme 1: Reminiscing about the PSD

According to the participants' descriptions, the bond between bereaved veterans and their deceased or relinquished PSDs seemed to continue long after they were gone. Participants held on to their PSDs' photos and possessions and reminisced about the lost dogs through storytelling and reliving positive memories. For example, Participant 1 had a pillow filled with [Dog A]'s fur, and Participant 2 and Participant 3 kept their PSDs' old vests. When asking Participant 4 how to cope with the loss, he answered, "Looking at her balls, for example, her toys and then the picture will come in, I am pretty sure."

Participant 1 also had a dream about [Dog A], and the dream made her feel better and helped her accept the new PSD. This dream acted as a means to remember her dog and also process some of her grief. She believed in reincarceration and believed she would be reunited with [Dog A] eventually:

> I went to bed one night and I had a dream about [Dog A]. In my dream, I remember I had [Dog A] in my arm and I was running, and [spouse] said I kept saying "no, not [Dog A], it's okay". And I remember [Dog A] said in my dream, "I'm not dead mommy." And I said "No you're not dead. I will protect you." And I woke up the next morning, and I told [spouse] and she said, "I know I heard you". And I said I think I feel okay. And then that afternoon, I was playing with [new PSD]. He has a little ball, he does what he always does, throws it in the air. Then I thought "you are beautiful!" And that was it! (Participant 1)

Memories played a vital role in the participants' journey through grief. They often remarked how their PSD was still with them in spirit and they used physical objects or storytelling to remember their bond. The participants also noted how important they felt it was to share these stories with others, including this research project and stated that by sharing their stories they were able to memorialize and pay tribute to their PSD.

Sub-Theme 2: Familial and friendship supports

Participants received support and comfort from their family members and friends, which helped them cope with the loss. For example, Participant 4 received supportive calls and texts from his family. When asking if support from family was helpful, Participant 4 agreed: "Word got around in the family so they all either called or texted... I knew I had support yes." Support from others comforted participants and represented the acknowledgment of the grief and recognition of the strong bond between participants and their PSD. Participant 4 went on to explain: "I don't think people would say [get over it] because they know me and they know me with dogs so I don't think they would go there."

Overarchingly, the participants felt they needed to cope with the loss by themselves: "I just, kinda went through [the grief] myself" (Participant 1).

Sub-Theme 3: Lack of formal support

Although participants received support from family and friends, they experienced an overall lack of support from service providers. When asked if they received support from other health and wellness providers, the participants gave a negative answer. The participants shared their frustration by this. As shared by Participant 2, "There's nothing there [for] when you lose your service dog. There's absolutely nobody other than your immediate family." When asked if they received any support, Participant 1 expressed: "No, no. Just ask how I was doing but ....

I'm doing good, and 'pick another dog.' And that was it."

Generally, there was a lack of knowledge on the part of the service providers of the important role of PSDs in veterans' lives and the importance of the human–animal bond.

Participant 1 commented that staff in the service dog organization seemed not to talk about her past PSD because they were afraid to have this conversation: "I think people were afraid to start you know. It was more like, 'Hi, how you're doing", 'Doing okay', and that was it. Stop talking to you.' Talking with others about the lost PSD could be a meaningful way to support the veterans and help them accept the loss. Participant 1 tried to have a conversation with and provided support to another person who lost his PSD because she had the same experience and understood the feeling.

> I think it would have been nice, if you had somebody that would sit down and talk to you. We had a guy, I did take him out to eat and his dog was poisoned and passed on. And when I found out through... He caught me... and told me he lost his dog. So, couple of days later, I went out and I recognized him and said, "how're you doing, and everything,' and we talked about it, and just checking in with them, because I know how I felt. So, I just kept checking in. Now he has a new dog and he's doing better with his dog. But, if there had been something like that [peer support]. I didn't do it for any other reason except for, I know how I felt. So, I thought if he doesn't feel that way, he's gonna tell me, "hey [Participant 1] I'm fine." But, if he does, he's gonna open up and talk about it. And I think he might, because he needs that. Because I needed that. I think it would be a good idea because, it's nice to be able to sit down and tell someone the story of [Dog A], and his character. And you know it makes some part of you feel better. And I think it's easier to like, not like let go, but to accept. (Participant 1)

These participant experiences highlight the unique relationship between the veteran and their PSD and how few others are able to understand. The participants noted that only others who had lost a PSD could truly understand the impact of the loss which created challenges in being able to receive adequate support.

Theme 4: Transitional Period

All of the participants brought a new PSD into their life after the death or relinquishment of their PSD. The process of accepting a new PSD into their lives and hearts highlights this.

Before the participants were able to build a strong bond with their new PSD, they had to traverse a transitional period. This period included expressions that the participants needed companionship through their grief, time was required to build a bond with a new PSD, and the transition to a new PSD was best when it came from within the veteran rather than being forced from an outside source.

Sub-Theme 1: Need for companionship

All participants shared it would have been helpful during the grief process if there were an animal companion available to them while they were grieving. In many instances, the veterans noted that their PSD was able to give support and companionship beyond what humans were able or willing to provide. A dog companion could provide support to participants as they went through the loss of their previous PSDs, perhaps reducing some of the impacts of experiencing this grief alone. As shared by Participant 4:

> I am well peer supported by the dogs and people obviously. I mean from the time that she passed away to [now] I was well surrounded with dogs.... [B]ut I think what I want to mention is I am kind of lucky in a way to have had other service dogs around me. I wouldn't want to imagine how it would be for someone who has one dog and it is their service dog because I imagine the same connection. But why I say I was lucky was because I had these dogs to touch and so maybe I don't know when someone loses their dog... maybe we should have, someone who is on their own have [a dog] there with them. (Participant 4)

Participant 2 had another PSD and started the training process before [Dog C] passed away. The new PSD distracted Participant 2's attention from the loss. The presence and companionship of the dog helped Participant 2 go through the transitional period.

> When I had to put [Dog C] down, [new PSD] was only 3 months old. So, the only thankful thing that I had, we had already started [new PSD]'s 12-week training point. So, again my whole focus, you know there's a couple of weeks, I was back on my meds. It was a lot stronger, you know things like that, for sleep. It was just all screwed up like totally. And the only out I had was [new PSD]. I was training him as much as I could... so, basically, my whole focus went on [new PSD]. (Participant 2)

The participants expressed the isolation they felt after the loss of the PSD and how having other canine companionship was helpful for them while they experienced this grief. Those living with PTSD are likely to experience isolation and the participants seemed to express that following the loss of a PSD, this isolation can greatly increase therefore supports are needed to prevent further isolation where possible.

Sub-Theme 2: It takes time to build bond with another PSD

Because participants relied on PSDs for daily functioning and emotional support, they acquired a new PSD after the loss. The deep bond between veterans and their former PSD influenced their relationship with the next PSD. It took months for the participants to move on from the grief and build a relationship with the new PSD.

> [B]ut to be honest, [New PSD] took me six, seven months, before my heart went to [New PSD]. Everybody was telling me he was beautiful. I never thought, just, I thought he was ugly. [B] ut I knew I needed a dog so I was willing to work with him and make him a partner. But it was never gonna be mine, it was just gonna be my partner.... It took me about 8 months, and my heart opened up and I'm like, "oh I love you, bud." But I couldn't let him in because I couldn't let [Dog A] out. Yeah, there was no room for both of them. (Participant 1)

Then when asking Participant 1 if she now had room in her heart for both of the service dogs, she answered, "Yeah, I do, for sure. Yeah." Participant 1 went on to say, "I think that part of me honestly, [didn't] wanna go through [the grief again].... I think it's gonna take a while."

Participant 2 felt that [Dog C] could predict their panic attacks, but his new PSD could not yet since the new dog was still young and they had not been together long. There was hope, however, that this would develop over time.

> [New PSD] is like, he's coming, but [New PSD] is not [Dog C]. I'll tell you right now that, [New PSD] has not been able to get the bond yet, he doesn't tell me when something's gonna happen. (Participant 2)

The participants' responses suggest that the change from their trained PSD to a new PSD can be difficult and frustrating. Given the deep bond they had with their previous PSD, it may be stressful to train a new PSD and not have the same level of support their previous PSD was able to provide. The emotions felt throughout the transition period may be difficult for the veteran and may require further supports from their friends, family, and support organizations.

Sub-Theme 3: Introduction of a new PSD and veteran readiness

Participants had a strong connection with their PSD, and they experienced intense sorrow and pain over the loss of their PSD. Although participants ended up acquiring another PSD, participants had negative feelings when an outside force pressured them to get a new PSD. For example, a trainer gave Participant 3 another dog shortly after she returned Dog D. It felt somewhat forced, and Participant 3 expressed a sense of betrayal, "I collapsed at the hotel and [name] picked me [up] and for me, she betrayed me, because she told me she... had already arranged a new dog and to me it was betrayal." (Participant 3)

Participants needed time to cope with the grief and go through the transitional period. It is crucial for service providers to check if veterans are ready to have a new PSD or would benefit from another dog's companionship. Therefore, veterans may be more likely to accept a new dog when they themselves make the decision, and it is not "forced" from the outside.

Discussion

The purpose of this study was to explore veterans' experiences of grief following the loss of their psychiatric service dogs. The findings from this exploratory study suggest that a cycle of grief reflects the building of a bond between the veteran and their PSD which is interrupted when the PSD passes away or is relinquished. In the case of the veteran participants in this study, grief at this loss of their dog was experienced as both losing a companion animal and also the loss of their "lifeline". This grief led to coping and healing strategies for the veterans often including reminiscing about their dog and accessing support from others. The integration of a new PSD into the veterans' lives led to a transition period before being able to develop a bond critical to a partnership. The findings from this study suggest that the grief participants experienced and the cyclical nature of this grief when multiple PSDs are part of that veterans' life, are important contributions for informing the practice of service providers working with clients with PSDs.

The reasons for the participants' grief were complex and support other research findings where losing a service animal can be devastating given that the animal provides both emotional support and vital functional day-to-day living support (Cohen and Clark, 2019; Fine, 2019). Further, grief at the loss of an animal companion can be exacerbated when the individual gives significant meaning to the animal in their life, have high levels of attachment to the animal, and are isolated, relying on the animal as a lifeline (Field *et al.*, 2009; Chur-Hansen, 2010; Cohen and Clark, 2019; Thomas, 2014; Messam and Hart, 2019; Yamamoto and Hart, 2020). In the case of veterans with PTSD, the findings from this study suggest they hold their PSD in high regard, as lifelines to the outside world, and often have a history of experiencing significant isolation due to their PTSD symptoms.

This study's findings reflect veterans' experiences of disenfranchised grief with the loss of their PSD. The participants often reported they felt they weren't supported or others simply did not understand the loss they were experiencing. This can be further detrimental to veteran health as the social norms around grief or even the perceived responses of others to their grief, may cause the veteran to grieve in isolation and feel they are "not allowed" to show outward displays of mourning (Doka, 1989; Thomas, 2014). In the case of the death of a companion animal and an assistance animal, there are no socially accepted rituals or mechanisms to grieve or mourn the loss, which can lead to further social isolation (Doka, 1989; Stewart *et al.*, 1989; Spain *et al.*, 2019). Disenfranchised grief also seems to be present in situations where the veterans in this study had to relinquish their PSD. A paucity of literature acknowledges grief when rehoming a companion animal or relinquishing an assistance animal, but the grief experienced should be acknowledged as an individual may go through challenging circumstances before ultimately relinquishing their animal (Thomas, 2014). There is a significant dearth of literature on this topic and should be explored in future research.

In instances of euthanasia, the veterans seemed to also experience anticipatory grief. Making decisions on behalf of their PSD was extremely difficult for the veterans, especially upon reflection of how much the PSD had given the veteran over their time together. Anticipatory grief can be profound and may also lead to immense feelings of guilt in having to make the decision to euthanize (Morley and Fook, 2005; Laing and Maylea, 2018). Recognizing disenfranchised and anticipatory grief is important for any and all healthcare professionals supporting veterans with PSDs.

Veterans with PSDs are often connected to a variety of service providers including service dog organizations, mental health professionals, and social workers. Education and training of these organizations and health care providers on the role PSDs is essential to supporting veterans' mental health (Johnson *et al.*, 2002). Therefore, these professionals need to understand the grief veterans are likely to experience at the loss of their PSD. Overarchingly, service providers need to reinforce the social acceptance of grief following the loss of a companion animal or PSD and provide means to affirm and validate feelings of grief to reduce the impact of their clients' grief (Stewart *et al.*, 1989; Thomas, 2014; Miller, 2021; Wilson *et al.*, 2021). Further, mental health professionals are uniquely placed to support their clients when experiencing grief and need to recognize the anthropocentric nature of acceptable grief and how their clients may not feel they are able to grief outwardly (Laing and Maylea, 2018). Miller (2021) suggests a three-tier model wherein: 1) the general population is made aware of the impacts of the loss of animals in our lives, 2) individuals at high risk of difficult grief are targeted, and 3) individualized therapies for those experiencing chronic grief. Further, professionals need to acknowledge what other factors may be influencing the grief the griever is experiencing which may include age, previous losses (human or non-human), gender, familial supports, and living situation (Stewart *et al.*, 1989; Wilson *et al.*, 2021). Health care providers also should acknowledge how they can prepare their clients for the eventual loss of their PSD. While it may be difficult, the intensity of a clients' grief can be mitigated when pre-emptive conversations are held on how they will memorialize their dog when they pass, quality of life they want their dog to experience and how this may relate to euthanasia options, and how the loss of the dog is beyond the control of the client despite their best efforts, investments, and emotions (Stewart *et al.*, 1989; Thomas, 2014; Cohen and Clark, 2019; Messam and Hart, 2019). Socially acceptable animal grief traditions have suggested the cutting of ties after a loss, but as we have seen from the veteran experiences, memorialization and memories are important to coping. The importance of continuing bonds in coping has been documented to support individuals who have lost pets and should be understood and supported by service providers (Thomas, 2014; Rémillard *et al.*, 2017; Kogan *et al.*, 2021; Wilson *et al.*, 2021).

Organizations who train and provide PSDs to veterans and other clients should also be aware of the grief their clients may experience at the loss or relinquishment of their PSD. These organizations play a vital role in communicating with and supplying access to PSDs and may become a support in their clients' grief. It is therefore important for service dog organizations to recognize their role in supporting their clients and how they can support the memorialization process, continuing bonds, and recognition of the unique form of loss that is the death or relinquishment of a PSD (Johnson *et al.*, 2002; Wenthold and Savage, 2007; Miller, 2021; Wilson *et al.*, 2021).

The participants of this study suggested the integration of animal supports after a loss, especially for individuals who did not have other pets in their home. The stressful nature of a pet death can be somewhat mitigated by the introduction of a new pet and the support an animal companion can provide which is often different from human supports (Stewart *et al.*, 1989). Service providers, and service dog organizations in particular, should explore the options of dog fostering or temporary companion dogs to stay with clients as they grieve. While this is an exploratory study, the authors of this study acknowledge there is a need to conduct more research to better understand how much time is required before the introduction of another animal into the household (Chur-Hansen, 2010).

Limitations

Given the small sample size, the qualitative findings from this study may not be generalizable to a larger population. However, this study acts as an important contribution given the paucity of literature available on veterans' experiences of grief associated with the loss of their psychiatric service dog. Future research should continue to explore the unique aspects and forms of grief experienced by those who have a PSD.

The current literature suggests grief at the loss of a companion animal appears to be experienced differently between men and women (Wrobel and Dye, 2003; Chur-Hansen, 2010; Messam and Hart, 2019). However, gender-based differences in the grief experienced by the participants could not be derived due to the small sample size nor was the intent. Future research should consider gender differences and the social norms associated with gender and grieving processes related to the loss of PSDs (Wrobel and Dye, 2003; Carper *et al.*, 2016; Packman *et al.*, 2016).

Given the duration of grief was not mentioned by participants, we are unable to assess if the grief experienced by the participants could be considered prolonged grief (Lund, 2020). Length of grief was not part of this study but may be important in future research to better understand how the grief is being experienced, when professional interventions should take place, and other unique aspects around the loss of a PSD.

The participants of this project were all Caucasian, so this paper was unable to explore the possible grief responses of those with other cultures or identities. Grief can be experienced and lost loved ones can be mourned differently in different cultural and identity groups (Doka, 2014; Messam and Hart, 2019; Cohen and Clark, 2019). Future research should consider the impact culture plays on grief and experiences of loss for veterans with PSDs.

Conclusion

Little research exists on the experiences of veterans with PTSD when they lose their psychiatric service dog. This exploratory study suggests that veterans experience significant grief at the loss of their PSD and this can be compounded by disenfranchised and anticipatory grief. The grief experienced by the participants in this study was a reflection of the depth of the human–animal bond they shared with their PSD and the lifeline the PSD represented for the veterans to carry on with their lives and access to the outside world. The PSD acted as an emotional and functional support; therefore, the loss was complex and impacts multiple realms of the veterans' lives. All veterans acknowledged a lack of support for them while they experienced this grief, suggesting a dire need for healthcare provider and service dog organization supports to better understand and support veterans with PTSD as they experience grief from the loss of their PSD.

Acknowledgements

We would like to acknowledge the courage of our participants for sharing their stories with us and reviewing our manuscript. Without you, this article would not be possible. We would also like to thank Linzi Williamson, PhD for her review of this work.

Conflict of Interest

We have no known conflicts of interest to disclose.

References

Accessible Transportation for Persons with Disabilities Regulations (2022) Government of Canada. Available at: https://laws-lois.justice.gc.ca/PDF/SOR-2019-244.pdf

Americans with Disabilities Act (2010) ADA 2010 Revised Requirements: Service Animals. Available at: https://www.ada.gov/service_animals_2010.htm

Assistance Dogs International (n.d.) Terms & Definitions. Available at: https://assistancedogsinternational.org/resources/adi-terms-definitions/ (accessed 18 June 2021).

Braun, V. and Clarke, V. (2013) Successful qualitative research: A practical guide for beginners. In: *Successful Qualitative Research a Practical Guide for Beginners (First)*. SAGE Publications. Available at: http://www.uk.sagepub.com/books/Book233059

Canadian Foundation for Animal Assisted Support Services (CFAASS) (2020) A Canadian service dog industry and marketplace study: Unleashing potential phase I. Available at: https://www.cf4aass.org/uploads/1/8/3/2/18329873/cnd_service_dog_industry_study_nov_2 020.pdf

Carper, T.L., Bartone, A.S. and Petty, F.C. (2016) Animal companions and military veterans: How dogs can help america's heroes. In: Blazina, C. and Kogan, L. (eds) *Men and Their Dogs: A New Understanding of Man's Best Friend*. Springer International Publishing, pp. 195–214. Available at: https://doi.org/10.1007/978-3-319-30097-9_10

Chur-Hansen, A. (2010) Grief and bereavement issues and the loss of a companion animal: People living with a companion animal, owners of livestock, and animal support workers. *Clinical Psychologist* 14(1), 14–21. DOI: 10.1080/13284201003662800.

Cohen, S. and Clark, A. (2019) Loss, grief, and bereavement in the context of human-animal relationships. In: Philip Tedeschi, M.A., Foreword, J. and Perry, B.D. (eds) *Transforming Trauma: Resilience and Healing through Our Connections with Animals*. Purdue University Press, pp. 395–422.

Cordaro, M. (2012) Pet loss and disenfranchised grief: Implications for mental health counseling practice. *Journal of Mental Health Counseling* 34(4), 283–294. DOI: 10.17744/mehc.34.4.41q0248450t98072.

Creswell, J.W. and Poth, C.N. (2018) *Qualitative Inquiry and Research Design Choosing among Five Approaches*, 4th edn. SAGE Publications Inc.

Dell, C.A., Arratoon, C., Lapointe, M. and Lohnes, C. (2017) Impact of service dogs for veterans with PTSD and substance abuse. *Canadian Vet Magazine* 12.

Doka, K.J. (2014) Disenfranchised grief in historical and cultural perspective. In: *Handbook of Bereavement Research and Practice: Advances in Theory and Intervention*. American Psychological Association. DOI: 10.1037/14498-011.

Doka, K.J. (1989) Disenfranchised grief. In: Doka, K.J. (ed.) *Disenfranchised Grief: Recongizing Hidden Sorrow*, Vol. 18. Lexington Books, pp. 3–12.

Field, N.P., Orsini, L., Gavish, R. and Packman, W. (2009) Role of attachment in response to pet loss. *Death Studies* 33(4), 334–355. DOI: 10.1080/07481180802705783.

Fine, A.H. (2019) The human-animal bond over the lifespan: A primer for mental health professionals. In: Kogan, L. and Blazina, C. (eds) *Clinician's Guide to Treating Companion Animal Issues*. Elsevier, pp. 2–20. DOI: 10.1016/C2016-0-04244-4.

Fischler, B. (2014) What Happens to Guide Dogs When They Retire? Dogster. Available at: https://www.dogster.com/lifestyle/guide-service-dogs-what-happens-retire

Glenk, L.M. (2017) Current perspectives on therapy dog welfare in animal-assisted interventions. *Animals* 7(2). DOI: 10.3390/ani7020007.

Hiby, E.F., Rooney, N.J. and Bradshaw, J.W.S. (2004) Dog training methods: their use, effectiveness and interaction with behaviour and welfare. *Animal Welfare* 13(1), 63–39.

Huggard, P.D. (2014) Caring for the carers: Compassion fatigue and disenfranchised grief. *The Importance of People* 67–71. Available at: www.proqol.org

Human Animal Bond Research Institute (2021) What is the Human-Animal Bond? Available at: https://habri.org/about/

Husband, A., Ahmed, A. and Dell, C.A. (2019) An exploratory case study of the impact of psychiatric service dogs on problematic substance use among PTSD-diagnosed veterans 25(2), 113–117. DOI: 10.1080/14659891.2019.1664663.

Jin, S. (2017) The effect of medical cannabis on alcohol and tobacco use in veterans with post-traumatic stress disorder (PTSD). *Journal of Pain Management* 24, 422–440. Available at: https://www.researchgate.net/publication/324088904_The_effect_of_medical_cannabis_on_alcohol_and_tobacco_use_in_veterans_with_post-traumatic_stress_disorder_PTSD

Johnson, R.A., Odendaal, J.S. and Meadows, R.L. (2002) Animal-assisted interventions research issues and answers. *Western Journal of Nursing Research* 24, 422–440.

Kogan, L.R., Packman, W., Currin-McCulloch, J., Bussolari, C. and Erdman, P. (2021) The loss of a service dog through death or retirement: Experiences and impact on partners. *Illness Crisis and Loss*. DOI: 10.1177/10541373211054168.

Kwong, M.J. and Bartholomew, K. (2011) "Not just a dog": An attachment perspective on relationships with assistance dogs. *Attachment and Human Development* 13(5), 421–436. DOI: 10.1080/14616734.2011.584410.

LaFollette, M.R., Rodriguez, K.E., Ogata, N. and O'Haire, M.E. (2019) Military veterans and their PTSD service dogs: associations between training methods, PTSD severity, dog behavior, and the human-animal bond. *Frontiers in Veterinary Science* 6(FEB), 23. DOI: 10.3389/fvets.2019.00023.

Laing, M. and Maylea, C. (2018) They burn brightly, but only for a short time": The role of social workers in companion animal grief and loss. *Anthrozoos* 31(2), 221–232. DOI: 10.1080/08927936.2018.1434062.

Lavorgna, B.F. and Hutton, V.E. (2019) Grief severity: A comparison between human and companion animal death. *Death Studies* 43(8), 521–526. DOI: 10.1080/07481187.2018.1491485.

Lund, P.C. (2020) Deconstructing grief: A sociological analysis of prolong grief disorder. *Social Theory & Health*. DOI: 10.1057/s41285-020-00135-z.

McCall, C.E., Rodrigues, K.E., MacDermid Wadsworth, S.M., Meis, L.A. and O'Haire, M.E. (2020) Effects of psychiatric service dogs on quality of life and relationship functioning in military-connected couples. *Military Behavioral Health* 8(4), 410–423. https://doi.org/21635781.2020.1825243.

Menna, L.F., Santaniello, A., Todisco, M., Amato, A., Borrelli, L. *et al.* (2019) The human-animal relationship as the focus of animal-assisted interventions: A one health approach. *International Journal of Environmental Research and Public Health* 16, 19. DOI: 10.3390/ijerph16193660.

Messam, L.L.M. and Hart, L.A. (2019) Persons experiencing prolonged grief after the loss of a pet. In: Kogan, L. and Blazine, C. (eds) *Clinician's Guide to Treating Companion Animal Issues*. Elsevier, pp. 267–280. DOI: 10.1016/b978-0-12-812962-3.00015-0.

Miller, T. (2021, Sept 29) Grief After the Loss of a Pet: A Three Tier Model. Available at: https://www.youtube.com/watch?v=gJKP5zIwPpI&ab_channel=LoriKogan

Morley, C. and Fook, J. (2005) The importance of pet loss and some implications for services. *Mortality* 10(2), 127–143. DOI: 10.1080/13576270412331329849.

Morris, P. (2016) Managing pet owners' guilt and grief in veterinary euthanasia encounters. *Journal of Contemporary Ethnography* 41(3), 337–365. DOI: 10.1177/0891241611435099.
Ng, Z. (2021) Strategies to assessing and enhancing animal welfare in animal-assisted interventions. In: *The Welfare of Animals in Animal-Assisted Interventions*. DOI: 10.1007/978-3-030-69587-3_6.
Nicholson, J., Kemp-Wheeler, S. and Griffiths, D. (1995) Distress arising from the end of a guide dog partnership. *Anthrozoös* 8(2), 100–110. DOI: 10.2752/089279395787156419.
Packman, W., Carmack, B.J., Katz, R., Carlos, F., Thérapeute, T. *et al.* (2014) Online survey as empathic bridging for the disenfranchised grief of pet loss. *Omega (United States)* 69(4), 333–356. DOI: 10.2190/OM.69.4.a.
Packman, W., Bussolari, C., Katz, R. and Carmack, B.J. (2016) Continuing bonds research with animal companions: Implications for men grieving the loss of a dog. In: Blazina, C. and Kogan, L. (eds) *Men and Their Dogs: A New Understanding of Man's Best Friend*. Springer International Publishing, pp. 303–320. DOI: 10.1007/978-3-319-30097-9_15.
PDQ Supportive and Palliative Care Editorial Board (2020) Grief, Bereavement, and Coping With Loss (PDQ®). PDQ Cancer Information Summaries. Available at: https://www.ncbi.nlm.nih.gov/books/NBK66052/
Prinold, H. (2021) Considerations for the Use and Training of Service Dogs in Canada: Information for Dog Trainers and People with Disabilities, Including Their Support Teams and Service/Care Providers. Available at: https://drive.google.com/file/d/1nYFxT-ikdxdWwiBqmhsNEyT5f4Y9WTcf/view
Rémillard, L.W., Meehan, M.P., Kelton, D.F. and Coe, J.B. (2017) Exploring the grief experience among callers to a pet loss support hotline. *Anthrozoos* 30(1), 149–161. DOI: 10.1080/08927936.2017.1270600.
Risley-Curtiss, C., Holley, L.C. and Kodiene, S. (2011) "They're there for you": Men's relationships with companion animals. In: *Families in Society*, Vol. 4. SAGE Publications, CA, Los Angeles, pp. 412–418. DOI: 10.1606/1044-3894.4152.
Schneider, K.S. (2005) The winding valley of grief: When a dog guide retires or dies. *Journal of Visual Impairment and Blindness* 99(6), 368–370. DOI: 10.1177/0145482x0509900606.
Sharkin, B.S. and Knox, D. (2003) Pet loss: Issues and implications for the psychologist. *Professional Psychology: Research and Practice* 34(4), 414–421. DOI: 10.1037/0735-7028.34.4.414.
Shubert, J. (2012) Dogs and human health/mental health: From the pleasure of their company to the benefits of their assistance. *The United States Army Medical Department Journal: Canine-Assisted Therapy in Military Medicine* 32(4), 21–29. DOI: 10.1080/08927936.2019.1621545.
Spain, B., O'Dwyer, L. and Moston, S., S. (2019) Pet loss: Understanding disenfranchised grief, memorial use, and posttraumatic growth. *Anthrozoos* 32(4), 555–568. DOI: 10.1080/08927936.2019.1621545.
Sterniczuk, R. and Whelan, J. (2016) Cannabis use among Canadian armed forces veterans. *Journal of Military, Veteran and Family Health* 2(2), 43–52. DOI: 10.3138/jmvfh.3836.
Stewart, C., Thrush, J. and Paulus, G. (1989) Disenfranchised bereavement and loss of a companion animal: Implications for caring communities. In: Doka, K.J. (ed.) *Disenfranchised Grief: Recongizing Hidden Sorrow*. Lexington Books, pp. 147–160.
Thomas, A.E. (2014) Liquid love — Grief, loss, animal companions and the social worker. In: Ryan, T. (ed.) *Animals in Social Work: Why and How They Matter*. Palgrave Macmillan, London, pp. 199–214. DOI: 10.1057/9781137372291_13.
Veterans Affairs Canada [VAC] (2019a) Post-Traumatic Stress Disorder (PTSD) and war-related stress - Veterans Affairs Canada. Available at: https://www.veterans.gc.ca/eng/health-support/mental-health-and-wellness/understanding-mental-health/ptsd-warstress
Veterans Affairs Canada [VAC] (2019b) Service Dogs - Veterans Affairs Canada. Available at: https://www.veterans.gc.ca/eng/about-vac/research/research-directorate/info-briefs/service-dogs
Volsche, S. (2019) Understanding cross-species parenting: A case for pets as children. In: Kogan, L. and Blazina, C. (eds) *Clinician's Guide to Treating Companion Animal Issues*. Academic Press, pp. 129–141. DOI: 10.1016/c2016-0-04244-4.
Weisman, A.D. (1995) Bereavement and companion animals. *OMEGA-Journal of Death and Dying* 22(4), 241–248. DOI: 10.2190/C54Y-UGMH-QGR4-CWTL.
Wenthold, N. and Savage, T.A. (2007) Ethical issues with service animals. *Topics in Stroke Rehabilitation* 14(2), 68–74. DOI: 10.1310/tsr1402-68.
Williamson, L., Dell, C.A., Osgood, N., Chalmers, D., Lohnes, C. *et al.* (2021a) Examining changes in posttraumatic stress disorder symptoms and substance use among a sample of canadian veterans working with service dogs: An exploratory patient-oriented longitudinal study. *Journal of Veterans Studies* 7(1). DOI: 10.21061/jvs.v7i1.194.

Williamson, L.E., Dell, C.A., Chalmers, D., Cruz, M. and Groot, P. (2021b) Strengthening zooeyia: Understanding the human-animal bond between veterans living with comorbid substance use and posttraumatic stress disorder and their service dogs. *Human-Animal Interaction Bulletin* 10(2), 20–47. Available at: https://www.apa-hai.org/haib/download-info/strengthening-zooeyia-understanding-the-human-animal-bond-between-veterans-living-with-comorbid-substance-use-and-posttraumatic-stress-disorder-and-their-service-dogs/?fbclid=IwAR0TnagBReg91g89Y72sxAZ_6yLSSg8QQOvyHG6rSEuS4saYsCcjxbh2 P2Q

Wilson, D., Underwood, L., Carr, E., Gross, D., Kane, M. *et al.* (2021) Older women's experiences of companion animal death: Impacts on well-being and aging-in-place. *BMC Geriatrics* 21(1). DOI: 10.1186/S12877-021-02410-8.

Wrobel, T.A. and Dye, A.L. (2003) Grieving pet death: Normative, gender, and attachment issues. *OMEGA - Journal of Death and Dying* 47(4), 385–393. DOI: 10.2190/qyv5-llj1-t043-u0f9.

Yamamoto, M. and Hart, L. (2020) Separation from assistance dogs: The complicated psychological burden during loss of the relationship. In: Kogan, L. and Erdman, P. (eds) *Pet Loss, Grief, and Therapeutic Interventions: Practitioners Vavigating the Human-Animal Bond*. Routledge, pp. 188–208.

Yarborough, B.H., Owen-Smith, A.A., Stumbo, S.P., Yarborough, M.T., Perrin, N.A. *et al.* (2017) An observational study of service dogs for veterans with posttraumatic stress disorder. *Psychiatric Services* 68(7), 730–734. DOI: 10.1176/appi.ps.201500383.

18 Animal Loss and Grief in Zoos: Qualitative Insights to Inform Organizational Support for Zoo Professionals and Volunteers

Nichole Louise Nageotte[1]*, Jennifer Currin-McCulloch[2], Shelby McDonald[2], Abigail Walker[2] and Lori R. Kogan[3]

[1]Department of Community Research and Evaluation, Denver Zoo Conservation Alliance, Denver, CO, USA; [2]School of Social Work, Colorado State University, Fort Collins, CO, USA; [3]Department of Clinical Sciences, Colorado State University, Fort Collins, CO, USA

Abstract

Zoo professionals and volunteers frequently face significant emotional strain due to animal losses, yet structured organizational support for processing grief remains limited. This study explores the perspectives of US-based zoo professionals and volunteers on organizational responses to animal-related grief, aiming to identify areas to enhance support and foster a grief-affirming culture. Data were collected through an anonymous online survey with open-ended questions regarding organizational-level grief support. A purposive sample of 1695 zoo professionals and volunteers was recruited, with responses from 182 participants (135 animal care and health professionals, 12 volunteers, and 35 other staff) selected for qualitative analysis. Thematic analysis identified three primary themes: creating an organizational culture supportive of grief expression, increasing organizational response mechanisms and resources, and enriching human resource policies to support grieving zoo professionals and volunteers. Many participants reported that insufficient grief support led to feelings of isolation, shame, and burnout. Findings underscore the importance for zoos to prioritize the development of comprehensive grief-affirming policies, including grief training for leadership, expanded access to mental health resources, and development of communication protocols for timely, compassionate responses to animal loss. These recommendations aim to foster empathetic organizational cultures that support staff and volunteer well-being and effective animal care.

Keywords: organizational culture, animal loss, zoo, grief and loss

Introduction

The well-being of zoo animals and those who care for them is interconnected (Mellen, 1991; Wielebnowski *et al.*, 2002; Carlstead *et al.*, 2019; Carlstead and Brown, 2024), yet support systems for zoo professionals coping with animal-related losses remain

*Corresponding author: NNageotte@denverzoo.org

underdeveloped (Brando *et al.*, 2023a; Currin-McCulloch *et al.*, 2024; McDonald *et al.*, 2024). Zoo professionals, especially animal care and health professionals (ACHPs), and volunteers often encounter significant animal losses, leading to complex emotional responses and stress (Fraser *et al.*, 2013; Brando *et al.*, 2023a, b; Currin-McCulloch *et al.*, 2024; McDonald *et al.*, 2024). These losses are often exacerbated by disenfranchised grief – grief that is not socially acknowledged or supported – due to societal and organizational norms that downplay the emotional significance of animal loss in professional contexts (Doka, 2008; Doka, 2017). Recent research indicates high levels of burnout, depression, and anxiety among ACHPs working in zoo settings, with animal loss representing a notable source of occupational stress (Brando *et al.*, 2023a, b; Currin-McCulloch *et al.*, 2024; McDonald *et al.*, 2024). One recent study revealed that within the past year, 80% of zoo professionals faced at least one unanticipated animal death, and 74% experienced an expected loss, with over half indicating these losses had occurred in the previous 3 months (McDonald *et al.*, 2024).

ACHPs, along with other zoo professionals and volunteers, often develop meaningful bonds with animals in their care. While fulfilling, these connections can intensify feelings of grief and burnout when animals are lost, whether due to natural death, health issues, transfers, or rehabilitation releases. Each type of loss has the potential to leave a lasting emotional impact (Fraser *et al.*, 2013; Brando *et al.*, 2023a, b; Currin-McCulloch *et al.*, 2024; McDonald *et al.*, 2024). At the same time, emerging research highlights that fostering these bonds benefits both personnel and animals, contributing to animal well-being through outcomes such as reduced stress and improved reproductive success in some species (Mellen, 1991; Wielebnowski *et al.*, 2002; Carlstead *et al.*, 2019; Carlstead and Brown, 2024). To balance these benefits with the emotional demands of caregiving, it has been suggested that zoos cultivate an organizational culture that encourages meaningful human–animal connections while also providing grief support systems to help zoo professionals and volunteers manage loss and adopt healthy coping mechanisms (Currin-McCulloch *et al.*, 2024; McDonald *et al.*, 2024).

Despite high levels of burnout in the zoo industry and growing awareness of the emotional challenges faced by ACHPs and other zoo professionals and volunteers, preliminary evidence suggests that organizational and industry-level support systems for grief and loss remain limited (Fraser *et al.*, 2013; Brando *et al.*, 2023a, b; Currin-McCulloch *et al.*, 2024; McDonald *et al.*, 2024). Research specific to US zoos suggests that most facilities lack structured grief rituals or policies, and many professionals feel compelled to suppress their grief to avoid perceived unprofessionalism (Brando *et al.*, 2023a, b; Currin-McCulloch *et al.*, 2024; McDonald *et al.*, 2024). Studies in other caregiving fields, such as healthcare and veterinary medicine, demonstrate that a lack of formalized grief support can create a 'culture of silence' where professionals feel unable to express and appropriately deal with their grief which can negatively impact job satisfaction, organizational commitment, and contribute to burnout (Furman, 2002; Brosche, 2003; Brunelli, 2005; Anderson *et al.*, 2010; Durall, 2011; Marcella and Kelley, 2015; Gilbert *et al.*, 2021; Frangieh *et al.*, 2023). This lack of acknowledgment correlates with decreased professional fulfillment and perceived organizational support and is linked to heightened burnout and depression among zoo-based ACHPs (McDonald *et al.*, 2024). Conversely, grief rituals – such as ceremonies or memorials honoring animals' lives, providing time, space, and opportunities for healing – are associated with better mental health outcomes among zoo professionals, underscoring the potential value of structured grief practices for ACHPs and other allied professionals (Barooah *et al.*, 2015; Puyat *et al.*, 2019; Ådland *et al.*, 2022; Ansari, 2022; McDonald *et al.*, 2024).

Current study

In light of these findings, there is a growing call within the zoo industry for a more compassionate and responsive approach to supporting staff and volunteers through experiences of animal loss and related grief. This study responds to gaps in prior research by examining zoo professionals' and volunteers' perspectives on how organizations currently respond to animal loss. Specifically, we aim (1) to identify how zoos can enhance support systems for zoo professionals and volunteers coping with these losses; and (2) to outline key actions zoo leaders can take to foster a culture that acknowledges grief and promotes adaptive coping strategies. Through these objectives, we aim to provide actionable recommendations that encourage grief acknowledgment and validate the complex emotional experiences of zoo personnel.

Methods

Positionality statement

We share the following positionality statement to transparently portray the backgrounds of the authors. NN is a zoo social science researcher with a background in zookeeping, informal science learning, and conservation behavior change, and JC-M is an academic researcher with 20 years of social work practice working alongside those experiencing life-limiting illnesses and their care partners. SEM is an academic researcher who focuses on human–animal interactions and was previously employed as a researcher in a zoo setting; AW is a social work graduate student and research assistant; and LK is an academic researcher who focuses on human–animal interactions. Throughout this research study, we integrated processes to reflect on and address potential personal and professional biases.

Study design

This qualitative research study originated from a larger mixed-methods study that explored US zoo professionals' and volunteers' experiences of anxiety, depression, burnout, professional fulfillment, and animal-related loss. The larger study invited participants to complete an anonymous online survey with both qualitative and quantitative items (Currin-McCulloch *et al.*, 2024; McDonald *et al.*, 2024).

The qualitative portion of the survey consisted of five open-ended questions:

1. In thinking back on your time at the zoo, please describe the most significant death loss you have experienced with an animal at the zoo.
2. What and/or who offered you the most support in coping with the death of animals in your zoo?
3. Please describe how your zoo community could better support you in coping with animal-related losses (e.g., animal transfers, deaths) at the zoo.
4. If you could give one piece of advice for leaders at the zoo on how best to support you leading up to or after the loss of an animal at the zoo, what would you say?
5. Please share other thoughts that you have in reflecting on your experiences of grief and animal-related loss in your role at the zoo.

This article specifically addresses questions three to five and aims to describe participants' perspectives on how their organization and/or the zoo industry can best support individual and communal well-being both pre- and post-zoo animal loss.

Recruitment strategies included purposive sampling of zoo professionals and volunteers through professional association listservs, community discussion forums (e.g., Association of Zoos and Aquariums [AZA]), and social media platforms. Participants completed online surveys (Alchemer survey platform) between July and October 2023. The average time for survey completion was 15 min. To acknowledge the potential emotional discomfort that participants may encounter while reflecting on their experiences of zoo animal loss, we added the following statement to the informed consent document:

> The survey includes some questions pertaining to feelings of loss and grief surrounding the death or transfer of zoo animals. If you experience any emotional discomfort from taking the survey, you can contact your zoo's human resource department to access your mental health benefits or con-tact Lap of Love Available at: https://www.lapoflove.com/ (accessed 28 March 2024) – they offer free support for animal loss and grief.

Sample

Surveys were completed by 1695 individuals, however, not every participant completed all qualitative items. Within the larger sample, most participants identified as white (91%) and female, feminine or woman (79%). Approximately 20% identified as LGBTQIA + and the mean age was 37. The survey included 19 distinct roles from which participants could identify their staff or volunteer position(s). From their responses, we created three categories of roles: volunteers, ACHPs, and other staff. The ACHP category included individuals directly responsible for the care and wellness of animals, such as zookeepers, curators, veterinarians, veterinary technicians, and nutritionists. The "Other Staff" category included paid staff not directly responsible for zoo animals' care and well-being, such as those working in education, guest services roles, or marketing. Our process for determining the sample for the present study entailed an initial filtering of participants, leaving only those who responded to all open-ended survey items. We then utilized IBM SPSS, version 28 to perform a random selection of 10% of these individuals from each of the three role categories. If participants were discarded from analysis due to not answering at least one of the five questions, additional participants were randomly selected until 10% of each group was represented. This process resulted in a sample of 182 participants (12 Volunteers, 135 ACHPs, and 35 Other Staff) for qualitative analysis.

Data analysis

We integrated Guest *et al.*'s (2011) applied thematic analysis method to inductively analyze participants' responses to three of the survey's open-ended questions which specifically inquired about participants' perceptions of how organizations and the overall zoo industry can best respond to zoo animal loss. As we engaged with narrative responses from zoo employees and volunteers, we inductively determined themes, rather than approaching the data with predetermined themes. As a team of three coders (JC-M, NN, AW), we used a systematic approach to coding data. The five steps included: (1) the individual reading of each response and the development of initial codes to represent participants' suggestions for enhancing organizational and industry responses to zoo animal loss and grief; (2) gathering as a team to determine codes, coding definitions, and themes; (3) discussing disparities in coding processes until we reached consensus; (4) creating a codebook to support the application of themes across the entire data set; and (5) choosing salient quotes to represent each theme. To protect the confidentiality of zoo professionals and volunteers, we intentionally removed identifying information from participants' quotes, including only their study identification number and their role (e.g., volunteer, ACHP or other staff).

Trustworthiness

Throughout the data analysis process, we incorporated several strategies to enhance trustworthiness. As coders, we met on 15 occasions to review participants' survey responses, line by line, and from there co-developed the codebook structure. At each meeting, we created memos to track thematic and analytic decision making processes. These memos became our audit trail to trace continual refining of code names, definitions, and examples of how to apply codes, as well as the emergence of code and meaning saturation (Hennink *et al.*, 2017). At the conclusion of data analysis and thematic synthesis, all authors met to discuss findings and to develop implications, based on our professional and personal knowledge. Microsoft Excel software was utilized to organize individual codes and the integration of team codes into the final codebook structure.

Results

Zoo professionals and volunteers expressed an understanding that there may be no singular way to address grief given the variability among individuals' experiences. Each participant offered suggestions for ways leaders and organizations could better support their employees and volunteers when dealing with the death or transfer of zoo animals. Participants acknowledged that while grief resources at an organizational level are essential, they also recognized that successful organizational support depends on an overall culture shift within the zoo industry toward one that openly discusses and validates expressions of grief. In terms of specific desired support, we discerned three main themes from participants' narratives: *zoo grief culture; increased organizational response and resources;* and *enhanced human resource policies and support.*

Zoo grief culture

Cultures of shame

Participants from a variety of organizations shared their experiences regarding their organization's culture around grief and loss. Workplace cultures that discourage expressions of grief were mentioned frequently by participants from multiple organizations, suggesting an industry-wide norm. An ACHP described their leader's expectation to hide feelings of grief: "My assistant director is not always the most sympathetic. He thinks tears are unprofessional and is straight to business very shortly after any death" (P2299, ACHP). Other participants used language such as "shame," "judged," and "guilt" when describing how they felt when they displayed grief. This cultural norm led some employees and volunteers to feel as though they needed to suppress their feelings at work:

> Often there isn't time to grieve, or the grieving is done on your own time at a later time. We are pushing down the feelings, putting on a brave face to do demos, and keeper chats. We are still responsible for making sure the other animals in the area are taken care of often while trying to not break down (P175, ACHP).

Participants expressed the need for a supportive environment within their organization to openly discuss loss and grief. They longed for systems that "Mak[e] it more culturally acceptable to cry and grieve the death or other loss of an animal instead of "toughening up" because they're 'just birds/ animals" (P825, ACHP). Some long-time employees noted a growing acceptance of expressions of grief. This cultural shift offered hope that there is movement away from shame and disenfranchised coping:

> I am grateful this is becoming a non-taboo topic to discuss. Even 10 years ago I feel like the culture was "suck it up and just get through it" and I am happy for a new generation of caretakers to not have to be met with a callous and unempathetic environment and to be empowered and encouraged to seek support for their grief (P381, Other Staff).

Those who experienced community and the ability to mourn publicly felt more supported in times of grief and described generally positive views of their position and leadership. This included being open about death and grief, as well as creating memorials for animals that had passed. One ACHP explained how differing zoo cultures can influence one's sense of belonging at their zoo:

> The most support I ever felt was from the first department I was a part of. I started as a volunteer there and that's how I got my foot in the door for [paid employment]. That department had the best sense of com-munity that I have ever felt at the zoo. It had hundreds of teen volunteers and wonderful staff, and you always had the sense that we were there for each other and when an animal was lost, we were all there to support and mourn together. Every animal that passed had a memorial set up in our break area. Every animal was respected there. Since that time, I've found myself in the main zoo working in our [taxa] department and I have never felt supported by managers when an animal had passed or was put down. If anything, I've just developed a sense of dread that a death was my fault and I would be blamed for it in some capacity, even if the animal died just by simply being old (P2217, ACHP).

This ACHP's experience highlights the variety of grief responses and ways that unsupportive cultures can foster employee dread and anxiety. In addition to those providing direct care to animals, individuals in managerial roles also felt grief when zoo animals died. One manager described the challenge of balancing their needs with those of their supervisees:

> Personally, when I am experiencing the loss, I am quiet and need space while I process through my feelings. This is challenging in my role as a manager when I know I have individuals who need direct sup-port from me in the moment. I often feel I have to park my emotions for after-hours so I can provide them with their needs to

> cope with the situ-ation at hand even though I am experiencing it as well. (P664, ACHP).

Departmental leaders also felt constraints in implementing grief resources due to upper management roadblocks. One middle manager, for example, explained that they attempted to provide resources to their staff, but were prevented from doing so by a more senior leader (P1574, ACHP). Others explained they find themselves caught in the middle, navigating their own feelings and leadership demands, while also trying to provide support to those they supervise.

Limited leadership infrastructure for empathic grief response

Participants called for leaders to hold empathy for their losses and to create infrastructure to support their emotional well-being. They shared examples of their loss not being acknowledged, disrespectful language, and uncaring responses. For example, one ACHP shared their experience of having their feelings disregarded:

> Recognize that we truly loved [the animal]; they were not just a thing to us but were a soul and body that we cared for every single day and poured ourselves out to, especially when there is a decline before they're passing. We've sat with them every day for the last week (or whatever time period depending on the animal) and begged them to eat, and take their meds, and get up and walk around, and just be bet-ter, and then we lose them. It is gut wrenching, and it feels like no one truly understands it, especially when we are immediately forced back into our daily tasks (P1633, ACHP).

Even if their feelings were not truly understood by others, it was important for participants that leadership not brush off their experiences. One person shared, "Some acknowledgement of our feelings from upper management would be meaningful. Rather than being treated like any show of emotion is over the top and we are not entitled to those feelings" (P607, ACHP). Another participant described their experiences with managers "... making fun of keepers for showing emotion at the death of an animal" (P2217, ACHP). Individuals commonly portrayed actions of leaders as hurtful. As one participant succinctly explained, they would like for leadership to "actually care" (P1820, ACHP).

One suggestion as a way for leaders to validate the feelings and experiences of others was to demonstrate trust in the expert knowledge of those who provide daily care for the animals:

> Keepers should be more involved in the planning of transfers/acquisitions/ euthanasia. There seems to be a trend across multiple institutions where upper management makes all of these decisions with little to no context as to an animal's health/history because they cannot even be bothered to check with the people who actually care for said animals (P324, ACHP).

Although the study asked participants to share their experiences with significant zoo animal death, many participants felt compelled to share about transfer losses – another form of loss that they felt significantly impacted their lives. Thus, we also received requests for leadership to proactively aid teams in preparing for and responding to animal transfers.

Several participants commented on actions that leadership could take to demonstrate their care, compassion, and understanding. One person suggested, "Administrative staff reaching out personally to share their condolences, giving us at least an hour to let us recognize our emotions before immediately getting back to work" (P2340, ACHP). Another shared, "I think just reaching out to say, to say sorry for your loss, giving us time and space to grieve" (P2343, ACHP). In addition to checking in following a loss, some asked for leaders to remember that grief is a process, and that people may need support in the weeks and months following the loss.

In addition, participants noted that increased empathy and compassion from leadership should be accompanied by similar support from colleagues, both within one's team and from other departments. For example, one participant saw an opportunity for someone with more life experience to mentor those newer in the profession: "Older coworkers need to have more compassion for those who are new and not used to the zoo life and how things are" (P1346, Other Staff).

Opportunities for increased organizational response and resources

Creating channels for open communication

While some participants expressed a desire for more communication in general, others offered suggestions for grief communication protocols. For example, creating communication protocols after a necropsy was offered as one way to help with closure after an animal died: "I think knowing as much as possible about the animal's health and cause of death can help with closure and healing" (P1244, ACHP). A volunteer shared, "Please give us as much information as possible about the death. Please follow up with autopsy results when they come in. It's frustrating to not hear the outcome of tests" (P189, Volunteer). Zoo professionals shared that knowing the cause of death could reduce their feelings of guilt, knowing that they made the right care decision:

> We should always have a meeting after euthanizing an animal and getting back necropsy results to make sure we did the right thing at the right time. Oftentimes I feel like we made the decision too late, and the animal suffered (P1923, ACHP).

Some participants felt that they could benefit from learning from the necropsy results and potentially integrate this knowledge to improve the care of animals in the future:

> But if an animal death felt preventable it is important to address this as quickly as possible to prevent a similar incident in the future. In cases like that, if no action is taken, people will feel powerless and like their pain isn't being taken seriously. It is so important to hear what people are saying and take those things into account when moving forward (P371, ACHP).

Both volunteers and zoo professionals requested more communication before and after transfers to enhance their ability to understand the reasoning behind the transfer and better prepare for the loss. One staff member suggested, "Notification zoo-wide via email or meetings, or both, in preparation for transfer or death, so we all have time to spend with the animal, take pics, etc. and have a team dedicated to the process" (P353, Other Staff). The sharing of pictures and updates following animal transfers can help people adjust to their loss by allowing a continued bond through connection in their new zoo home:

> Some curators are good about following up with animal transfers and re-laying positive information about an animal adjusting well, or having new, successful social pairings. I've found this info helpful in easing the feeling of missing a transferred animal (P339, ACHP).

Stories highlighting positive pre-loss experiences centered on open communication, creating the best possible quality of life for animals, and opportunities for those close to the animal to be a part of the final moments of life. Open communication about an animal's decline and pending euthanasia enabled employees and volunteers to feel that they could have a part in the animal's ability to have a "good death." This time enabled one ACHP team to orchestrate a positive dying experience: "We spoiled her with whipped cream and her favorite food. She then trained for anesthesia for her own euthanasia. She kept coming back for more attention until the meds kicked in. It was a beautiful gift to give her but also very difficult to lose one of my all-time favorite animals" (P2266, ACHP). Being present at death and holding animals close also fostered meaning in the dying experience. The veterinary staff at one facility were lauded for their exemplar end-of-life practices:

> Our vet staff is truly wonderful and have a lot on their plates. They do always provide the best care and are so gracious when it comes to helping keepers process and giving us time with the animal. We get footprints when we ask and we always know they exhaust every option before calling it (P2299, ACHP).

Other examples of how participants were able to continue bonds with animals after their death or transfer included clipping of small hair samples, taking nose or paw prints, or sharing photos of animals.

Enhanced equity

Participants called for leadership to respect the losses of smaller and less charismatic animals. Those who worked with animals such as birds, reptiles, small mammals, amphibians, or fish felt as though organizations often overlooked these deaths. They shared how organizations would provide communications about the deaths of large mammals such as tigers or elephants, but not for the smaller animals. Likewise, they would share that the keeper staff of these larger animals may receive resources or empathy but keeper staff for smaller animals may not. Requests for equitable acknowledgment of loss included animals of all ages, sizes, and taxa, as described by an ACHP:

> I have found it increasingly frustrating that the higher ups don't seem to care about animal deaths unless they are large mammals. The bird department and aquatic department don't even receive an "I'm sorry' when an animal dies, but the mammal department gets food and comforting from the high ups when one of the animals they care for dies (P841, ACHP).

When the deaths of smaller animals were acknowledged, the timing also felt important to participants. Waiting to respond to some losses and not others created a sense of disparity in how much one was valued in their role. One suggested solution for creating cultures that more equitably honor the lives of all animals was better communication among all types of animal losses, not just certain species. A call for equity appeared as follows: "So, if anything, treating all the animals with the same respect when it comes to death, no matter if it is an elephant or a secretary bird or a warthog, death sucks for the keepers every time" (P1885, ACHP). This lack of equity in response to loss was also mentioned by volunteers. One volunteer requested that zoo leaders and staff

> recognize that we are people too. We bond with the animals! We bond with them out of our own free time and will. No one made us care. We just did and to just send out an email weeks later is insulting (P520, Volunteer).

Enhanced human resource policies and support

In addition to calls for individual leaders to increase their attention to employee and volunteer loss, participants urged organizations to adapt human resource policies and resources to foster a grief-affirming culture. This included the development of programs, supportive policies, and enhanced grief resources, as well as recommendations for flexible job duties, designated grieving time during the workday, and support from other departments to assist teams that experienced a loss.

Time off and time flexibility

Offering time off to grieve was commonly mentioned by participants as an essential step forward for organizations. Some participants suggested that paid time off for grieving would allow employees time to process their loss. When time off is not feasible, participants felt it would be helpful to have a reduced workload or flexible tasks on the day of a loss. The option for adjusted responsibilities or a lighter workload would "... allow keepers to 'take it easy' on days where losses occur and would take a lot of weight off on those days" (P775, ACHP). Having time to recenter was viewed as crucial to allow employees to focus on the needs of the other animals under their care.

Some participants also shared that allowing time for grieving could be essential to ensuring the safety of zoo professionals, visitors, and animals:

> I think it would also be valuable to look at how people feel working the rest of the day or week after a loss, because this job is very dangerous and after loss, people might be more distracted or unfocused, and how does that impact occupational safety... (P1759, ACHP).

For example, those working with predatory animals experienced increased concerns about returning to work immediately after an animal loss: "I work with carnivores, so safety is huge. You need to right your mind quickly so that you can keep yourself, coworkers, guests, and the animals safe" (P175, ACHP).

Another related suggestion was for other teams to assist with the daily tasks of teams experiencing a loss. For example, individuals from other departments or a manager could provide supports:

> Not expecting keepers to just go back into their normal routine after such a significant event. The stress of not being well mentally but still needing to take care of all of the other animals I worked with, not leaving a lock unlocked etc., makes the whole thing even harder. Having someone come and help from another area

> would have been helpful. Even just having bosses help (P2270, ACHP).

Participants also shared that having a break from work or support from others would show they are valued:

> Show us you see us as humans worth your thoughts and efforts. We [are] not robots, we need time to heal. The ability to take a day off without the rest of the keeper staff being left shorthanded. Show up and help make a few diets so we can sit and cry it out for just a moment without getting behind (P232, ACHP).

Several participants cited other teams as their main source of support following animal loss, including assisting in tasks and offering gestures of comfort:

> We're often offered support from other teams around the zoo (animal and non-animal staff) that can look like taking out our trash, sending us cof-fee, calling us to a meeting then just handing us ferrets to hold, delivering pre-made enrichment. I've also had docents and regular zoo guests offer good support including food, hugs, cards, stories, etc. (P371, ACHP).

When staffing constraints prevent ACHPs from taking time off or getting help from other departments for tasks, participants suggested adjustments to visitor-facing programs. Options included temporarily closing animal exhibits where an animal died or canceling educational programs. Many zoos have scheduled programs where staff interact with guests, and participants described the challenges of these interactions immediately after death. One participant proposed that leadership respond by "Giving staff a break. Canceling programming to give them time to grieve for at least the day" (P2021, ACHP). Shifting care responsibilities, closing exhibits, and providing time for staff to pause and reflect after a loss were all viewed as ways to help ACHPs and other staff manage their feelings following an animal's death.

Creating ritual around loss

Across all zoo roles, participants identified opportunities for communal rituals and acknowledgment around death or transfer losses. Suggestions included ways to systematically communicate about the loss through emails, newsletters or social media posts. Some, however, felt that recognition beyond an email was necessary to honor the life of an animal:

> When an animal passes, it should not be a footnote in an email. Often-times, these animals have spent their entire lives at a zoo, and their absence is obvious to staff and guests alike. Any animal that passes deserves to be recognized and should not be overlooked in the hopes that the public will not notice the absence (P324, ACHP).

Suggestions for honoring an animal's legacy included creating a memorial on-site (e.g., plaques) or through social media. Some participants suggested quarterly or annual memorials as a way to honor every animal, regardless of species, size or charismatic appeal. A staff member shared about an activity that fostered shared expression at their organization:

> My colleagues and I have, in the best of scenarios, held a large group celebration of life for the animals that recently passed away which was a great way to allow everyone to grieve and reminisce together and support one another. We also started making an ofrenda that we put up every year around the time of Dia de Muertos that has pictures of animals we lost during the past year. That has been a fun way to honor and celebrate the animals that were lost (P1755, Other Staff).

Likewise, volunteers also suggested creating ways to celebrate the lives of animals that died or were transferred such as "Having a goodbye party for those being transferred, and a quiet ceremony or even just an area to leave notes or small tokens for those who died. A space for quiet reflection. Perhaps with photos and written memories" (P1156, Volunteer).

Participants described other personalized ways to honor animals including artifacts and tokens, such as footprints, nose prints, or hair samples. For transfers, participants also suggested distributing prints or mementos:

> For animal transfers, there could be prints made and distributed, which is not something we do at all. Making a more concerted effort to get and distribute periodical updates about animals at a new institution would help. For deaths I think making print distribution a job responsibility for one department or staff would be a good idea, and to standardize when, how many and what kind of prints get distributed. I think volunteers

> would cherish even photocopied prints, but this isn't offered to them (P192, Other staff).

Participants noted that tailoring rituals to individual needs allowed for personalized expressions of grief. One participant explained that their organization's use of ritual resulted from staff suggestions:

> We have an incredible toolbox of resources available. This is a direct result of the focus group we have being comprised of a diverse body of vets, ACHPs, and education staff. Each team who experiences these losses have a voice in these conversations and are represented in the efforts made to support staff after loss (P381, Other Staff).

Team-based memorialization activities offered participants the ability to reflect on their bond, tell stories, and share in the emotional weight of their loss.

Increased mental health resources

Zoo professionals and volunteers offered several suggestions for enhancing mental health resources. Many participants recommended that zoos provide no- or low-cost counseling to staff. They also emphasized that financial limitations often restrict their ability to access these resources: "Quit saying 'it comes with the job' when we don't get paid enough to deal with it despite being educated and experienced individuals" (P84, ACHP).

For those working in organizations that provide mental health services, such as employee assistance programs (EAPs), there was gratitude for access to these resources: "Management does try to help staff, especially keepers. After a sudden, unexpected loss of an animal last year, they brought in a grief counselor. Notifying us of resources and even this survey are other examples of assistance from them" (P2495, Other Staff). However, not all participants found these resources beneficial. They emphasized that mental health professionals brought in for support should have experience with zoo animal loss to better "[...] understand our [zoo] business and the multitude of different emotions that occur with an animal loss" (P983, ACHP). In the animal care profession, feelings of grief can be compounded by feelings of guilt, underscoring the need for professionals with a nuanced understanding of zoo-related grief. Without expertise in this area, counseling may be less effective, for example, one participant stated, "The zoo did bring in grief counselors as well. They didn't really help because it's hard to explain an animal setting compared to the outside world but at least they tried" (P2343, ACHP). Providing mental health and counseling resources relevant to the type of loss was often seen as an important consideration.

In addition, some participants suggested it would be helpful to have mental health resources on-site and readily accessible. One ACHP proposed: "I think there can be better resources on grounds for ACHPS. A group of people you can turn to and chat with on site, not needing to rely on counselors off grounds" (P1759, ACHP). Throughout their suggestions for mental health support, participants highlighted the importance of eliminating time and cost barriers that may limit access to these vital mental health resources and supports.

Discussion

This study gathered knowledge from zoo professionals and volunteers about ways to foster adaptive coping following zoo animal deaths and transfers. Participants identified both systemic and cultural problems and described encounters that resulted in experiences of hurt, shame, isolation, oppression, and/or anxiety. They also highlighted examples of grief-affirming cultures and offered concrete strategies for needed cultural shifts in the zoo industry to enhance organizational and industry responses both pre- and post-loss. Building on research related to zoo professionals' and volunteer burnout (McDonald *et al.*, 2024), and individual and interpersonal experiences of significant animal loss (Currin-McCulloch *et al.*, 2024), we integrated participants' voices into practical strategies and resources that zoos and industry leaders can implement to enhance individual and collective well-being.

Overarching among participants' suggestions was a desire to change their organizations' overall grief culture. They offered several strategies to enhance culture, policies, and norms that influence interpersonal reactions and organizational actions following animal deaths and transfers. Participants' narratives about culture commonly focused on the need for both organizational and industry-wide culture shifts to encourage more open, affirming dialogues and policies around loss and grief. Several participants noted positive practices and recognized individuals within their organizations who provided safe spaces to discuss loss and grief. Yet, others expressed a desire for a culture where they could openly ask for support, take a moment to catch their breath and have access to grief resources tailored to the needs of zoo professionals and volunteers.

Many participants shared visions for policies and processes to create cultures that promoted better care leading up to an animal's death or transfer, and memorialization rituals. They desired opportunities for team members to participate in planning for a "good death" or transfer. Specific examples allowed interested individuals the chance to say "goodbye," take photos, or gather samples of fur, feathers or paw/footprints; thus enabling zoo professionals and volunteers to cultivate a continuing bond with animals no longer under their care.

Based on the narratives of participants and the professional experiences of the authors, we offer several examples of no- to moderate-cost strategies to foster organizational and industry-level changes that support open, affirming grief cultures (see Table 18.1). Studies of zoo professionals that draw attention to high burnout, depression and anxiety levels among ACHPs (McDonald *et al.*, 2024) underscore the need for zoos to invest in policies, procedures, and programs to support validated expressions of grief. Research demonstrates that organizational investment in employees' mental health, including bereavement support, can result in increased employee well-being and productivity, and lower healthcare costs and absenteeism (Hall *et al.*, 2013; Gilbert *et al.*, 2021).

Organizational level response

An overarching call throughout the responses was for organizational members and leaders to be present for and supportive of each other during times of loss. Suggested supportive actions included allowing time and space to

Table 18.1. Suggested organizational interventions, sorted by cost.

No cost interventions	Low cost interventions	Moderate investment
Celebration of life rituals at regularly scheduled employee and volunteer meetings	Shifting of tasks so that others can be of support following a death	Contract zoo therapists or counselors to have on site
Leadership stopping by to check on people after any loss	Take teams who have experienced a loss to lunch, send a card, or bring in baked goods	Paid time off for employees as grief time following the death of an animal under their primary care
Saving of paw prints, hair or feathers	Create peer-led mutual aid groups to debrief after losses	Closing exhibit areas and/or tours immediately following a death
Communication about pending transfers or deaths so that people close to the animal can say "goodbye"	Develop a decision making tree around internal and external communication about animal losses	Send a team of employees to crisis response training to support staff after a loss has occurred
Communication across the zoo before and after a death and prior to external communication	Create a shared resource drive where zoo professionals and volunteers can access grief and loss psychoeducation materials	Offer coaching for managers to provide empathic, trauma-informed responses to their team
Sharing of photos and memories of animals	Develop policies and resources for debriefing following deaths such as necropsy debriefings or Schwartz Rounds	Host an annual memorial for all zoo members, including a reading of the names of all animals that have died that year at the zoo

grieve, including days off, solitary moments, or being with others who knew the animal well. To support time for zoo professionals to reflect on the death of an animal in their exhibit, organizations could develop policies that provide time away from the exhibit area for people to gather their thoughts before returning to their work. Zoos could develop internal grief response teams trained in crisis response who are alerted to assist when an animal is actively dying or following a death. Additionally, a support team could step in to aid with tasks such as meal preparation, habitat cleaning, or supply stocking, allowing zoo keepers more time to process their grief. In addition, temporarily closing exhibits after a death could reduce public-facing strain on grieving zoo professionals and volunteers. Policies could also be established to create standards for paid time off following significant animal loss, whether it be leaving work early or taking day(s) off.

Our findings suggest that communication strategies and policies should be created to allow timely notification of animal deaths and transfers. Access to this information should be available in a way that individuals can access it when they are emotionally prepared. Further, organizations should consider developing external communication protocols that balance staff and volunteers' needs for external validation of the loss (e.g., from friends, family, peers, colleagues) alongside organizations' privacy needs. Circumstances and reasoning around confidentiality and privacy decisions should be clearly communicated with staff and volunteers.

In addition, a variety of free, easily accessible, grief and loss resources such as peer mutual aid groups, grief psychoeducational resources, and grief counselors (particularly those with expertise in zoo animal loss and zoo cultures) would be of value. Zoos could create designated quiet spaces for members of their work community to access, either individually or collectively, and reflect or memorialize an animal loss. These spaces might include memorial artifacts, music, or journals and craft supplies to promote reflection.

Guidance for zoo leaders

Zoo professionals and volunteers sought guidance and support from their leaders to reduce the psychosocial distress they experienced following zoo animal deaths and transfers. They indicated a desire for leaders to create more affirming grief cultures. Our findings indicate there are many opportunities for personal growth among zoo leaders and a widespread need for strategic leadership coaching centered on leading with empathy (Tehan and Thompson, 2013; Gilbert *et al.*, 2021). Some other examples of actions leaders could take include seeking out training on trauma-informed leadership and empathic grief responses. Notably, leaders in middle-management roles requested coaching on how to balance their own grief while supporting the needs of their staff.

To respond to requests for transparency following traumatic deaths, leaders could offer time and space for their teams to debrief about the events leading up to the death, while also allowing people time and space to process their feelings individually if desired. One example of a way for all members of the exhibit team to debrief following a death could be to follow examples of human hospital care through Schwartz Rounds (Adamson *et al.*, 2018; Ng *et al.*, 2023). In Schwartz Rounds style, all members of the care team from the volunteers, custodial staff, zoo keepers, other staff and leadership team would be invited to share stories about the animal that was lost and have a collective community to process their loss. Of note, this would be up to each team to plan and determine how the experience would best fit their needs and foster a safe expression of grief.

Industry level response

Drawing on insights from zoo professionals and volunteers, we propose a few strategies for the zoo industry to build supportive infrastructure and resources that enhance the well-being and retention of its workforce. An initial step could be the creation of a zoo animal grief special interest or advisory group that meets regularly to discuss industry grief culture, share resources, and promote self-compassion around loss. This could begin with the creation of a dedicated session at the next AZA conference, allowing interested individuals to come together to exchange ideas, establish frameworks for regular meetings, and develop a repository of grief resources that could be shared among AZA zoos. Within this group, experienced members might mentor newcomers less familiar with zoo animal death and transfers, providing guidance and support. Additionally, this group could partner with mental health professionals to offer training to support leaders and other interested zoo professionals through workshops, classes, or webinars.

Another valuable activity of this special interest group could be the creation of an online database of grief resources that could be made available at no cost to AZA members. Within this online repository, zoos could share best practice examples of memorial activities, such as photographs of meditation spaces; activities that people use for rituals, poems, music, and programs from memorial services; and memorial activities that integrate the public into the grieving process or ritual. It could also feature a directory of zoo counselors, grief support organizations, mutual aid groups, and individuals interested in mentoring others experiencing zoo animal loss.

Limitations and future research directions

This study has several limitations that should be considered in interpreting and applying its findings. First, the sample was limited to AZA-accredited zoos in the United States and may not reflect the diversity of experiences within all zoological settings, particularly smaller, less-resourced facilities. Future research should aim to include a broader range of institutions to understand how grief processes and related organizational supports vary across different organizational types and settings. Additionally, this study relied on personal narratives, which, while rich in qualitative insight, may be influenced by social desirability or recall bias. Future studies could incorporate longitudinal designs, observing the implementation of grief-support initiatives over time to measure their impact on employee and volunteer well-being and retention. Such approaches could yield insights into the long-term benefits of grief support practices and help identify which strategies are most effective. Finally, while this study offers an important foundation for understanding grief in zoo settings, further research is needed to examine how individual differences, such as prior grief experiences, personality traits, or cultural backgrounds, influence coping strategies. Studies in this vein would deepen our understanding of how diverse zoo staff and volunteers experience and navigate grief, allowing for the development of more personalized support systems.

Despite these limitations, our findings provide valuable insights and strategies for grief support in zoo settings, laying the groundwork for sustainable, collaborative approaches. Through sharing the narratives of zoo professionals and volunteers, this study emphasizes the importance of participatory action, empowering staff to co-create grief responses, work cultures, and policies that meet their unique needs (Israel *et al.*, 2005; Greenwood and Levin, 2006; Kemmis and McTaggart, 2014). For instance, zoo professionals and volunteers could participate in developing grief support training, designing memorial spaces, and identifying team-specific rituals that align with departmental culture. Integrating these participatory strategies cultivates a sense of ownership among zoo professionals and volunteers, fostering a supportive community that collectively values and validates the role of grief in their work.

Engaging in participatory action research (PAR) (Baum *et al.*, 2006) could also play a crucial role in evaluating and refining the effectiveness of implemented grief support strategies. For instance, organizations could use PAR to assess how well new grief protocols are working, gather feedback from staff, and adapt policies over time, ensuring that grief support initiatives remain relevant and responsive to the evolving needs of the zoo community (Kemmis and McTaggart, 2014). In alignment with PAR's principles of collaborative adaptation, this approach builds a resilient organizational culture that enhances zoo professionals' capacity to fulfill conservation goals. A supportive environment not only benefits staff but also strengthens their ability to care for animals and foster visitor connections, furthering the zoo's conservation mission and inspiring broader empathy toward animals, people, and the environment.

Conflict of Interest

The authors have no conflict of interest to declare.

Funding

This research project was funded by an organizational fund at the Denver Zoo Conservation Alliance.

Ethics Statement

The study received approval from the Institutional Review Board at (university name redacted for blind study).

Author Contributions

All authors contributed equally to the development of this article.

Acknowledgments

The authors would like to acknowledge the zoo professionals and volunteers who shared their experiences of zoo animal grief and loss and their ideas for how to enhance the ways that organizations and the zoo industry respond to zoo animal loss. The authors also wish to thank the peer review committee at Denver Zoo Conservation Alliance for reviewing and approving this manuscript.

References

Adamson, K., Searl, N., Sengsavang, S., Yardley, J., George, M. *et al.* (2018) Caring for the healthcare professional: A description of the Schwartz rounds™ implementation. *Journal of Health Organization and Management* 32(3), 402–415. DOI: 10.1108/JHOM-05-2017-0103.

Ådland, A.K., Gripsrud, B.H., Lavik, M.H. and Ramvi, E. (2022) "They stay with you": Nursing home staff's emotional experiences of being in a close relationship with a resident in long-term care who died. *Journal of Holistic Nursing* 40(2), 108–122. DOI: 10.1177/08980101211017766.

Anderson, K.A., Ewen, H.H. and Miles, E.A. (2010) The grief support in healthcare scale: Development and testing. *Nursing Research* 59(6), 372. DOI: 10.1097/NNR.0b013e3181fca9de.

Ansari, D. (2022) An accumulation of distress: Grief, loss, and isolation among healthcare providers during the COVID-19 pandemic. *SSM-Mental Health* 2, 100146. DOI: 10.1016/j.ssmmh.2022.100146.

Barooah, A., Boerner, K., van Riesenbeck, I. and Burack, O.R. (2015) Nursing home practices following resident death: The experience of certified nursing assistants. *Geriatric Nursing* 36(2), 120–125. DOI: 10.1016/j.gerinurse.2014.11.005.

Baum, F., Mac Dougall, C. and Smith, D. (2006) Participatory action research. *Journal of Epidemiology and Community Health* 60(10), 854–857. DOI: 10.1136/jech.2004.028662.

Brando, S., Gjerris, M., Field, S. and Hart, V. (2023a) The impact of animal loss on zoo professionals: A qualitative study. *Zoo Biology* 42, 103–117.

Brando, S., Gjerris, M., Field, N. and Hart, L. (2023b) Caring for elderly wild animals: The human experience. In: *Optimal Wellbeing of Ageing Wild Animals in Human Care*. Springer International Publishing, Cham, pp. 235–251.

Brosche, T.A. (2003) Death, dying, and the ICU nurse. *Dimensions of Critical Care Nursing: DCCN* 22(4), 173–179. DOI: 10.1097/00003465-200307000-00006.

Brunelli, T. (2005) A concept analysis: The grieving process for nurses. *Nursing Forum* 40(4), 123–128. DOI: 10.1111/j.1744-6198.2005.00024.x.

Carlstead, K. and Brown, J.L. (2024) Relationships between patterns of fecal corticoid excretion and behavior, reproduction, and environmental factors in captive black (*Diceros bicornis*) and white (*Ceratotherium simum*) rhinoceros. *Zoo Biology* 24, 215–232.

Carlstead, K., Paris, S. and Brown, J.L. (2019) Good keeper-elephant relationships in North American zoos are mutually beneficial to welfare. *The Journal of Applied Animal Behavioral Science* 211, 103–111. DOI: 10.1016/j.applanim.2018.11.003.

Currin-McCulloch, J., Nageotte, N.L., Walker, A., McDonald, S. and Kogan, L. (2024) Experiences of animal loss and grief among aoo professionals and volunteers: A qualitative study. *Animals* 14, 2925. DOI: 10.3390/ani14202925.

Doka, K.J. (2008) Disenfranchised grief in historical and cultural perspective. In: *Handbook of Bereavement Research and Practice: Advances in Theory and Intervention*. American Psychological Association, pp. 223–240. DOI: 10.1037/14498-011.

Doka, K.J. (2017) Disenfranchised grief and trauma. In: *Handbook of Traumatic Loss*. Routledge, London, pp. 401–410. DOI: 10.4324/9781315627274.

Durall, A. (2011) Care of the caretaker: Managing the grief process of health care professionals. *Pediatric Annals* 40(5), 266–273. DOI: 10.3928/00904481-20110412-08.

Frangieh, J., Jones, T., Kinser, P.A., Wood, R. and Baker, K. (2023) “You can’t pour from an empty cup”: A qualitative exploration of formal and informal social support as experienced by frontline nurse leaders. *Nurse Leader* 21(5), 590–596. DOI: 10.1016/j.mnl.2023.07.002.

Fraser, J., Pantesco, V., Plemons, K., Gupta, R. and Rank, S.J. (2013) Sustaining the conservationist. *Ecopsychology* 5(2), 70–79. DOI: 10.1089/eco.2012.0076.

Furman, J. (2002) What you should know about chronic grief. *Nursing* 32(2), 56–57. DOI: 10.1097/00152193-200202000-00053.

Gilbert, S., Mullen, J., Kelloway, E.K., Dimoff, J., Teed, M. *et al.* (2021) The CARE model of employee bereavement support. *Journal of Occupational Health Psychology* 26, 405.

Greenwood, D.J. and Levin, M. (2006) *Introduction to Action Research: Social Research for Social Change*. SAGE, Thousand Oaks, CA.

Guest, G., MacQueen, K.M. and Namey, E.E. (2011) *Applied Thematic Analysis*. Sage Publications.

Hall, D., Shucksmith, J. and Russell, S. (2013) Building a compassionate community: Developing an informed and caring workplace in response to employee bereavement. *Bereavement Care* 32(1), 4–10. DOI: 10.1080/02682621.2013.779819.

Hennink, M.M., Kaiser, B.N. and Marconi, V.C. (2017) Code saturation versus meaning saturation: How many interviews are enough. *Qualitative Health Research* 27(4), 591–608. DOI: 10.1177/1049732316665344.

Israel, B.A., Eng, E., Schulz, A.J. and Parker, E.A. (2005) Introduction to methods in community-based participatory research for health. Jossey-Bass, San Francisco, CA, pp. 3–38.

Kemmis, S.K. and McTaggart, R.M. (2014) *The Action Research Planner: Doing Critical Participatory Action Research*. Springer, Singapore.

Marcella, J. and Kelley, M.L. (2015) Death is part of the job in long-term care homes: Supporting direct care staff with their grief and bereavement. *SAGE Open* 5(1), 2158244015573912. DOI: 10.1177/2158244015573912.

McDonald, S.E., Kogan, L., Nageotte, N.L., Currin-Mc Culloch, J. and Dickler-Mann, R. (2024) Zoo professionals and volunteers in the U.S.: Experiences and prevalence of burnout, mental health, and animal loss. *Frontiers in Psychiatry* 15, 1373525. DOI: 10.3389/fpsyt.2024.1373525.

Mellen, J.D. (1991) Factors influencing reproductive success in small captive exotic felids (Felis spp.): A multiple regression analysis. *Zoo Biology* 10, 95–110.

Ng, L., Schache, K., Young, M. and Sinclair, J. (2023) Value of Schwartz Rounds in promoting the emotional well-being of healthcare workers: A qualitative study. *BMJ Open* 13(4), e064144. DOI: 10.1136/bmjopen-2022-064144.

Puyat, J.H., Leclerc, A., Song, A., Chan, K., Pott, K. *et al*. (2019) Exposure to deaths and dying and risks of burnout among long-term care staff: A cross-sectional survey. *Palliative Medicine* 33(6), 717–720. DOI: 10.1177/0269216319833248.

Tehan, M. and Thompson, N. (2013) Loss and grief in the workplace: The challenge of leadership. *OMEGA-Journal of Death and Dying* 66(3), 265–280. DOI: 10.2190/OM.66.3.d.

Wielebnowski, N.C., Fletchall, N., Carlstead, K., Busso, J.M. and Brown, J.L. (2002) Noninvasive assessment of adrenal activity associated with husbandry and behavioral factors in the North American clouded leopard population. *Zoo Biology* 21, 77–98. DOI: 10.1002/zoo.10005.

Conclusion

Lori R. Kogan
Colorado State University, USA

Throughout this volume, companion animal end-of-life (EOL) care and loss emerge as relational, ethically complex processes that extend beyond the moment of death. The chapters demonstrate that EOL experiences are shaped not only by medical trajectories, but also by communication quality, relational dynamics, institutional cultures, and emotional and structural support (Moses *et al.*, 2018; Nogueira Borden *et al.*, 2019; Kogan and Cooney, 2023). Together, these contributions portray companion animal EOL and loss as fundamental issues at the intersection of animal welfare and human well-being (Walsh, 2009; Ellis *et al.*, 2024).

Pet owners, animal caretakers, and veterinary professionals alike often navigate moral ambiguity, ethically complex decisions, and situations in which no clear answers exist (Fournier and Mustful, 2019; Scotney *et al.*, 2019). Companion animal death is now widely recognized as a significant life event with meaningful implications for mental health and family functioning (Behler, 2020; Crossley and Rolland, 2022; Brown *et al.*, 2023). The intensity and trajectory of grief, however, are shaped by numerous factors, including attachment strength, anthropomorphism, guilt, shame, social support, and the circumstances surrounding the death (Field *et al.*, 2009; Packman *et al.*, 2014; Testoni *et al.*, 2019; Siess *et al.*, 2021). A central theme across the volume is the emotional labor inherent in EOL caregiving and the consequences that arise when this labor is unrecognized or unsupported.

When grief and emotional labor are minimized, rushed, or silenced, suffering is compounded, increasing the risk of guilt, moral distress, compassion fatigue, and burnout (Moses *et al.*, 2018; Leonhardt-Parr and Rumble, 2024). Yet, the findings presented throughout this volume make clear that these outcomes are not inevitable consequences of caring for animals. Rather, they reflect gaps in preparation, communication, and structural support. The caregiving-focused chapters illustrate how veterinary hospice and palliative care models, technician-led approaches, mobile EOL practice, and ritualized caregiving strategies can mitigate distress while honoring both animal welfare and human emotional needs (Ellis *et al.*, 2024; Kogan and Rishniw, 2024; Piche, 2025; Truman, 2025). Despite these promising models, EOL care and grief preparation remain limited within educational curricula and institutional policies, underscoring an urgent need for systemic change (Florian *et al.*, 2024; Corrigan *et al.*, 2025).

A central contribution of this volume is the reframing of companion animal EOL care and loss as ongoing processes rather than discrete events. Whether experienced by veterinarians guiding families through EOL decisions, caregivers navigating grief, service dog partners adjusting to retirement or death, or zoo professionals coping with cumulative animal loss, EOL experiences unfold across time. They often begin with diagnosis and shifting expectations, continue through caregiving and decision-making, and extend into bereavement and meaning-making (Packman *et al.*, 2011; Kogan *et al.*, 2022; Hudock, 2025). Recognizing EOL as a process rather than a singular outcome carries important implications for professional communication, as well as organizational resource allocation.

This volume further expands scholarship on companion animal loss beyond private caregiving contexts into professional, service, and organizational domains. Service dogs, assistance dogs, and therapy animals are not only companions – they are emotionally significant partners and integral contributors to safety, independence, treatment, and education (Brooks *et al.*, 2018; Currin-McCulloch *et al.*, 2022). Their loss therefore represents both a relational and functional disruption, frequently accompanied by ambiguous loss and institutional pressure to adapt quickly or continue performing (Currin-McCulloch *et al.*, 2022; Gibson *et al.*, 2022; DeSantis and Gerlach, 2025).

Across these diverse contexts, a unifying insight emerges: grief is not solely an individual psychological response, but a relational and social experience shaped by norms, roles, and institutional structures. Disenfranchisement, whether rooted in species hierarchies, professional expectations, or organizational silence, often intensifies suffering (Doka, 1989; Bussolari *et al.*, 2021; McDonald *et al.*, 2024) as well as individual differences in self-compassion and use of continuing bonds. By documenting these dynamics through empirical and narrative approaches, this volume calls for a more expansive framework for understanding loss within human–animal relationships.

Looking forward, the contributions in this volume identify several priorities for advancing scholarship, practice, and policy related to companion animal EOL and loss. First, education and training must evolve to treat EOL care, grief literacy, and emotionally attuned communication as core competencies across veterinary medicine, mental health, animal care, and allied professions (Florian *et al.*, 2024; Corrigan *et al.*, 2025). Integrating EOL education longitudinally, rather than confining it to isolated modules or electives, is a critical step toward normalizing these topics and reducing distress for both professionals and those they serve.

Second, organizational policies and leadership practices must move beyond ad hoc, reactive responses toward intentional, grief-affirming infrastructures. Chapters addressing assistance dog organizations, service dog partnerships, and zoo settings illustrate how institutional culture can either buffer or exacerbate loss-related distress (McDonald *et al.*, 2024; DeSantis and Gerlach, 2025). Organizations that prioritize anticipatory guidance, transparent communication, time and space to grieve, and meaningful ritual practices foster greater well-being, trust, and ethical integrity (McDonald *et al.*, 2024; Truman, 2025).

Third, research agendas must continue to integrate lived experience with empirical rigor. Quantitative studies clarify predictors and outcomes, while qualitative and narrative approaches capture complexity and contextual nuances (Packman *et al.*, 2011; Kogan *et al.*, 2023). Expanding attention to underrepresented populations, cross-cultural contexts, and longitudinal trajectories will further strengthen the research in this field (Northrope *et al.*, 2025).

Finally, policy and accreditation bodies play a pivotal role in shaping norms around EOL care and loss. Formalizing expectations for EOL preparation, caregiver support, and workforce well-being can lead to sustained, system-level education and support programs (Ellis *et al.*, 2024; Florian *et al.*, 2024). By viewing compassion not merely as an individual sentiment but as a skill set, an institutional responsibility, and a policy priority, this book offers a roadmap for advancing a more humane, equitable, and sustainable approach to companion animal EOL care and loss.

References

Behler, A.M.C. (2020). "We Lost a Member of the Family": Predictors of the grief experience surrounding the loss of a pet. *Human Animal Interaction Bulletin*, *8*(3), 18.

Brooks, H.L., Rushton, K., Lovell, K., Bee, P., Walker, L. *et al.* (2018). The power of support from companion animals for people living with mental health problems: A systematic review and narrative synthesis of the evidence. *BMC Psychiatry*, *18*(1), 31. DOI: 10.1186/s12888-018-1613-2.

Brown, C.A., Wilson, D.M., Carr, E., Gross, D.P., Miciak, M. *et al.* (2023). Older adults and companion animal death: A survey of bereavement and disenfranchised grief. *Human-Animal Interactions, 2023.*

Bussolari, C., Habarth, J.M., Phillips, S., Katz, R. and Packman, W. (2021). Self-compassion, social constraints, and psychosocial outcomes in a pet bereavement sample. *OMEGA - Journal of Death and Dying*, *82*(3), 389–408. DOI: 10.1177/0030222818814050.

Corrigan, V., Cooney, K. and Foster, R. (2025). Compassionate end-of-life care: Development, implementation, and evaluation of a comprehensive euthanasia course in veterinary education from 2019–2024. *Human-Animal Interactions*. DOI: 10.1079/hai.2025.0025.

Crossley, M.K. and Rolland, C. (2022). Overcoming the social stigma of losing a pet: Considerations for counseling professionals. *Human-Animal Interactions*, *2022*. DOI: 10.1079/hai.2022.0022.

Currin-McCulloch, J., Bussolari, C., Packman, W., Kogan, L. and Erdman, P. (2022). The loss of a service dog through retirement: Experiences and impact on human partners. *Human-Animal Interaction Bulletin*, *2022*. DOI: 10.1079/hai.2022.0017.

DeSantis, D. and Gerlach, J.H. (2025). Supporting clients through loss: A qualitative review of current practices of accredited assistance dog organizations. *Human-Animal Interactions*, *13*(1), 0009. DOI: 10.1079/hai.2025.0009.

Doka, K. (1989). *Disenfranchised Grief: Recognizing Hidden Sorrow*. Lexington Books. https://www.worldcat.org/title/disenfranchised-grief-recognizing-hidden-sorrow/oclc/20015907.

Ellis, C., Littrell, K., Carmack, T. and Christopher, K. (2024). The evolution, challenges and future of veterinary hospice and palliative care. *Human-Animal Interactions*, *12*(1). DOI: 10.1079/hai.2024.0033.

Field, N. P., Orsini, L., Gavish, R. and Packman, W. (2009). Role of attachment in response to pet loss. *Death Studies*, *33*(4), 334–355. DOI: 10.1080/07481180802705783.

Florian, M., Skurková, L., Mesarčová, L., Slivková, M. and Kottferová, J. (2024). Decision-making and moral distress in veterinary practice: What can be done to optimize welfare within the veterinary profession? *Journal of Veterinary Medical Education*, *51*(3), 292–301. DOI: 10.3138/jvme-2022-0073.

Fournier, A.K. and Mustful, B. (2019). Chapter 27 - Compassion Fatigue: Presenting Issues and Practical Applications for Animal-Caring Professionals. In L. Kogan and C. Blazina (Eds.), *Clinician's Guide to Treating Companion Animal Issues* (pp. 511–534). Academic Press. DOI: 10.1016/B978-0-12-812962-3.00027-7.

Gibson, M., Chalmers, D. and Ru, S. (2022). "My Lifeline is Gone": An exploration of the experiences of veterans following the loss of their psychiatric service dog(s). *Human-Animal Interaction Bulletin*, *2022*. DOI: 10.1079/hai.2022.0009.

Hudock, A. (2025). One owner's perspective after a pet hospice journey. *Human-Animal Interactions*. DOI: 10.1079/hai.2025.0027.

Kogan, L.R. and Cooney, K.A. (2023). Defining a "Good Death": Exploring veterinarians' perceptions of companion animal euthanasia. *Animals : An Open Access Journal from MDPI*, *13*(13), 2117. DOI: 10.3390/ani13132117.

Kogan, L.R., Packman, W., Bussolari, C., Currin-McCulloch, J. and Erdman, P. (2022). Pet death and owners' memorialization choices. *Illness, Crisis & Loss*, 10541373221143046. DOI: 10.1177/10541373221143046.

Kogan, L.R., Packman, W., Currin-McCulloch, J., Bussolari, C. and Erdman, P. (2023). The loss of a service dog through death or retirement: Experiences and impact on partners. *Illness, Crisis & Loss*, *31*(2), 244–270. DOI: 10.1177/10541373211054168.

Kogan, L.R. and Rishniw, M. (2024). Relief and mobile veterinary careers may offer a path towards improved quality of life. *Journal of the American Veterinary Medical Association*, *262*(2), 209–215. DOI: 10.2460/javma.23.07.0422.

Leonhardt-Parr, E. and Rumble, B. (2024). Coping with animal companion loss: A thematic analysis of pet bereavement counselling. *Omega*, *89*(1), 362–378. DOI: 10.1177/00302228211073217.

McDonald, S.E., Kogan, L.R., Nageotte, N.L., Currin-McCulloch, J. and Dickler-Mann, R. (2024). Zoo professionals and volunteers in the U.S: Experiences and prevalence of burnout, mental health, and animal loss. *Frontiers in Psychiatry*, *15*. DOI: 10.3389/fpsyt.2024.1373525.

Moses, L., Malowney, M.J. and Boyd, J.W. (2018). Ethical conflict and moral distress in veterinary practice: A survey of North American veterinarians. *Journal of Veterinary Internal Medicine*, *32*(6), 2115–2122. DOI: 10.1111/jvim.15315.

Nogueira Borden, L.J., Adams, C.L., Bonnett, B.N., Ribble, C.S. and Shaw, J.R. (2019). Comparison of veterinarian and standardized client perceptions of communication during euthanasia discussions. *Journal of the American Veterinary Medical Association*, *254*(9), 1073–1085. DOI: 10.2460/javma.254.9.1073

Northrope, K., Shnookal, J., Ruby, M.B. and Howell, T.J. (2025). The relationship between attachment to pets and mental health and wellbeing: A systematic review. *Animals*, *15*(8), 1143. DOI: 10.3390/ani15081143.

Packman, W., Carmack, B.J., Katz, R., Carlos, F., Field, N.P. *et al*. (2014). Online survey as empathic bridging for the disenfranchised grief of pet loss. *OMEGA - Journal of Death and Dying*, *69*(4), 333–356. DOI: 10.2190/OM.69.4.a.

Packman, W., Field, N.P., Carmack, B.J. and Ronen, R. (2011). Continuing bonds and psychosocial adjustment in pet loss. *Journal of Loss and Trauma*, *16*(4), 341–357. DOI: 10.1080/15325024.2011.572046.

Piche, E. (2025). The untapped potential of Registered Veterinary Technicians in hospice care. *Human-Animal Interactions*. DOI: 10.1079/hai.2025.0034.

Scotney, R.L., McLaughlin, D. and Keates, H.L. (2019). An investigation of the prevalence of compassion fatigue, compassion satisfaction and burnout in those working in animal-related occupations using the Professional Quality of Life (ProQoL) Scale. *The Veterinary Nurse*, *10*(5). https://www.magonlinelibrary.com/doi/abs/10.12968/vetn.2019.10.5.276

Siess, S., Kramer, G.A., Ozer, D., Gaudette, N., Williams, B. *et al*. (2021). Predictors of opting for advanced medical care versus euthanasia for companion animals with severe cardiac disease. *Human-Animal Interaction Bulletin*, *11*(3), 1–22.

Testoni, I., De Cataldo, L., Ronconi, L., Colombo, E.S., Stefanini, C. *et al*. (2019). Pet grief: Tools to assess owners' bereavement and veterinary communication skills. *Animals : An Open Access Journal from MDPI*, *9*(2), 67. DOI: 10.3390/ani9020067.

Truman, L. (2025). How to care for the caregiver: The power of ritual. *Human-Animal Interactions*, *13*(1), 0022. DOI: 10.1079/hai.2025.0022.

Walsh, F. (2009). Human-Animal Bonds II: The role of pets in family systems and family therapy. *Family Process*, *48*(4), 481–499. DOI: 10.1111/j.1545-5300.2009.01297.x.

Index

Printed and bound by CPI Group (UK) Ltd, Croydon, CR0 4YY

18/08/2026

14944364-0001